Beyond Antibiotics

Other Books by Michael A. Schmidt:

Brain-Building Nutrition: How Dietary Fats and Oils Affect Mental, Physical, and Emotional Intelligence

Childhood Ear Infections: A Parent's Guide to Alternative Treatments

Bio-Age: Ten Steps to a Younger You

Tired of Being Tired: Overcoming Chronic Fatigue and Low Energy

Beyond Antibiotics

Strategies for Living in a World of Emerging Infections and Antibiotic-Resistant Bacteria

Michael A. Schmidt, PhD

THIRD EDITION

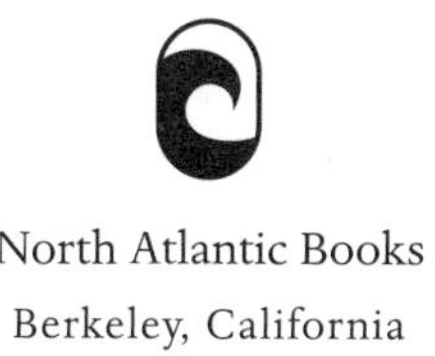

North Atlantic Books
Berkeley, California

Published by
North Atlantic Books
P.O. Box 12327
Berkeley, California 94712

About the Cover Images: The four cover images are color-enhanced views of bacterial cultures, used with permission from the laboratory of Eshel Ben-Jacob. These images represent bacterial colony cooperation under different stress conditions.

Cover and book design by Brad Greene
Printed in the United States of America

Beyond Antibiotics: Strategies for Living in a World of Emerging Infections and Antibiotic-Resistant Bacteria is sponsored by the Society for the Study of Native Arts and Sciences, a nonprofit educational corporation whose goals are to develop an educational and cross-cultural perspective linking various scientific, social, and artistic fields; to nurture a holistic view of arts, sciences, humanities, and healing; and to publish and distribute literature on the relationship of mind, body, and nature.

North Atlantic Books' publications are available through most bookstores. For further information, visit our Web site at www.northatlanticbooks.com or call 800-733-3000.

Library of Congress Cataloging-in-Publication Data

Schmidt, Michael A., 1958–
Beyond antibiotics : strategies for living in a world of emerging infections and antibiotic-resistant bacteria / Michael A. Schmidt.
p. cm.
Includes bibliographical references and index.
Summary: "A self-help guide for readers seeking to take control of their own health at a time when antibiotic use is less of a viable option"—Provided by publisher.
ISBN 978-1-55643-777-9 (alk. paper)
1. Natural immunity—Popular works. 2. Antibiotics—Health aspects—Popular works. 3. Naturopathy—Popular works. 4. Health—Popular works. 5. Infection—Prevention—Popular works. I. Title.
QR185.2.S35 2008
616.07'9—dc22

2008025475

1 2 3 4 5 6 7 8 9 SHERIDAN 14 13 12 11 10 09

To my son Julian,
trusted companion on life's journey

MEDICAL DISCLAIMER: The following information is intended for general information purposes only. Individuals should always see their health care provider before administering any suggestions made in this book. Any application of the material set forth in the following pages is at the reader's discretion and is his or her sole responsibility.

Acknowledgments

As no person's work stands alone, I would like to thank all those in science and medicine who have gone before. These contributions to my own understanding have been tremendous.

I would like to acknowledge the late Linus Pauling, who shared his comments with me on the first edition of this book. His insights helped me deepen the vision of what this message must become. To Ralph Pelligra, MD, at NASA—Thanks for your openness, humor, and wisdom. To an early mentor of mine, Dr. Jeffrey Bland—Thank you for your inspired rigor. My appreciation to Dr. Roy Goodacre at the University of Manchester—Thank you for being a friend and advisor. I would also like to thank all my colleagues at the University of Cambridge who have been so helpful, including those at Addenbrooke's Hospital, the Wolfson Centre for Brain Imaging, the Department of Biochemistry, and the Department of Neurosurgery. I would also like to thank Drs. Doug Kell and Rick Dunn at the University of Manchester for their insights into metabolomics and systems biology.

I would also like to thank Drs. David Manning and Tim Donovan at the University of Lancaster. Thank you for your kindness, insight, and thoughtful manner. To Nichole and Rick Reisdorph at the University of Colorado, thank you for your insights in metabolomics. To Tom Goodwin at NASA, thank you for your ideas on the manuscript and for the many fascinating discussions. My sincere gratitude also to Drs. Bill Toscano and Pat Cowings.

I would like to thank JW Wilson, whose positive and thoughtful demeanor inspire those around him. I appreciate all your insights on the cover design. My thanks to Dr. Bob Hubbard, the warrior sage.

Thank you also to Dr. Andy Meyer. I appreciate your friendship, insight, and wisdom.

Thank you to the *Milbank Memorial Fund Quarterly* for permission to reprint the graphs in Chapter 3. Thank you also to the National Geographic Society. I am grateful to the Natural Medicines Comprehensive Database for permission to reprint the table on antibiotic-nutrient interactions. I would also like to extend my thanks to Dr. Eshel Ben-Jacob, who provided the brilliant cover images of microbial communities in cooperation. A special thanks to Jerry Caires for the fine illustrations.

I would finally like to thank Jessica Sevey at North Atlantic Books, who helped nurture this book from early to late stages. I would like to thank Anne Connolly for help in adding clarity and for her diligence. I would also like to thank Brad Greene and Paula Morrison, also at North Atlantic Books. A special thanks to Richard Grossinger, who has published my books for almost twenty years.

Table of Contents

Illustrations

Figures

Tables

Author's Note

This book contains a discussion of the crisis in antibiotic resistance, the complications that may arise from antibiotic use (or overuse), and factors that are known to be important in our defense against infectious microbes. It is based upon a careful review of thousands of papers from the scientific and medical literature. However, anyone using this book should do so with full knowledge that there is not yet a consensus of opinion regarding interpretation of the scientific data in this field.

While the evidence is compelling with regard to the role of nutrition, lifestyle, and behavioral change in improving immune defenses, opinions exist that are different than mine. For this reason, it is important that you consider all relevant viewpoints and review the relevant data for yourself. Moreover, before attempting to utilize information contained in this book, it is advisable to consult your licensed health care professional. You and your physician or licensed health care professional must take full responsibility for the uses made of this book.

Introduction

The War on Germs cannot be won. And each of us is now affected. Remarkably, we did not see this as a war that could not be won. Now, at a time when emerging infections and antibiotic-resistant bacteria are rising sharply, our development of new antibiotic drugs is nearly drying up. A recent study of the largest drug companies in the world revealed that only **6** of 506 new drugs in development were antibiotics. This is extraordinary. As infections are becoming more threatening, the supply of new drugs to treat them has fallen to a trickle.

Where does this leave those of us who want to protect ourselves and our families?

What can each of us do to curtail our use of antibiotics so this problem does not accelerate?

What new set of tools must each of us have so that we can live safely in the **bacteria's world**?

And what if prior antibiotic use has led to poor health? Is there a straightforward path to recovery?

Before we answer these questions, we must understand why we have lost the war on germs and why we cannot win. We are living in a world where the bacterial "enemy" comprises some 90 percent of all living matter on earth. We are living in ***their*** world. We also failed to consider that our bodies are cloaked in a blanket of bacteria so pervasive that the bacterial cells outnumber our "human" cells by a factor of ten. The sheer numbers of bacteria are so vast that "victory," however we might define it, is impossible.

The war on germs most certainly grew from noble roots. It expanded from treating the very sick, to treating the not-so-sick, to treating those who might get sick. Their use spread to animals, then to fruit trees, then to the fish we eat. As we learned about growing microbial threats, we took the war on germs into everyday life—dish soap, shampoo, toothpaste, and deodorant. Through all this, we did not know that we were training the "enemy."

Suddenly, though not without warning, we were awash in a sea of microbes with an astonishing ability to resist our most potent drugs and to pass that capability for resistance to neighboring bugs. The casualties of our undeclared war on germs have clearly emerged. *We* are now the casualties of the war on germs. We have reached a point where some of us will become seriously ill or die because of antibiotic-resistant bacteria.

We don't expect that it will be one of us, but we cannot predict whether we will be in an accident, sustain a cut, develop pneumonia, have a knee replaced, be weakened by diabetes, mourn the loss of a loved one, or encounter antibiotic-resistant bacteria that threaten our own lives.

Microbes, for all their tiny simplicity, behave as complex, adapting, and cooperative creatures, not unlike bees or ants. They are much more adaptable than we give them credit for and they are surely more adaptable than we are. When we use antibiotics unwisely, we are merely training this endless universe of bacteria to get better at what they do. Much as a musician or an athlete goes through endless hours of training to hone his craft, antibiotics provide the training ground for microbes in our midst to accelerate their training in how to best handle . . . **antibiotics**. If we want to train the next Beethoven of the bacterial world, we will surely do so unless we curtail our approach to antibiotic use—which is why the war on germs must end.

We must move *beyond antibiotics,* because nature has forced us to do so. Our tools have begun to fail and the bacteria have shown they will win. This has brought us to the **Post-Antibiotic Era**, in which untreatable infections are now commonplace. But what lies in this new world *beyond antibiotics*? To thrive in this new world, I propose we now describe it as the **Era of Host Defenses**—where our first thought is of the host, the complex defenses of each one of us. We must marshal the vast body of research in the fields of nutrition, biochemistry, immunology, genetics, toxicology, psychology, exercise physiology, and related fields that permit us to propose a strategy of **personalized medicine** that can be used to build and balance the system of immune defense, energy, and repair.

We have surely entered an era of expanding scientific knowledge. With these great advances, however, we have still not solved the riddle of how we ultimately may defeat the microbes in our midst. It may be strongly argued that we will never do so. *Beyond Antibiotics,* then, is the emerging story of how we are to live *with them.* It is the story of how we will raise our defenses and coexist with the microbial world, while preserving the drugs of last resort that we so cherish.

Beyond Antibiotics is a roadmap, a way forward, and an important step in showing us how this can be accomplished.

Michael A. Schmidt, PhD
Boulder, Colorado

PART I

The Unseen

Chapter 1

Why the War on Germs Cannot Be Won

We have declared war on an unbeatable foe—the microbe. It is now clear that this war cannot be won.

But there is a way forward.

Over a quarter century ago, the U.S. Surgeon General made a stunning announcement before congress that it was "time to close the book on infectious diseases."[1] This heralded a kind of V-day (or perhaps B-day, for bacteria). It was a day long awaited, when we might declare victory against bacterial foes that had so devastated previous generations.

But a small chorus of stubborn dissenters would not join the celebration. Time quickly showed that our declaration was premature. A flurry of studies harkened the advance of emergent infections, more virulent microbes, and bugs that could thwart even our most potent antibiotic drugs.

In 1992, Dr. Harold Neu at Columbia University wrote a paper in the journal *Science* entitled "The Crisis in Antibiotic Resistance." In this article, he pointed out that in 1941, only forty thousand units of penicillin per day for four days were required to *cure* pneumococcal pneumonia. "Today," said Neu,

> a patient could receive 24 million units of penicillin a day and die of pneumococcal meningitis.

He added that bacteria that cause infection of the respiratory tract, skin, bladder, bowel and blood

> . . . are now resistant to virtually all of the older antibiotics. The extensive use of antibiotics in the community and hospitals has fueled this crisis.[2]

Doctor Neu was not alone. Also in 1992, Dr. Mitchell Cohen, a researcher with the National Center for Infectious Diseases at the Centers for Disease Control, issued this warning about antibiotics: "Unless currently effective antimicrobial agents can be successfully preserved and the transmission of drug-resistant organisms curtailed, the post-antimicrobial era may be rapidly approaching in which infectious disease wards housing untreatable conditions will again be seen."[3]

A mere twenty-five years after the triumphal announcement of the Surgeon General came an urgent warning in the *Annals of Internal Medicine* with the sobering title, "The Conquest of Infectious Disease: Who Are We Kidding."[4] This was just the beginning of our recognition that the war on germs had, in fact, not been won and, perhaps, *could not be won*. Indeed, on the eve of the twenty-first century the sitting U.S. Surgeon General declared that "We are seeing a global resurgence of infectious disease,"[5] while Nobel Laureate Joshua Lederberg, PhD, of Rockefeller University offered this scathing view of the present crisis in antibiotic-resistant bacteria: "We are on the road to an impending public health disaster." Placing antibiotic-resistant infections in context with the dreaded Ebola virus, Dr. Lederberg vividly stated: "The odds of Ebola breaking out are quite low, but the stakes are very high. With antibiotic resistance, the odds are certain and the stakes are just as high."[6]

Authors of a report by the Institute of Medicine stated, "Pathogenic microbes can be resilient, dangerous foes. Although it is impossible to predict their individual emergence in time and place, we can be confident that new microbial diseases will emerge."[7] Harvard professor and Nobel Laureate Dr. Walter Gilbert offered his dire assessment, warning that, "There may be a time down the road when 80 percent to 90 percent of infections will be resistant to all known antibiotics."[8] A chilling notion.

Infections Still Dominate Our World

In this modern day of sophisticated medicine, it is almost unthinkable that infection by microbes still dominates our world. It is a testament to the fantastic vigor of microbes to adapt to seemingly impossible conditions.

Consider that:

- Infection is still the number one killer worldwide.
- Hospital infections are now the fourth leading cause of death in the United States.
- Collectively, infection is the third leading cause of death annually in the United States.
- Foodborne microbial infections are responsible for an estimated **76 million** illnesses in the United States each year.[9]
- Infections are responsible for 30 percent of the deaths in senior citizens.[10]
- Infections are the most common cause of hospitalization in older adults.[11]
- Infections in children are the most common reasons for visits to the doctor.
- In the U.S., the estimated cost to employers of people with respiratory infections is over $112 billion, including costs of medical treatment and time lost from work.[12]

The Startling Rise of Antibiotic-Resistant Bacteria

MORE DEATHS FROM MRSA THAN FROM AIDS

This was the headline that dominated the news in late 2007. An article in the *Journal of the American Medical Association* revealed that of some 100,000 cases of MRSA in the U.S. each year, there are over 18,000 deaths—more deaths than are due to AIDS. Consider also that:

- According to the World Health Organization, infectious diseases like malaria, tuberculosis, and pneumonia could have "no effective therapies within the next ten years."
- Of the estimated 1.6 million nursing-home residents in the U.S., 250,000 have infections, and 27,000 of them have antibiotic-resistant infections.[13]
- In 1974, just 2 percent of the most common form of staph infections found in hospitals were resistant to the common antibiotic methicillin. Today, more than 60 percent are resistant to this drug.
- Today, 70 percent of hospital infections are now resistant to at least one antibiotic.
- For virtually every bug/drug combination, resistance has been increasing over the last four or five years.
- A strain of ear-infecting bacteria known as strain 19A has now been found that can only be killed by an antibiotic (levofloxacin, or Levaquin) approved for adults. This antibiotic has a warning on its label against use in children.
- The United States alone spends **$5 billion** annually to treat resistant bacteria.
- The cost of treating a patient with non-drug-resistant tuberculosis, about $12,000, rises to $180,000 for a patient with a multidrug-resistant strain of tuberculosis.
- Since 2003, three U.S. National Football League (NFL) teams have reported multiple infections of MRSA.
- 1 out of every 136 hospital patients becomes seriously ill as a result of acquiring an infection in the hospital. This is equivalent to 2 million cases and about 80,000 deaths a year.[14]

Bacteria Are More Intelligent Than We Realize

Bacteria are masters at adaptation and cooperation. When exposed to antibiotics that wipe out 90 percent of their population, the remaining 10 percent further adapt and form new colonies that can live in the presence of the antibiotic. In some cases, microbes can even subsist on chemicals we consider harmful to them.

Microbes are also genius at cooperation. They communicate with one another through many different "languages," which includes an array of molecular signals. For instance, through quorum sensing, they can tell when population numbers are getting too large and slow their reproductive rate accordingly. Microbes are well known to produce biofilms, where they layer themselves into protective niches so that harmful agents cannot penetrate and reach the central core.

One strain of microbe will even cooperate with another (as in the case of plaque in the mouth), forming biofilms that allow an entire colony of collaborating microbes of different species to thrive together. In this case, different species perform different tasks in support of the collective effort. New estimates suggest that as many as twenty different bacterial species collaborate to form the biofilm in dental plaque.

In the case of middle ear infection, for instance, bacteria seem to build cooperative biofilms that help them ward off threats in the middle ear, which may be one reason why antibiotics are ineffective in many earaches.

The microbes in a biofilm literally build castles as defenses out of specific molecules they manufacture from the raw materials in the host—the human. The bacteria use sugars (much like we would use bricks) and assemble them into multisugar branching chains to build up walls and towers (as we would assemble bricks into protective walls and towers). Bacteria even seem to organize scaffolding to raise the height of their towers—a remarkable feat. The cooperating bacteria in a biofilm encase themselves in a self-made fortress that keeps our bacteria-munching white cells and our chemical agents from permeating the barrier.* As for antibiotics, bacteria on the edges may be sensitive to our antibiotics, but those on the interior may be protected. The biofilms become all but impervious to antibiotics.[15]

Beyond their cooperation building castles and towers, bacteria are masters at swapping genes with one another. They quickly adapt to harsh conditions by receiving genes from other microbes that might possess the ability to adapt to a given condition. Moreover, when conditions become too harsh, certain microbes form spores that are small, bowling-ball-like, impenetrable one-microbe islands. In this state, microbes can go without food or water for vast stretches of time. One reason antibiotics trigger severe intestinal bleeding in some people is that *Clostridium dificile* (an excellent spore former) lies dormant in the gut, in its impervious, docile, sporulated state. When an antibiotic wipes out the competing helpful bacteria in the gut, the *Clostridium* emerges from its spore state with little competition, begins munching on abundant nutrients, and produces toxic proteins that ravage the gut lining. The bowling ball becomes a Tasmanian devil.

Microbes can also send out all sorts of signals that fool or blunt our immune response. Some even develop "cloaking" technology, allowing them to hide from our immune system. They can drift along almost unseen by our immune surveillance system, which normally patrols the tissues and bloodstream.

A real world example of such successful adaptation has now fully taken root. And we will most certainly regret if we take this one lightly.

---

*We will see later why strong host (human) defenses are important to establish as preventive measures, to ensure that bacterial invaders do not gain a foothold and that defenses mount before a biofilm can be formed.

Why Staph Aureus Is Winning

Our skin is covered with over a trillion bacteria, which generally protect us against the colonization of more harmful microbes. About 30 percent of us carry *Staph. aureus* on our skin right now. Most of us have had or will have *S. aureus* on our skin now or in the future. Before antibiotics, *S. aureus* posed no significant threat to the majority of healthy people.

Microbiologists have marveled that *S. aureus* possesses an arsenal unlike almost any other bacteria. However, the very capacities that strike awe in these scientists now elicit dread among doctors and hospital personnel. *S. aureus* secretes a range of proteins that prepare the human body for invasion, thwart the immune defenses, and invade white blood cells. Most frightening among its defenses is an uncanny ability to make a protein that binds to our own antibodies, fooling our defenses. Because of its many complex proteins, *S. aureus* participates in more varied types of disease processes than almost any other bacteria. This impressive arsenal also means that far fewer *S. aureus* bacteria are required to be lethal than many other bacteria.

It was a chance discovery of mold contamination in a culture surely containing *S. aureus* that led to discovery of penicillin. Herein lay one of medicine's greatest achievements—the advent of drugs to treat infectious disease. It was this moment that led to the stunning conquest of many infections of the past and brought about our disturbing vulnerability to infectious disease today.

S. aureus once posed its greatest threat to immune-compromised people, such as those undergoing surgery, burn victims, trauma victims, and transplant patients. In this respect, *S. aureus* became the number one infection in hospitals around the world. The good news had always been that a healthy immune system could confine *S. aureus* infections to the skin, but as it developed the tools of resistance, the infection became a growing threat to all hospitalized patients.

Enter Methicillin-Resistant Staff (MRSA)

Methicillin-resistant staphylococcus aureus (MRSA)*—this is a dreaded term, all too familiar to physicians, nurses, hospital personnel, and all patients who have met its scourge. For decades, *S. aureus* infections were responsive to penicillin. In the 1960s, a synthetic version of penicillin, methicillin, arrived to combat those *S. aureus* strains that were resistant to penicillin. Then, the rebellion began. *S. aureus* developed resistance to methicillin, earning the moniker MRSA. This rebellion was followed by resistance to chloramphenicol, clindamycin, erythromycin, gentamycin, ciproflaxin, trimethoprim, tetracycline, and others.

Today a previously unheralded drug, vancomycin, is the "agent of last resort" for many patients. Vancomycin is not more potent than other drugs. It is a last resort because it fell into less frequent use, so fewer microbes were able to develop resistance to the drug. At least 50 percent of staph infections in hospitals today are multi drug-resistant.

MRSA in Everyday Life

While MRSA can be life-threatening in the hospital, incursions into daily life is what has doctors most alarmed. Robust, healthy men, women, and children have fallen seriously ill to this infection. Some have been ravaged and disfigured. Others have died horrible deaths.

Clostridium difficile

Clostridium difficile is the most common cause of infections in the hospital. It is a common bacterium found in the air, water, soil, surfaces, feces, and intestinal tract of humans. In the hospital, these bacteria can

---

*The acronym MRSA is now also used to describe multidrug resistant staphylococcus aureus, or those resistant to multiple drugs, not just Methicillin. Thus MRSA could refer to Methicillin-Resistant Staph aureus or Multidrug-Resistant Staph aureus.

be found on hand rails, doorknobs, telephone, stethoscopes, and almost any surface. It normally causes little trouble until the colon is flooded with antibiotics.

As mentioned above, when antibiotics enter the colon, the normal healthy bacteria are dramatically altered, allowing *Clostridium difficile* to emerge from its spore form and take a virulent active state. Almost any antibiotic can trigger the awakening of this dangerous bug, but amoxicillin, ampicillin, cephalosporins, clindamycin, and fluoroquinolones are the most likely to cause trouble.

Clostridium difficile is a relative of *Clostriudium botulinum,* which makes the most potent toxin known to us (causing botulism). *Clostridium difficile* makes two highly toxic proteins of its own that damage the colon, causing bleeding and diarrhea. More recent forms have doctors deeply worried because the toxins are even more destructive. *Clostridium difficile* infections frequently recur once a person has left the hospital and are often more serious than the initial infection. Ironically, antibiotics are usually needed to eliminate *Clostridium difficile* (though probiotics have been shown to be helpful). In severe cases, surgery is needed.

These bacteria represent just brief examples of bacteria causing severe problems because of antibiotic use. While there are many others, these remind us of the potential dangers in making war with germs.

Running Out of Options

At a time when the frequency of infections caused by antibiotic-resistant bacteria is rising sharply, the pool of antibiotics in development by drug companies is drying up. Between 1988 and 1992, the FDA approved an average of three new antibiotics per year. Since 2003, that number has fallen to only one approval per year. Moreover, some of the largest drug companies, such as Wyeth, Eli Lilly, Procter & Gamble, Roche,

Abbott Laboratories, and Aventis, have either sharply reduced antibiotic research or gotten out of antibiotic research altogether.

According to Joseph R. Dalovisio, MD, of the Infectious Diseases Society of America, "Infectious disease physicians are alarmed by the prospect that effective antibiotics may not be available to treat seriously ill patients in the near future. There simply aren't enough new drugs in the pharmaceutical pipeline to keep pace with drug-resistant bacterial infections, so-called 'superbugs.'"[16]

Below is a graph of the numbers of antibiotics approved over the past two decades (figure 1.1). It is obvious that the trend is sharply downward. We can contrast this disturbing trend with graphs of rise in antibiotic-resistant bacteria and infection rates to a variety of different antibiotics (figures 1.2 and 1.3). These trends are clearly in the wrong direction.

The war on germs has led us to a point where there are now infections for which there are very few treatment options. Antibiotic development remains down while research on other drugs is rising. This is largely because pharmaceutical companies have shifted their emphasis to drugs with large markets and to chronic conditions like diabetes, high cholesterol, depression, and arthritis, for which patients must be on long-term therapy. In short, there is vastly more money to be made from blockbuster drugs than from antibiotics that can only be used sporadically by patients.

What Next?

We have arrived at a fork in the road. Go left, and we are on the path well-traveled. Here we continue with our focus on killing the microbe, and do so at our peril. This is the path of emerging infections, antibiotic-resistant bacteria, and few new antibiotics on the horizon.

To the right is the road less traveled. This path holds the same threat—emerging infections, antibiotic-resistant bacteria, and few new antibiotics on the horizon. However, this path is strewn with promis-

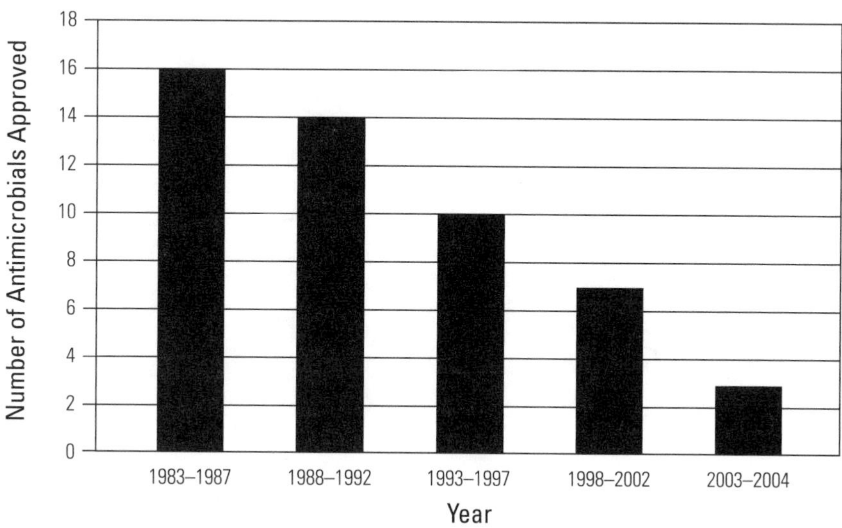

■ **Figure 1.1. Antibacterial Agents Approved 1983–2004.** The number of new antibacterial agents approved for human use has declined steadily since 1983.

ing signposts not seen on the left. These messages point to the power of the host, the wisdom of garnering the profound adaptive and defensive resiliency of the human being. The trail to our right has abandoned the microbe-first manner of thinking. While attention to the microbe must remain in sharp focus, our thinking, our research, our treatments, and our core philosophy places the *host* squarely in the center.

Should we choose the path of the host, we begin to marshal a growing body of research that suggests an entirely new way of coping with the microbial world, perhaps even thriving in the midst of our microbe-riddled surroundings.

This path requires that we better understand those things that influence our coexistence with microbes, our defense against them, and our recovery from failed encounters with them. Our discussion now shifts to that path. We become explorers of the complex world of the human and the myriad influences on our cohabitation with the microbes all around.

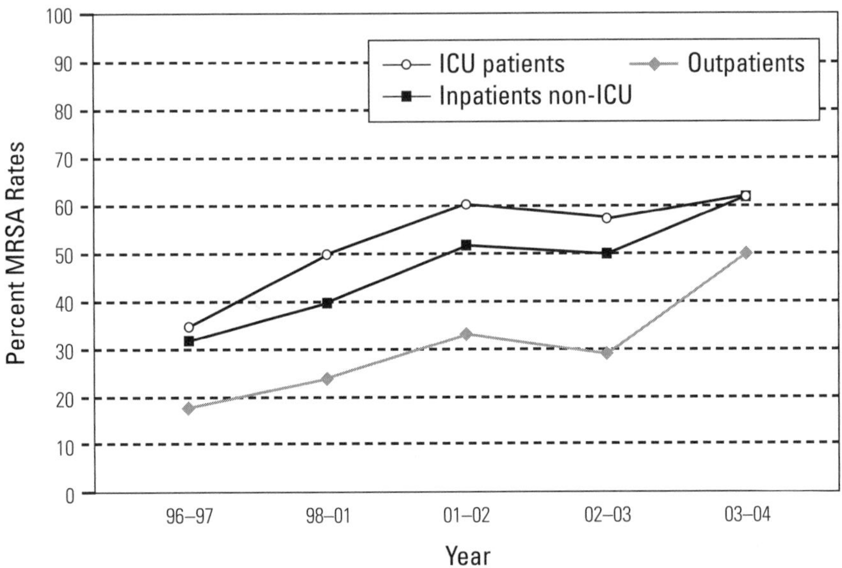

■ **Figure 1.2. Rise in MRSA Rates 1984–2004**. Temporal trends of MRSA rates according to data from the NNIS System. MRSA: methicillin-resistant S. aureus; NNIS: National Nosocomial Infection Surveillance; ICU: intensive care unit.

Why Did We Fail in the War on Germs?

Our efforts at gaining ascendancy over the microbial world have shown impressive individual results, but near catastrophic consequences when taken as a whole. The primary reason for our failure lies with the microbe. Microbes are nearly everywhere and their ability to adapt is stunning. It was natural for us to perceive ourselves as living in *our world,* where annoying or dreaded microbes occasionally surfaced, to our dread. We have conducted our daily lives oblivious to the untold numbers of microbes around us. How could it have been otherwise? We could not see them. Even the most learned of our scientists encountered microbes largely through microscopes, culture dishes, and gene sequencers.

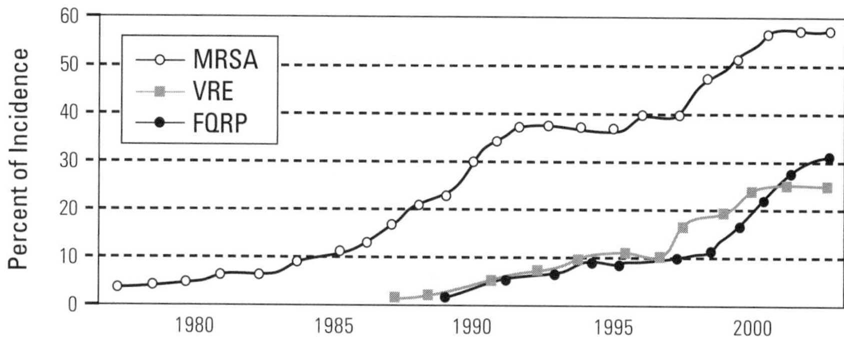

Source: Centers for Disease Control and Prevention

MRSA = Methicillin-resistant Staphylococcus Aureus

VRE = Vancomycin-resistant Enterococci

FQRP = Floroquinolone-resistant Pseudomonas aeruginosa

■ **Figure 1.3. Rates of Antibiotic Resistant Strains of MRSA, VRE, FQRP.** The percentage of antibiotic resistant strains of three common microbes has risen steadily since 1980.

But our old notion is a fantasy. Microbes, by their sheer numbers, ubiquity, and complexity are the true denizens of this world. We are sharing *their world.* It is estimated that microbes constitute approximately 90 percent of all living matter on this earth.

Professor William Whitman at the University of Georgia has calculated that the number of bacteria in all the nooks and crannies of earth, above and below ground, is an astonishing 5×10^{30}. That number is a little hard to fathom—a five followed by thirty zeros. To put it in some perspective, the number of bacteria on earth is almost one billion times more than the total number of stars in the universe (about 10^{21}, or a 10 followed by 21 zeros).

The Grand Prismatic Hot Spring located in West Yellowstone is highlighted by a hue of extraordinary colors that fade from red, to green, to blue, to purple. These regions of the hot spring are colored this way because of different species of bacteria, such as *Chloroflexus* (green) and *Chromatium* (purple). The bacteria in a single three-by-three-inch chunk from the hot spring outnumber the total number of people on earth.

Even the coloration (or discoloration) of some of our most revered ancient paintings owe their look to bacteria. For example, the famous frescoes in the Crypt of Original Sin (Matera, Italy) owe their rosy discoloration to a bacterium known as *Rubrobacter radiotolerans.*[17]

Beyond such exotic features as hot springs and medieval paintings, the dirt under our feet is teeming with some one billion microbes in every gram of soil. And this soil is a virtual war zone. In order for soil microbes to survive, they must produce their own antibiotic compounds or they will be overrun by their neighbors. It is an ancient game of chemical warfare carried out invisibly beneath our feet every day.

These dirt-bound warrior microbes are the very same ones with which our children play out in the backyard and the ones tracked beneath our shoes into our nicely carpeted homes. To our benefit, it is exposure to these microbes that helps prime our immune system as we grow up. In many cases, it is the antimicrobial defenses of these dirt-bound microbes that have given rise to some of our own medical antibiotics. With all due respect, soil microbes are our allies.

But these same soil microbes also possess a spectacular, if not disturbing, trait. They literally eat antibiotics for breakfast. Not only can they live off natural antibiotics, but they have even evolved to live off our modern synthetic antibiotics. Scientists have been humbled by the sheer number of bacterial species able to accomplish this feat, their presence in many different soil types, and the large number of antibiotics they can use.[18] That bacteria can actually consume antibiotics as a food source expands our concerns well beyond the issue of antibiotic resistance. The fact that many of these antibiotic-loving soil microbes are closely related to human disease-causing bacteria only adds to the dilemma we now face.

We have been living with a comforting (and outdated) notion that we can somehow conquer microbial infections by carefully crafted molecular agents. While our drugs have saved countless lives and future drugs are expected to do likewise, it now seems unwise to frame our encounter with the microbial world as a war. In this chapter, I use the phrase "war on germs" because our approach to infections has been treated as a war and our terminology is that of war. Even our description of the immune system has embraced war metaphors. Indeed, during epidemics in which thousands, if not millions, of innocent people died, it must have seemed like war.

But our war metaphor must now yield to a maturing vision. If we are at war, we are outnumbered by odds so vast that we can surely not win. Consider the virulence odds. It takes only five hundred cells of the food-contaminating bacterium *Campylobacter jejunii* to make a person ill. This means approximately two organisms per milliliter of an 180-milliliter serving of milk, or about three-fourths of a cup of milk.[19]

It takes only 200 cells of *Shigella dysentarii* to bring down a 200-pound man with a bout of dysentery. *Vibrio cholera* takes only 1,000 bacteria to cause illness, while *E. coli* 0157:H7 requires only 10 to 100 microbes. It takes roughly 100 *Staph aureus* per gram of food to produce enough toxin to cause illness. In someone with weakened immunity, the number of bacteria required to cause illness is even smaller.

The botulinum toxin, produced by *Clostridium botulinum* (and associated with a serious form of food poisoning), is the most potent naturally occurring toxin known to humankind. The toxin is lethal at a femtamolar dose of 10^{-9}g/kg, which makes it some 15,000 to 100,000 times more potent than sarin gas. More simply, a single gram (about one-fourth of a teaspoon) would kill more than one million people. After the 1991 Persian Gulf War, there were 19,000 kilograms of botulinum toxin produced by the Iraqi regime unaccounted for. This was estimated to be roughly three times the amount needed to kill the entire human population by inhalation.[20]

If we are not overwhelmed by the potency of bacteria and their toxins, we must certainly stand in awe of the rate at which bacteria can multiply, reproducing every twenty minutes. Their ability to swap genes renders them able to adapt in ways that would ordinarily take millions of years if left to natural processes.

Fortunately, much of the microbial world is of little direct threat to us. Indeed, without most of it, the world of reforestation, soil enrichment, plant growth, and animal life would simply not exist. We are living in a world largely driven by microbes, but we see only the tapestry. We see the web, but we cannot see the weaver.

This leads us to the second reason for our failure in the war on germs, which lies with us—the host, the human being. While the world around us is teeming with microbes, we have only begun to understand the vast microbial world that lies on and within us. Remarkably, the weaver has woven *us* into the web. The microbial threads have been so finely stitched into the fabric of our own bodies that separation is not possible.

Chapter 2

You're Not Who You Think

We are living in the microbe's world. We cannot outnumber them, we cannot outwit them, we cannot defeat them, and we will not outlive them. But if we accept the humbling notion that we are living in the microbe's world, we are on our way to thriving in that world. In order to do so, however, we must surrender another sacred belief—our belief about what it means to be human.

Our Bacterial Selves

Before birth, our bodies are free from bacteria. During the process of our birth, each of us (unless born by cesarean section) travels down the birth canal, bathing in the microbial inhabitants of our mother. It is by transit through the birth canal that we begin the process of our inoculation by exposure to the resident vaginal bacterial strains (which are generally, but not always, beneficial). Our mouths become painted in microbes. We swallow the microbes, inoculating our gut. Our nose, eyes, our skin, our scalp, and every other external part of us are inoculated by the bacteria of the mother's body. If we breast-feed, we immediately begin to ingest the beneficial bifidobacteria and the like, which are transferred from the mother's breast. Within the first hours of our lives, we become blanketed in bacteria. This begins the long journey of our exposure to microbes, many of which become residents of our bodies.

As we were exposed to other adults, we accumulated their microbes. As we encountered new foods, we gathered still more microbes. When

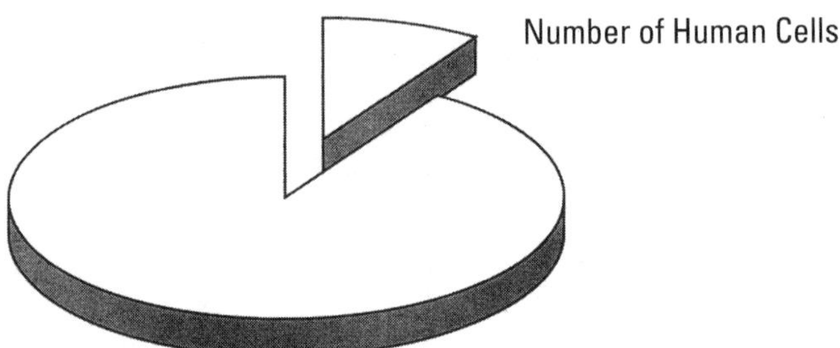

■ **Figure 2.1. The Number of Bacterial Cells vs. Human Cells in a Human Being.** The number of bacterial cells on and within a human being outnumber the number of human cells by ten times. Based on new DNA analysis, there are estimated to be from 1,000 to 5,000 different bacterial phylotypes in the gut alone.

we played in the dirt, we confronted novel bacteria. The toys we were so fond of chewing disseminated their own population of microbes into our growing bodies.

We have grown quite comfortable with our unique place in the world and with the preeminence of our complex cellular makeup. We reason that it is this complexity that places us atop the hierarchy of beings on this planet. But things are not so simple. By adulthood, we have become cloaked in a blanket of bacteria so pervasive that the bacterial cells outnumber our "human" cells by ten times.* And they are no mere hitchhikers. These microbes contribute mightily to our defenses, to our metabolism, and to the essence of who we are. The bacteria that live

---

*Scientists put the total number of cells in the human body at roughly 10^{13}. That's a 10 followed by 13 zeros, or 10,000,000,000,000. The total number of microbial cells living on and within the human body is 10^{14}, which is a 10 followed by 14 zeros, or 100,000,000,000,000. While the estimate of 10^{14} bacterial cells noted above is impressive, we may find this number to be far greater as our efforts to detect them gain in sophistication. For now, the current list of microbes that serve as our cohabitators, or whatever we'd like to call them, is surely an impressive one.

on and within us account for roughly 90 percent of the cells of a human being—leading some to now call us a human-microbe hybrid.

The Microbiome

The microbial part of us (the human-microbe hybrid) is collectively referred to as the **microbiome.** The microbiome has garnered so much interest of late that the U.S. National Institutes of Health has launched a five-year initiative to study the comprehensive profile of all the microbes of the human body. Until the arrival of sophisticated genomic techniques, our ability to culture and fully identify our coinhabitants has been limited. The general classes of bacteria are listed below, followed by the specific body regions and some of their microbial cohorts.

Table 2.1. Bacterial Classes Living within Humans

Potentially Harmful	Neutral	Potentially Beneficial
Clostridia	Bacteroides	Bifidobacteria
Veillonelia	Eubacteria	Lactobacilli
Staphylococci	Anaerobic G + Cocci	Methanogens
Proteus	E. coli	Fusobacteria
P. aeruginosa	Enterobacteria	
E.coli (some strains)	Sulfate reducers	

Mouth

The mouth is home to some six hundred different aerobic (oxygen-loving) and anaerobic (those living without oxygen) bacteria.[21] In health, the mouth is occupied by predominantly gram-positive bacteria, while in disease the population shifts to gram-negative bacteria. The group of bacteria in the mouth most associated with disease includes *Tannerella forsythia, Treponema denticola,* and *Porphyromonas gingivalis.*[22] *Streptococcus mutans (S. mutans)* is the microbe associated with plaque and gingivitis. Once it gets a foothold, it metabolizes dietary sugars to produce lactic acid. This acid is not only hard on teeth, but it creates such harsh surroundings that other bacteria begin to fail. Once this occurs, it is surprisingly hard for other bacteria to displace *S. mutans* as the "alpha-bug" of the mouth.

Nose and Throat

The nose and throat are home to a vast web of microbes. Some of these microbes are now known to keep more harmful microbes at bay. As defenses falter, the more troublesome microbes in the nose and throat prevail, causing illness. A partial list of the microbes of the nose and throat is below.

Actinomycetes
Enterobacteriaceae (E. coli)
Enterococcus faecalis
Haemophilus influenzae
Lactobacillus sp.
Mycobacteria
Mycoplasmas
Neisseria sp.
Neisseria meningitidis
Proteus sp.
Pseudomonas aeruginosa
Spirochetes
Staphylococcus epidermidis
Staphylococcus aureus
Streptococcus mitis
Streptococcus salivarius
Streptococcus mutans
Streptococcus intermedius
Streptococcus pneumoniae
Streptococcus pyogenes

Stomach

The harsh environs of the stomach were once thought too severe to contain bacteria. It is clear now that some bacteria live in the stomach. The stomach can harbor strep, staph, lactobacilli, fungi, and other organisms. There have been estimates of 10,000 bacteria per milliliter of stomach contents. After a meal, this number can rise to 100,000 bacteria per milliliter of stomach contents. The numbers of bacteria in the stomach can grow even higher in the elderly, whose production of protective stomach acid lessens with age. *Helicobacter pylori,* a spiral-shaped bacterium, can cause erosion of the stomach lining and it is considered one of the primary causes of stomach ulcers.

Duodenum

The duodenum is the uppermost portion of the small intestine, home to an estimated 1,000 to 10,000 colony-forming units of bacteria per gram of contents. The jejunum is the middle portion of the small intestine, where nutrient absorption is at its highest. The jejunum contains 100,000 to 10,000,000 colony-forming units of bacteria per gram. Both have similar populations in a healthy state, including Bacteroides, *Candida albicans,* Lactobacillus, and Streptococcus.

Ileum

The ileum is the terminal part of the small intestine and it is the most densely colonized region of the small intestine (10,000,000 to 100,000,000 cfu/gram). Microbes in the healthy ileum include:

Bacteroides
Clostridium
Enterobacteriacaea
Enterococcus
Lactobacillus
Veillonella

Colon

The colon harbors the richest concentration of bacterial cells in the human body. It is estimated that there are 100 billion to 10 trillion bacteria for every gram of dry stool. One gram of feces contains about twenty times more microbes than the number of human beings on earth.[23] There are two main phyla of bacteria in the gut: Bacteroidetes and Firmicutes.* There is also another form called Archaea, which are ancient, tiny, single-celled organisms that consume hydrogen and gen-

*This is the single largest grouping of bacteria in humans. It includes microbes like *Lactobacillus, Mycoplasma, Bacillus, Clostridium* and *Streptomyces*. The Firmicutes are all gram-positive.

erate methane. Within these groups, the common organisms are generally listed as:[24]

Bacteroides
Bifidobacteria
Clostridium
Escherichia
Eubacteria
Fusobacterium
Lactobacillus
Peptococcus
Peptostreptococcus
Veillonella

Vagina

The normal vaginal flora is predominated by lactobacilli. In healthy women, the lactobacilli species are the closely related *L. iners, L. acidophilus, L. gasseri,* and *L. vaginalis.* However, there is wide variation between women and also between women of different ethnic groups. In women with bacterial vaginosis, lactobacillus numbers are often lower, which may cause lowered defenses. In their place, other species emerge, including *Gardnerella vaginalis, Atopobium vaginae, Leptotrichia* sp., *Prevotella* sp., *Megasphaera* sp., *Chloroflexi, Clostridium* sp., *Streptococcus* sp., *Staphylococcus* sp., and *Veillonella* sp. In vaginal candidiasis, the lactobacilli are not always depleted, but it appears that *L. acidophilus, L. gasseri,* and *L. vaginalis* (which are strong hydrogen peroxide producers), could be more protective against candida infection that *L. iners* (which is not a strong hydrogen peroxide producer).[25] Common vaginal bacteria include:[26]

Lactobacillus crispatus
Lactobacillus acidophilus
Lactobacillus gasseri
Lactobacillus iners
Atopobium vaginae
Megasphaera sp.
Leptotrichia sp.
Gardnerella sp.
Peptostreptococcus sp.
Veillonella sp.
Enterococcus faecalis
Aerococcus sp.

Skin

Until recently, a full description of the bacteria living on human skin has been elusive. However, a newer genetic technique called 16S rRNA sequencing has revealed an astonishing number of microbes. In one recent study, scientists identified 240 bacterial species on six healthy volunteers.[27] Follow-up investigations detected 360 species in twelve subjects.

The most universally vexing of these species would seem to be *Propionibacterium acnes,* associated with acne. *Staphylococcus aureus* has become a rogue element due to its high prevalence of antibiotic resistance—enter MRSA infections. Likewise with *Streptococcus pyogenes,* a potentially lethal organism associated with virulent disorders of the skin. *Streptococcus pyogenes* infections typically begin in the throat or skin, contributing to "strep throat" or scarlet fever (due to toxins released by the bacterium). In severe cases, a form of flesh-eating skin disease called necrotizing fasciitis can occur, which requires surgical treatment.

Beneficial microbes on the skin can produce a host of chemicals that prevent harmful microbes from gaining a foothold. These are noted below.

Table 2.2. Antimicrobial Compounds Produced by Beneficial Microbes on the Skin[28]

Antibacterial Compound	Example of Effects on Harmful Bacteria
Carbon Dioxide	Inhibits dermatophytes
Lysozyme	Kills Brevibacterium, micrococci, Corynebacterium
Proteases	Kills some staphylococci
Propionic acid	Inhibits many other bacteria, acidic
Acetic acid	Inhibits many other bacteria, acidic
Fatty acids	Kill streptococci and Gram-negative species
Hydrogen peroxide	Kills many bacterial species
Bacteriocins	Kill many bacterial species on skin

Adapted from: Wilson, M. Microbial Inhabitants of Humans: Their Ecology and Role in Health and Disease. Cambridge, UK: Cambridge University Press, 2005:91.

Scalp and Forehead

The scalp and forehead are also awash in microbes. In part because they are oily and ripe for bacterial growth, they are dominated by pripionobacteria and staphylococcus.

The Eye

Even the eyes appear to contain bacteria. Our eyes receive bacterial exposure when they are inoculated through vaginal birth. It is believed that much of the bacteria found in the eyes of adults comes from and is similar to that of the skin. In 80 percent of newborns delivered by cesarean section, the conjunctivae were sterile, compared with only 20 percent in babies delivered by the vaginal route.

A Whole New Genome Living Inside Us

The number of genes associated with our gut bacteria outnumber our own genes by one hundred times. And they make an extraordinary amount of "stuff." Most certainly, the products of all this gene activity are related to helping our gut bacteria survive. But it appears that our lives have become so entangled with these gut microbes that the products of *their* genes also help *us* survive.

Dr. Steven Gill at Stanford University has begun to carefully analyze the effect of these gut bacteria gene products and to sort through how they relate to the products of our own genes. For instance, his group found that our gut bacteria contain genes that code for some eighty enzyme families for metabolizing carbohydrates, many of which *we humans do not possess.*[29]

This and similar work by Drs. Brent Finlay, Jeffrey Gordon, and others has led to the clear understanding that the human gut microbiome encodes numerous metabolic pathways important for normal human metabolism. This discovery is not new, but it gets more interesting.

Writing in *Nature Medicine,* Finlay comes to the conclusion that "The [gut] microbiome encodes *a larger proportion* of these pathways that are important for human life than the human genome itself."[30] [emphasis added]

This is astonishing. Is it really possible that this massive genome of our gut bacterial community contributes more to our metabolism than does our own genome? If true, this new understanding will surely change everything about the way in which we view our gut bacteria, and will add a stark note of caution to the idea of antibiotic use. We will have to consider that every time we use antibiotic drugs, we run the risk of altering our gut bacteria to the point of changing our metabolism in fundamental ways.

To give a sense of scale to what these doctors are describing, Dr. Gill notes one example where the gut bacterial genome codes for a molecule called IPP (isopenteryl phyrophosphate), which can give rise to some twenty-five thousand known compounds. Some of these molecules, and many others of bacterial origin, are absorbed into the human bloodstream, merging with our human metabolic network in complex ways. Such evidence leads to the conclusion that we are literally awash in a soup of gut bacterial metabolites.

Marinating in the Microbial Soup

Not only have these microbes gained such robust access to nearly every quarter of what we once thought to be our private domain—ourselves (whatever that now means), but we are also literally bathing, each and every day, in the biochemical products of their immense metabolic activity. The metabolic activity of our *gut* bacteria alone is comparable to that of the human liver, which is *the* most metabolically active organ in the human body.

This bacterial soup in which we marinate daily is no small thing. Many of our cells, in the colon for instance, rely on the chemicals in this soup for their very survival. Bacterial products include acetic acid, valeric acid, and butyric acid. Butyric acid, for instance, is used for fuel by the cells that make up the wall of our colon. In fact, the cells lining the colon begin to fail when starved of butyric acid. It has been estimated that the cells lining the intestinal tract get up to 70 percent of their energy from the butyrate made by our intestinal bacteria.[31] It also appears that cells within the body, such as muscle and liver cells, may derive up to 10 percent of their total energy requirement from these gut-derived fatty acids.[32]

Our biochemical marinade is not confined to the colon. These microbial products routinely travel across the gut lining to be absorbed into the bloodstream. Here, they circulate far and wide, bathing our cells with small molecules of known and unknown effects, depending upon their chemical nature.

Our resident microbial allies also produce beneficial proteins. Select microbes on our skin secrete antimicrobial peptides, which keep threatening skin bacteria at bay. Helpful microbes cloaking our tonsils secrete antimicrobial peptides that keep the more odious residents of our throat from rummaging freely about. The gut bacterium *Lactococcus lactis* produces a protein called nisin, which kills harmful microbes by "poking holes in them." Other gut bacteria produce vitamins K, B12, biotin, and several B-vitamins.

Some biochemical products of gut microbial metabolism are not beneficial. When yeast or fungal populations expand in the colon, toxic by-products of their metabolism such as *D*-arabinitol can be found in the blood. In fact, overgrowth of harmful organisms in the gut can lead to compounds circulating in the blood such as tartaric acid, tricarbalylate, *p*-phenyllactate, beta-ketoglutarate, and a wide array of others. Tartaric acid is noteworthy because it is a known poison of the energy system of mitochondria. Tricarbalylate (another product of harmful gut microbes) binds to magnesium and may reduce the availability of dietary magnesium.[33]

Cresol (*p*-cresol) is related to phenol and represents another noxious compound produced by gut bacteria, which can find its way into circulation. This compound can accumulate to toxic levels in patients with chronic illness, especially kidney disease or celiac disease.[34]

Shaping Behavior

Microbes may even have the power to change us by altering our behavior. This is well-documented with microbes like *Toxoplasma gondii.* When *Toxoplasma gondii* infects rats, it appears to alter their behavior in a manner that causes them to seek out their most lethal enemy—the cat. We are only beginning to understand such effects in humans. But we do know that bacteria can alter our behavior, mood, and coping abilities by virtue of compounds found in the microbial soup. Also, the endotoxins (bacterial cell wall fragments) appear to change our minds (so to speak), by virtue of the inflammatory proteins we produce in response (to be explored later). Gut bacteria may even influence developmental brain disorders, such as autism.

Is Our Energy System Driven by Ancient Bacteria?

Not only do the bacteria living in and on us outnumber our "human" cells some ten-fold, but the very means by which each of our cells generates energy may be driven by bacterial ancestors living within. This is referred to as the **endosymbiosis** theory. The theory begins with the knowledge that our cells owe their prodigious ability to generate energy to microscopic structures within them called mitochondria. The energy that powers the beating of our hearts, the movement of our limbs, and the generation of our thoughts derives from these tiny structures embedded in our cells. Mitochondria take fragments of the raw material from our diets and use them as fuel to produce this vital energy. Without it, we would quickly fail.

Each of our cells contains from 50 to 500 mitochondria. Cells with high energy demands, such as those in the muscles of a well-trained athlete, contain as many as 2,000 or more mitochondria per cell. Skin and blood cells contain very few, if any. In all, there are an estimated 10 million billion mitochondria in the human body, accounting for nearly 10 percent of our weight.

Scientists have studied mitochondria relentlessly for decades. This work has led to somewhat of an enigma. Mitochondria seem to have much more in common with bacteria than they do with the human host cells they inhabit. Mitochondria are similar in size to bacteria; they have a two-layered cell membrane, like bacteria; and they reproduce by dividing in two, like bacteria. Like bacteria, mitochondria even have their own circular DNA (mitochondria contain thirty-seven genes, though bacteria can contain more or less), separate from the DNA with which we're all familiar, that resides in the nucleus of the cell.

The endosymbiosis theory suggests that mitochondria are, in fact, ancient bacteria that found some benefit in entering into partnership with human cells. Scientists further agree that humans have managed to forge a mutually beneficial relationship with these bacteria-like mitochondria. We are now dependent upon them, and they on us. We provide the habitat in which mitochondria can grow, reproduce, and thrive. In return, they provide the currency of life—energy.

Mitochondria are also often similar to bacteria in their response to antibiotics. For instance, the drug cycloheximide blocks a key function of RNA (a close relative of DNA) in "human" cells (called eukaryotic cells). However, this drug does not affect bacteria *or* human mitochondria. In other cases, drugs such as tetracycline and erythromycin block protein synthesis in bacteria *and* in mitochondria. However, these drugs do not block protein synthesis in ordinary human cells.[35] In short, the response of mitochondria to certain antibiotics seems to have more in common with the response of bacteria than with the response of human cells. This similarity of mitochondria to bacteria is problematic for doctors, since antibiotic prescribing can then harm our mitochondria and threaten this energy system.

Life and Death Decisions

Another feature of mitochondria is their role of the gatekeeper of cell death. Every cell in the body is programmed to undergo a natural process of death, should something go awry. This process is called **apoptosis** or programmed cell death. It is one way in which we keep normal cells from turning cancerous and eliminate damaged cells. Remarkably, these mitochondria of ancient microbial origin have integrated themselves so fully into our cellular processes that they have come to be the agents that switch on the apoptosis (cell death) process.

Our Viral Heritage

If it were not enough that bacteria, bacterial end-products, and ancient bacteria have set up enclaves on and within us, we must also entertain the notion that our genome itself has been shaped by the world of infectious agents. This blending of the human and microbial world grows more fascinating as we contemplate the nature of what scientists have called "junk" DNA.

Junk DNA is the term used to describe vast regions of the genome that do not appear to have a well-defined function. By some estimates, junk DNA represents nearly 98 percent of the human genome. Careful analysis of the "junk" DNA led experts in virology to the startling conclusion that our genome is littered with DNA sequences derived from ancient viruses.* These fragments of viral DNA are called HERVs,

*We can easily detect and identify these sequences as viral (HERVs), because all infectious retroviruses contain at least three genes, which includes env (surface envelope

or human endogenous retroviruses, and they account for an astonishing 8 percent of our genome.

Viruses are masters at swapping genes. In fact, it is one of the tools they use to propagate their species. Over millennia, viruses have managed to insert their gene fragments into ours, akin to someone inserting sentences into your favorite novel while you slept. Imagine that you had handed this two-hundred-page novel down to your descendents through the ages. Only now, the book is some twenty pages longer, filled with sentences of uncertain meaning. So it is with ancient viruses, rewriting the book of our genes with sentences of uncertain meaning. Many scientists now contend that we are part viral (at least in our DNA).

It appears that our bodies have managed to silence these viral genes, so that they do not produce viral proteins and cause us harm—at least as far as we can tell at this time. However, there is suspicion that some of these retrovirus genes might code for proteins that help us, while others might code for proteins that harm us.

As a side note, bacterial gene sequences have been identified within the human genome. However, the matter of whether these are contaminants or whether they are true bacterial genes is hotly debated. We will have to wait a while before this debate is concluded, but it does raise the possibility that our genome is also peppered with bacterial genes. If true, it only adds to the mystery of how we've come to be this hybrid creature.

Why the War on Germs Cannot Be Won

We are literally a hybrid of human cells, microbial cells, microbial molecules, and viral genes that have all managed to merge into the fascinating being we now call the human. These new findings have caused us to ask new questions about who we are. If our hybrid selves are so

*[continued] proteins), gag (encoding structural proteins), and pol (viral enzymes). They also include something called long terminal repeats (LTRs).

linked to the world of the microbe, is it any wonder that we are failing in our attempts to wipe out the microbes that threaten us? Given how tightly woven are the biology of microbial and "human" cells, the adverse effects of antibiotics on human physiology would seem to be the expected outcome, since we have so fully joined with microbes in the game of mutual survival.

Nobel Laureate Joshua Lederberg has coined the term **superorganism** to describe this complicated weaving of life-forms into one dynamic entity we call the human being. Professor Roy Goodacre at the University of Manchester calls us a **human-bacteria hybrid** and reflects that, we may be born 100 percent human, but as we blend and merge with microbes over our lifetime, the number of cells we harbor will be 90 percent bacterial.[36] With a tapestry, we see the grand image, but we do not see the true nature of each thread. With the human tapestry, we see the grand image before us, but we cannot see the extent to which the microbe gives rise to this image.

As we move forward, then, we must pose a new question. That is, "What is the cost of waging indiscriminate war on 'invading' bacteria, if so much of the human is comprised of bacteria and bacteria-like functional units (mitochondria)?" If we are to wage war on the bacteria that threaten our well-being from without, we must find a way to preserve the harmony of our coexistence with our bacterial "selves" (those on and within). I use the term bacterial "selves" because we cannot easily separate the biological activity of our microbial compatriots from our own. Our fate cannot be separated from the fate of our body bacteria and our ancient, bacterialike mitochondria. They have become part of us and they serve us. They have become part of us to such an extent that it may be inaccurate to refer to the relationship as "us" and "them."

As we contemplate our relationship with microbes, for better or for worse, we must also revisit our relationship with antibiotics. They have brought us miracles and they have brought us hardship. It is no longer safe to leave it up to "others" (government, doctors, companies) to solve the problem of antibiotic resistance. Time is on the side of the bacteria. We must each do our part through education, wise decisions, and wise action. We can only make wise choices if we better understand the limitations of antibiotic drugs, the depth of our misunderstanding about them, and what to do in the face of their failures.

Chapter 3

Myths, Failures, and Consequences

In order to understand why antibiotics often fail and to describe the way forward, it is helpful to ask some basic questions:

- Are antibiotics the reason for past declines in infectious disease?
- What do medical organizations now say about the effectiveness of antibiotics for the most common conditions in which they are used?
- What are the adverse health effects of antibiotics as we now understand them?
- How will we preserve existing antibiotics for when we truly need them?

Louis Pasteur believed a germ could be found for every malady. He contended that if the germ could be isolated and a treatment devised to kill the germ, virtually all disease might someday be eradicated. Indeed, history has remembered Pasteur as the father of microbiology. Yet, in the final years of his life, Pasteur came to realize that his theories about germs were erroneous. Just prior to his death, he is said to have uttered the words "The terrain is everything, the bacteria is nothing."[37]

Pasteur recognized that it was not bacteria that were responsible for disease, but the "terrain" (the landscape, our bodies), or the inability of the host to combat them. If the host was "strong" (i.e., the defenses were active), the organisms could not get a foothold. If the host was weakened, the organisms could gain an advantage. Pasteur had come to the conclusion that myriad factors, including diet, nutrition, stress, heredity, environment, and state of mind, had a profound effect on resistance to microbes.

The view of infectious disease became divided into two camps: those who adhered to Pasteur's original germ theory and those who believed the health of the host was more important. The discovery of sulfa drugs and penicillin in the 1930s and 1940s launched medicine fully into the chemotherapeutic approach to infection and reduced our attention to host resistance. Thus was born the Antibiotic Era.

Antibiotics are rightly credited with having saved countless lives over the past seventy years that might have been lost to overwhelming infection. Sulfanilamide drugs antibiotics were effective against specific forms of bacterial infections such as pneumococcal pneumonia. This was followed by the introduction of penicillin, which proved to be nearly miraculous in its effect upon stubborn bacterial diseases. Today, antibiotics save lives and reduce suffering, and they will continue to do so.

Yet there is disagreement over whether antibiotics can be given credit for the general decline of infectious diseases. The incidence of tuberculosis, rheumatic fever, pneumonia, diphtheria, scarlet fever, whooping cough, and typhoid had declined substantially before the introduction of antibiotics. Antibiotics did not appear to cause further decline in these diseases. According to epidemiologist R. R. Porter, "Nearly 90 percent of the total decline in the death rate during this epoch [1860–1965] had occurred prior to the introduction of antibiotics."[38]

Dr. Thomas McKeown, physician and professor of social hygiene at the University of Birmingham in England, agreed that "Deaths from common infections were declining long before effective medical intervention was possible."[39] He goes on to say:

> . . . the decline in mortality in the second half of the 19th century was due wholly to a reduction of deaths from infectious diseases; there was no evidence of a decline in other causes of death. Examination of the diseases which contributed to the decline suggested that the main influ-

ences were: (a) rising standards of living, of which the most significant feature was a better diet; (b) improvements in hygiene; and (c) a favorable trend in the relationship between some micro-organisms and the human host. *Therapy* [medical treatment] *made no contributions,* and the effect of immunization was restricted to smallpox, which accounted for only about one twentieth of the reduction of the death rate.[40] [emphasis added]

McKeown cites tuberculosis as one example. He writes, "By the time streptomycin was introduced, mortality from the disease had fallen to a small fraction of its level during 1848 to 1854.... Its contribution to the decrease in the death rate since the early 19th century was only about 3 percent."[41]

In a presidential address to the Infectious Diseases Society of America in 1971, infectious disease expert Dr. E. H. Kass argued that most of the decline in mortality for most infectious conditions occurred prior to the discovery of either "the cause" of the disease or some purported "treatment" for it.[42] Dr. Kass appears to be saying that discovery of bacteria associated with a disease and the ensuing antibiotic treatment had little or no impact on the decline of infectious diseases. This is in agreement with many other researchers.

John B. McKinlay and Sonja M. McKinlay, while at Boston University, conducted an extensive analysis of the impact of medical treatment on infectious disease. Regarding ten common infectious diseases, their analysis suggests that "... at most, 3.5 percent of the total decline in mortality since 1900 could be ascribed to medical measures introduced for the diseases considered here." They conclude, "In general, medical measures (both chemotherapeutic and prophylactic) appear to have contributed little to the overall decline in mortality in the United States since about 1900—having in many instances been introduced several decades after a marked decline had already set in and having no detectable influence in most instances."[43]

Marc Lappé, PhD, while professor at the University of Illinois, sug-

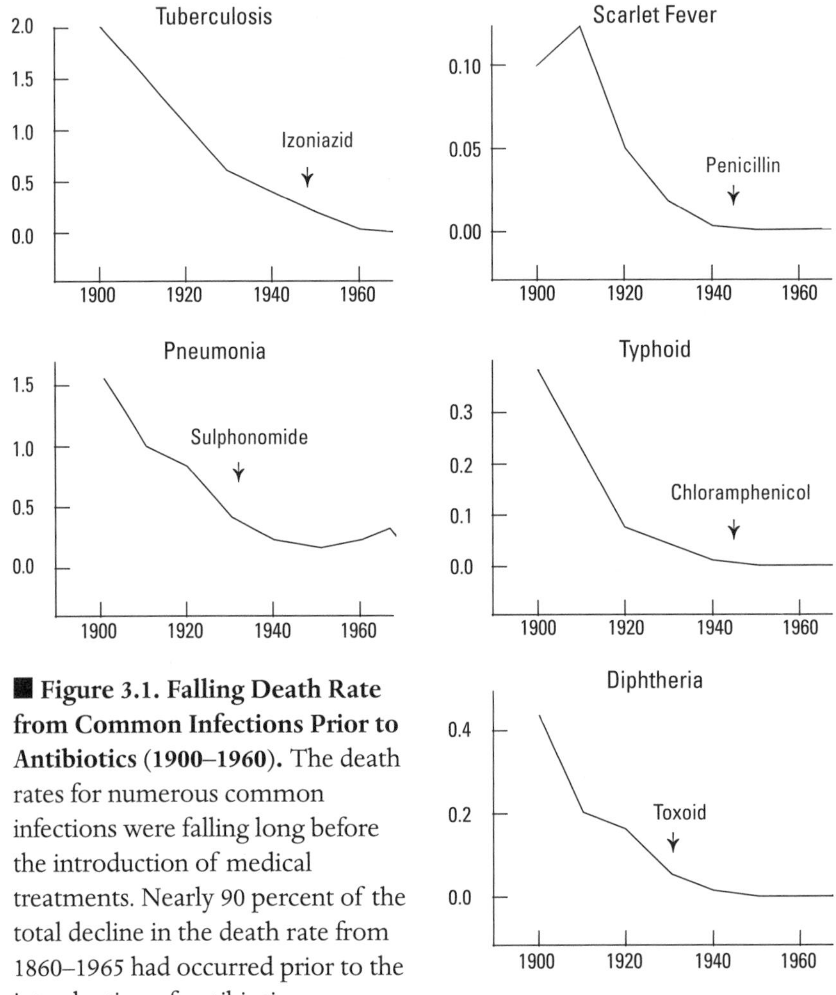

■ **Figure 3.1. Falling Death Rate from Common Infections Prior to Antibiotics (1900–1960).** The death rates for numerous common infections were falling long before the introduction of medical treatments. Nearly 90 percent of the total decline in the death rate from 1860–1965 had occurred prior to the introduction of antibiotics.

gested similarly that "no antibiotic can be said to have proven successful in truly eradicating any infectious disease in modern times."[44]

Writing in the *Journal of Infectious Disease,* Dr. L. Weinstein pointed out that despite the supposed value of antibiotics, the incidence and mortality of many infectious conditions (such as subacute bacterial endocarditis, streptococcal pharyngitis, pneumococcal pneumonia, gonorrhea, and syphilis) have actually increased. He notes, somewhat paradoxically, that the incidence and mortality of other diseases such as chickenpox have decreased in the absence of any treatment.[45] So what are we to make of this evidence?[46]

While the case has been made that antibiotics may not have been responsible for general decline of infectious disease in the past, it is important to recognize our victories. Trauma units of the past were filled with people with injuries of every imaginable type. Battlefield trauma was among the worst of such circumstances. Whether it was trauma from war, automobile accidents, or other calamity, one of the greatest risks encountered was that of infection. In many cases, the risk of death by infection was greater than the risk of death from the original trauma. There can be no question that antibiotics completely revolutionized the field of emergency medicine and trauma management.

Another area in which antibiotics revolutionized medicine was in the area of surgery. In fact, it can probably be said that surgery as we know it today would not be possible without antibiotics to fight opportunistic infections that would surely affect some percentage of surgical patients. Ironically, then, antibiotics have saved the lives of countless people with diseases whose origin was unrelated to microbial infection.

Cancer treatment and organ transplantation as we know it today might also not be possible if not for antibiotics. In the case of organ transplant, immunosuppressive drugs must be given, which naturally lower the defenses against our lowly microbial neighbors. Antibiotics have made use of such procedures and suppressive drugs possible, since they repel opportunistic infections so common in the immune-compromised patient.

We must also add life-threatening illnesses in infants to the list of circumstances where antibiotics have produced startling results. Diphtheria, whooping cough, tetanus, pneumococcal infections, and others once claimed the lives of countless young children whose immune systems were too immature to resist.

While antibiotics cannot be credited for the drop in most infectious diseases, they must be given credit for their stunning successes. Knowing this, we must move forward with respect for the wisdom of our defenses joined with the wise use of antibiotics, and tread with caution in using these drugs. This path seems the most reasoned as we grapple with the challenge of living in the microbe's world. The question of wise use begins with understanding where some of our most prized medicines have the most potential to fail.

Common Conditions: Are Antibiotics Warranted?

It may not be widely known that the Centers for Disease Control and Prevention (CDC) have a very aggressive plan in place to reduce the use of antibiotics. Their main objective is to reduce unnecessary use of these drugs so that antibiotics remain a viable tool in the future. Another reason for their aggressive campaign is to reduce needless adverse effects in patients who might receive these drugs unnecessarily. In Chapter 13, we will explore the most common conditions for which antibiotics are given, the likelihood of a condition being due to bacterial infection, the potential for success or failure in using antibiotics in these conditions, and the current recommendations from medical groups on best use of antibiotics.

The issue of appropriate use is only one concern. There are a range of other concerns related to antibiotics that deserve attention. Among these is how antibiotics may contribute to fungal infections.

Antibiotics and Fungal Infections

One of the most troubling effects of antibiotic use is the consequent rise of fungal organisms, such as *Candida albicans*. *Candida albicans* is a normal inhabitant of the human colon. It is usually of little concern, since its numbers are small. In addition, the beneficial bacteria in the colon are so abundant that they literally carpet the entire surface, making it difficult for *Candida albicans* to attach and proliferate.

One way in which antibiotics can have a negative effect is by removing beneficial bacteria from the colon, which allows *Candida albicans* and other candida species to multiply. If the person's defenses are weakened, the candida species can attach to the colon wall. Candida species are capable of infecting almost any other organ of the human body. As defenses weaken, candida sprout rootlike structures called hyphae, which allow it to penetrate any body cell, membrane, or tissue.

Candida is notoriously difficult to treat once it sets its roots. This is why judicious use of antibiotics and use of antifungals, where needed, is so important. Doctors have commonly used culture techniques to detect candida overgrowth. However, candida can be difficult to culture. Additional methods have come available that help detect a biochemical footprint of candida called arabinitol. One form of arabinitol, called L-arabinitol, is produced from a sugar in the diet called L-arabinose. *Candida albicans* causes the production of a mirror image of that form of arabinitol, called D-arabinitol. Doctors now measure D-arabinitol, and the ratio of D-arabinitol to L-arabinitol (D/L-arabinitol) to detect the presence of *Candida albicans* in the blood or urine.

Antibiotics and Candida Overgrowth

While antibiotics are well-known triggers of candida overgrowth, long-term antibiotic therapy is the most troublesome. In one study, 51 infants were taking antibiotics for 3 to 12 weeks. Urinary arabinitol levels were checked before and after antibiotic therapy. Children on long-term antibiotic therapy were found to have elevated D-arabinitol to L-arabinitol ratios, which rose from the beginning of antibiotic therapy to the end of the study. When the children were given the antifungal drug fluconazole, their D/L-arabinitol ratios were reduced, accompanied by improvement in their medical condition.[47]

Cancer and cancer treatment are also linked to lowered immunity. This too can lead to candida overgrowth. A group of children with cancer were studied to see how their condition was reflected in their D/L-arabinitol ratios. These researchers found that the ratios increased in urine 3 to 31 days before other evidence of a fungal infection appeared. The doctors suggested that regular monitoring of D/L-arabinitol ratios in urine holds great promise as a sensitive method for diagnosing invasive candidiasis in immune-compromised children with cancer.[48]

Infants in intensive care are at increased risk of candidiasis as well. In a study of 117 infants, the D/L-arabinitol ratio was more sensitive than fungal blood cultures in detecting candida infection.[49]

Antibiotics are well known for their adverse effects on vaginitis in women. In order to better quantify this effect, doctors in Australia recruited 233 women in whom vaginal swabs were taken before and after an 8-day course of antibiotics. Twenty-one percent of the women had detectable candida species at the beginning of the study. That number rose to 37 percent after antibiotic therapy.[50]

The Candida Controversy

Doctors have known for decades that antibiotics trigger fungal overgrowth in the bowel, in other body cavities, and on body surfaces. But during a period spanning the 1970s to the present, a number of physicians and writers brought this fact directly to the public. During this time, many claims about candida were made that were either not substantiated or difficult to substantiate. This created a backlash among physicians, such that many began to reject the idea that was once common knowledge and widely accepted. This rejection of *Candida* infection as a legitimate health threat, shockingly, still persists among many doctors in clinical practice.

It is important to note that the topic of *Candida* infection receives significant research attention and is taken seriously by physicians. A search of the National Library of Medicine using the terms "Candida," "symptoms," and "humans," yields more than eight thousand research citations. Broadening the search to "Candida," and "humans," yields more than twenty thousand research citations. It is clear that *Candida* infection remains a serious threat, is under constant research scrutiny, and is being assessed in many hospital and clinic environments. According to the Infectious Diseases Society of America,

> Candida species are the most common cause of fungal infections. Candida species produce infections that range from non–life-threatening mucocutaneous illnesses to invasive processes that may involve virtually any organ. Such a broad range of infections requires an equally broad range of diagnostic and therapeutic strategies.[51]

Other Fungal Infections

While candidiasis remains the most common fungal infection in humans, it is followed in frequency of infection by aspergillosis and a number of other fungal organisms below. These can also occur with antibiotic use, and they become more serious as barrier defenses and immune defenses weaken. Included are Aspergillosis, Blastomycosis, Coccidioidomycosis, Cryptococcosis, Histoplasmosis, Paracoccidiomycosis, Sporotrichosis, and Zygomycosis. Factors that render one susceptible to fungal infections include: underlying debilitating disease, chemotherapy, disruption of normal flora, use of antimicrobial drugs, use of steroid drugs, surgery, trauma, age, and poor nutrition.

Antibiotics and Development of Neurological Disease

A link between antibiotic use and neurological disorders has been reported by doctors for many years. One condition that has received attention in recent years is autistic spectrum disorder (ASD). Children with autism often have a history of multiple courses of antibiotics. One of the first to report this link was Dr. William Shaw, who was at Children's Mercy Medical Center in Kansas City at the time of his discovery. According to scientists like Shaw and Dr. E. R. Bolte, repeated antibiotic use likely disrupts the protective gut bacterial population, giving way to microbes that are toxin-producing.[52] One form of gut bacteria that can flourish in the face of antibiotic use is clostridium, which is a known neurotoxin-producing organism.

Scientists at the University of Reading in the United Kingdom have recently completed the first study looking at clostridium species in the stool of children with ASD. In their study, children with ASD were much more likely to have taken broad spectrum antibiotics. Children with ASD also had abnormal levels of *Clostridium histolytica* in their stools when compared with non-affected controls.[53] Since clostridium species are known producers of neurotoxins, this study has garnered greater interest in the role of gut bacteria and antibiotic use as it relates to autism.

These findings are not unprecedented, as a recent trial with rats clearly shows. Propionic acid is a short-chain fatty acid produced by gut bacteria. When rats were injected with propionic acid "they displayed social behavior impairments." Further, brain tissue taken from rats treated with propionic acid revealed "reactive astrogliosis," which indicates that inflammation was taking place within brain cells. According to the scientists, "These findings suggest that propionic acid can change both brain and behavior in the laboratory rat in a manner that is consistent with symptoms of human ASD."[54]

Other evidence of the effects of the gut on the brain comes from doctors studying musculoskeletal syndromes such as fibromyalgia. Fibromyalgia is characterized by bodywide muscle pain, digestive complaints, chronic fatigue, cognitive impairment, and mood changes. In one study, 42 out of 42 people with fibromyalgia had bacterial overgrowth of the small intestine.[55]

Antibiotics and Development of Allergic Disease

According to the Centers for Disease Control and Prevention, there has been a dramatic increase in allergy and asthma in many Westernized countries. For example, in the U.S., asthma rates increased 75 percent from 1960 to 1994, with a 160 percent increase in children aged 0 to 4 years.[56] Allergic disease incidence in the UK, Canada, and Australia are comparable. A number of studies have now linked the development of asthma and allergic airway diseases to the use of antibiotics and to alteration of gut bacteria.[57]

Researchers at the University of Michigan Medical School took a direct approach to studying whether and how antibiotics might be involved in this effect. They were well aware that antibiotic use can result in overgrowth of fungi like *Candida albicans* in the gut and that *Candida albicans* can trigger and alteration of the host immune response in a direction that favors inflammatory immune system changes—the sort that is common in asthma and allergy.

Through a series of studies, they showed that giving antibiotics led to overgrowth of *Candida albicans.* Those with the fungal infection, who were challenged with an allergen, were more likely to develop allergic airway (lung) disease. These researchers also made it clear that fungi like *Candida albicans* can produce inflammatory substances that traumatize body tissues, including the airways.

At the conclusion of their paper they wrote, "We propose that the link between antibiotic use and dysregulated pulmonary [lung] immunity is through antibiotic-induced long-term alterations in the bacterial and fungal GI [gastrointestinal] microbiota, which we predict disrupts the regulatory T-cell response."

These doctors also mentioned a correlation between altered gut bacteria and the development of allergies. A number of other studies have suggested a correlation between antibiotic use and allergies in humans. According to the doctors, "While it remains to be tested whether human allergies result from altered microbiota, we have demonstrated in an animal model that antibiotic use leading to altered bacterial and fungal microbiota can allow the development of an airway allergic response to subsequent allergen exposure via the nose."[58]

In short, they suggest that there is a progression that begins with antibiotic use, then leads to disruption of gut bacteria, candida overgrowth, a shift in the immune system that favors inflammation, and, finally, hypersensitivity of the airway to allergens.

Antibiotics and Tendon Damage

The U.S. FDA has received a growing number of reports that link fluoroquinolone antibiotics to tendon injury and ruptured tendons. Doctors at the Mayo Clinic have stated that taking fluoroquinolone antibiotics like Cipro® and Levaquin® may cause tendon inflammation or even tendon rupture. The FDA has now issued warning about this class of antibiotics, which includes Avelox®, Factive®, Proquin®, and Noroxin®. Generics would include drugs like ciproflaxin and ofloxacin.[59]

According to doctors, Achilles' tendon ruptures associated with fluoroquinolones are three to four times more frequent than ruptures among people not taking these drugs. In the general population, risk is understood to be about 1 in 100,000 users of this drug. The risk to damaged tendons is greater in people over 60 and people who are using other drugs like steroids. Some doctors suggest that the incidence of tendon rupture is low, considering that some 100 million prescriptions for drugs like Cipro® have been written in the past ten years. However, Dr. Riley Williams, an orthopedic surgeon at Manhattan's Hospital for Special Surgery, suggests that athletes putting excessive stress on tendons by activities like weight lifting may be at special risk.

He notes that tendons are in a constant state of remodeling, as tissues break down and build up again. Dr. Williams and his colleagues have exposed canine tendons to fluoroquinolones, which resulted in weakening of the tendons. He has replicated these findings on studies of human cells.

Dr. Williams speculates that a person taking ciprofloxacin may rupture a tendon, for example, while exercising. He suggests that the Achilles' tendon, knee, quadriceps and rotator cuff—tendons subjected to heavy stress—are most at risk.[60] Follow-up studies published in the *European Journal of Clinical Pharmacology* showed that, in one population of almost 500,000 people, fluoroquinolones tripled the risk of Achilles tendon ruptures (an increase of 12 ruptures per 100,000 people over the normal number of Achilles ruptures). Still, they commented that the overall incidence among users "is low."[61]

Antibiotics and Adverse Drug Reactions

Once a drug enters the body, it is transformed by a complex of enzymes called the cytochrome P450 system (CYP450). There are about thirty forms of these enzymes, but most drugs are metabolized via one of only six of them. About 50 percent of all prescription drugs are detoxified by a single enzyme, known as CYP3A4. Whenever a CYP enzyme is blocked or slowed, its ability to detoxify other drugs can be impaired. In short, use of drugs that inhibit CYP enzymes can cause the concentration of other drugs you may be taking to remain dangerously high.

Many antibiotics are potent inhibitors of the CYP detoxication enzymes. This means that if you are taking other medication that requires a specific CYP in order for it to be safely detoxified, the antibiotic may prevent this from happening, increasing the likelihood that you will have an adverse reaction to the drug.

For example, the antibiotics erythromycin and clarithromycin are potent inhibitors of CYP3A4 (the main drug-metabolizing enzyme). This means that the potential for these two antibiotics to trigger adverse reactions to other drugs you may be taking is very high. Examples of drugs that have to be detoxified by CYP3A4 and that would interact adversely with erythromycin or clarithromycin include (but are not limited to) several of the statins (atorvastatin, lovastatin, simvastatin), warfarin used as an anticlotting medicine, hydrocortisone, and theophylline.

A partial list of antibiotics that influence the detoxication enzymes include:

Ciproflaxin	Enoxacin
Oflaxacin	Norfloxacin
Isoniazid	Metronidazole
Sulfamethoxazole	Trimethoprim
Clarithromycin	Erythromycin

Since antibiotics contribute to overgrowth of fungi, such as *Candida albicans,* antifungals are frequently prescribed as a therapy. Antifungal drugs can also have significant effects on the CYP enzymes and cause adverse drug interactions. Whenever an antifungal drug is used, attention to the interaction with other drugs being taken should be foremost. Antifungal drugs that strongly influence the CYP enzymes include Fluconazole, Miconazole, Ketoconazole, and Itraconazole.

Herbs and food can also influence these enzymes. The most potent among these are hypericin (from the herb St. John's Wort) and grapefruit constituents. Hypericin stimulates the CYP3A4 enzyme, which *speeds up* drug detoxication and causes drugs to disappear quickly, losing much of their therapeutic benefit. Most pharmacists are aware of the significant effect of grapefruit on inhibiting CYP3A4 and they caution against this food with certain medications.

One reason (but certainly not the only reason) people experience adverse reactions to antibiotic drugs is due to the effects of CYP enzymes interacting with other prescription drugs. These drug interaction profiles are very complicated, but the profile of which drugs influence which detoxication pathways are fairly well described. An important way to reduce the likelihood of an adverse reaction when taking an antibiotic is to make sure that it is not likely to interfere with the detoxication of other drugs you may be taking. This can be done by referencing tables such as those published on the Web by the Indiana University School of Medicine Division of Clinical Pharmacology.* A simpler way is to discuss the drug interaction profile with your pharmacist, who will be able to interpret these tables for you.

Antibiotics and Nutrient Depletion

The study of drug–nutrient interactions is an important subdiscipline within the fields of nutrition and within pharmacology. When nutrients are depleted by a drug, all the metabolic functions served by those nutrients can be compromised. Since immune defense, energy, and repair are all metabolically intensive activities, the potential effect of antibiotic–nutrient interactions should be considered. Short-term antibiotic therapy does not always have a severe direct impact on nutrient status, but it can affect nutrient status for several reasons.

For example, when antibiotics cause diarrhea, the effects on nutrient status can be pronounced. In a study of children with recurrent infections, those who experienced diarrhea had lowered magnesium levels in their blood, and the duration of their illness was longer. According to an article published in the *Biological Trace Element Research,* diarrhea can result in significant loss of trace elements such as zinc.[62] For instance, in one kg of diarrhea—about 2 pounds, or one day's output—over 17 milligrams of zinc can be lost. Zinc is important in fighting both bacterial and viral infection, and plays an important role in regulating inflammation.

Broad-spectrum antibiotics or very potent narrow-spectrum antibiotics (even if used for very short periods) that disrupt gut bacteria or

*www.medicine.iupui.edu/flockhart/table.htm

foster fungal overgrowth can have wholesale effects on nutrient status that can persist for months or even years. Long-term antibiotic therapy or repeated courses of antibiotics can also have lasting effects on nutritional health. If damage to the intestinal lining (mucosa) occurs because of antibiotics, the inflammatory changes can alter nutrient absorption for many months or years.

Appendix A contains a brief table of known effects of antibiotics on key nutrients. It is important to note that antibiotic effects on the mucosa (gut lining), gut bacteria, or fungal infections can affect almost any nutrient. For instance, fat malabsorption has been observed in people on repeated rounds of antibiotics, which has led to fatty acid deficiency and alteration of the inflammatory cascade.

In Chapter 5, we will explore the role of nutrition in immune defense, energy, and repair. At this point, however, it is important to understand the effect that antibiotics might have on the nutrients that are important in our defense network.

Can Antibiotics Make Us Fat?

A new potential culprit in the cause of obesity has come under scrutiny in recent years—gut bacteria. This has, naturally, implicated antibiotic overuse.

To answer the question of whether antibiotics may lead to obesity in humans, we have to first look at our experience with animals. Do antibiotics make animals fat? Of course, antibiotics have been used to promote growth in animals for some fifty years.[63] According to Dibner and Richards, "The [increased growth] performance benefits of antibiotics have been demonstrated for all major livestock species. For example, a meta-analysis of more than a thousand growth experiments performed in swine over a twenty-five-year period, demonstrated that antibiotics improved growth rate in starter pigs (7-25 kg) by an average of 16.4 percent and feed efficiency by 6.9 percent. There are significant improvements in grower and finisher pigs as well."[64]

From the past fifty years of research, it is now well established that antibiotics cause animals to grow bigger and grow more quickly. Research has, therefore, turned to understanding the *means* by which antibiotics promote growth. Since the 1960s, studies have focused on research of gut microflora. The gut microflora was first implicated when scientists learned that antibiotics did not affect the growth of germ-free animals—animals whose guts had been experimentally sterilized of all gut bacteria. In other words, the gut bacteria were somehow needed in order for animals to experience the growth-promoting effects of antibiotics.[65] Research then moved on to describe the complex interaction between antibiotics, gut bacteria, and weight gain in animals. (See Appendix B for more information on antibiotics and obesity.)

Gut Bacteria and Obese Adults

The scientists at Washington University in St. Louis have also been among the leaders in studying this newly emerging question of gut bacteria and obesity in *humans*. In their recent study published in the journal *Nature,* they investigated the relation between gut bacteria and obesity in 12 obese humans. Subjects were divided into two groups and given either a low-fat diet or a low-carb diet. Similar to studies with mice, Bacteroidetes and Firmicutes were the dominant forms of bacteria detected, via this genetic identification method being used (16S rRNA sequencing).

At the beginning of the study (and before dietary intervention) obese people had fewer Bacteroidetes and more Firmicutes than did lean people being studied as controls. This was, incidentally, similar to the findings between lean and obese mice. Over time, the abundance of Bacteroidetes increased, while the abundance of Firmicutes decreased—regardless of the type of diet consumed. The increase in Bacteroidetes was correlated with the percentage loss of body weight.

According to the authors of the paper, "Obesity is, to our knowledge, the only condition in which a pronounced, division-wide change in [gut] microbial ecology is associated with host pathology."[66]

This study is consistent with another that looked at weight gain in pregnancy. Doctors found that women who were overweight before pregnancy had higher levels of *Bacteroides, Clostridium,* and *Staphylococcus* in their stool. Gut bacterial counts increased during pregnancy, with higher numbers of *Bacteroides* being linked to excessive weight gain during pregnancy. This led the authors to conclude that "Gut microbiota [gut bacteria] composition and weight are linked, and mother's weight gain is affected by microbiota. Microbiota modification before and during pregnancy may offer new directions for preventive and therapeutic measures to reduce the risk of overweight and obese conditions.[67]

Gut Bacteria and Obese Children

In order to better understand whether gut bacteria contribute to obesity, it would be helpful to follow young children and see whether those who develop obesity have different gut bacterial populations than those who remain at normal weight. Such a study was recently conducted at the University of Turku in Finland. Children were enrolled from birth and followed for seven years. Stool samples were collected at six months and twelve months and analyzed for their bacterial composition. The scientists also looked at antibiotic and probiotic use. Children who had higher numbers of bifidobacteria in their stools in the first year of life were more likely to remain at normal weight by age seven. This fits with studies that show breast-fed children have a 13 to 22 percent reduced likelihood of being obese owing to the higher numbers of bifidobacteria in breast-fed babies.[68]

In addition, normal weight at age seven was linked with lower numbers of *Staph aureus* in the stools of these children during infancy. *Staph aureus* is well known for producing toxins that trigger widespread inflammation. Authors of this study suggest that "*S. aureus* may indeed act as a trigger of low-grade inflammation, contributing to the development of obesity." In other words, more *Staph. aureus* in the guts of children was associated with more inflammation, which contributed to obesity. The researchers further remarked that "Aberrant compositional development of the gut microbiota precedes overweight, offering new possibilities for preventive and therapeutic applications in weight management."[69] Stated more succinctly, alteration of gut bacteria preceded obesity. This is truly a revolutionary finding.

These studies have launched a flurry of investigations to confirm and demonstrate the complex ways that gut bacteria might contribute to obesity. By extension, it is also likely to spur more research into the role that antibiotics might play in fostering obesity, since antibiotics are well known for their role in altering gut flora.

Certainly, more study is needed to confirm the proposed link between gut bacteria and obesity in humans. However, it should also be stated that several thousand studies have been done in livestock and poultry that have quite clearly shown the link between gut bacteria, weight gain, and growth. And these studies are large, including millions of animals. It could be said that this is one field of study in which the magnitude of the existing animal research overwhelmingly supports the basic premise, raising the high probability of a similar trend in humans.

Public Perception: The Myths of Antibiotic Use

Public perception about appropriate antibiotic use has improved, but significant misconceptions remain. These misconceptions, combined with pressures placed on doctors, can lead to overuse of antibiotics at a time when overuse is linked to grave consequences. In the 1970s, researchers at Mater Children's Hospital, South Brisbane, Australia asked 103 people a series of questions regarding antibiotic use. Their startling results are summarized below.[70]

What the public believed:

- Antibiotics kill viruses 55%
- Antibiotics kill bacteria 46%
- Antibiotics are a stronger form of aspirin 13%
- Penicillin is not an antibiotic 15%
- Antibiotics should be given for colds and flu 75%
- Antibiotics should be given for gastroenteritis 40%

Unfortunately, some of these perceptions have not changed a great deal today. In a 2003 study:[71]

- 66 percent of parents believed colds are caused by bacteria
- 53 percent of parents believed that antibiotics are needed to treat colds
- 60 percent said a cold would warrant a doctor's visit

Recently, doctors in the United Kingdom surveyed more than 7,000 people and learned that 38 percent of respondents did not know that antibiotics do not work against most coughs or colds. Forty-three percent did not know that "antibiotics can kill the bacteria that normally live on the skin and in the gut."[72]

Myths also abound in the childcare setting. Doctors studying child care centers in Massachusetts found that more than 80 percent of staff members believed (incorrectly) that antibiotics were required for green nasal discharge or for bronchitis. Equally worrisome, more than 25 percent of staff thought that antibiotics speed recovery from colds and flu, as well as being helpful in treating viral infections.[73,74]

Patient and Doctor Expectations

In another disturbing trend, parents are evidently more satisfied when they emerge from the clinic with an antibiotic prescription. Researchers interviewed 378 parents of children 2 to 10 years of age who were seen at a pediatric clinic for cough and cold symptoms. Nearly half (47 percent) received antibiotics at the initial visit, and their parents gave higher satisfaction scores (9.25 on a 10 point scale) compared with parents whose children did not receive antibiotics (8.95). When children received antibiotics at a subsequent visit, the parents' scores averaged 7.25, compared with 6.25 for parents of children who did not receive antibiotics.[75]

In a large study, the parents of 522 children with cold symptoms were studied to assess the doctor's perception of what the parents expected regarding antibiotics. When doctors perceived that the parents expected antibiotics, they were almost 32 percent more likely to inappropriately prescribe an antibiotic. Also, parents were 24 percent more likely to question the doctors' recommended treatment plan if the doctor *ruled out the need for* an antibiotic. This and other similar studies led the researchers to conclude that inappropriate antibiotic prescribing is primarily driven by physicians' perceptions that parents expect an antibiotic for their child.[76]

In another study, patient expectations seemed to drive the likelihood of an antibiotic prescription even higher. In a recent study by the Centers for Disease Control, doctors prescribe antibiotics 65 percent of the time if they perceive parents expect them and 12 percent of the time if they feel parents do not expect them.

Is Pain Relief What People Want?

There is reason to believe that the persistent problem of people pressuring doctors for antibiotics may be due to the fact that relief from pain is all they seek. In one study of 298 people with sore throat, the desire for pain relief was the strongest predictor of the hope to receive an antibiotic prescription.[77] If this is truly the case, doctors and patients will need to communicate their expectations and intentions more clearly in order to avoid needless exposure to antibiotic drugs.

The Way Forward

Many doctors have used the term Post-Antibiotic Era to describe the period in which we now live. Others are more conservative and note that we are merely entering the Post-Antibiotic Era. Regardless of how one views the matter, a seismic change in philosophy, vision, and practice is in order.

While the name Post-Antibiotic Era is useful, I propose that we surrender the name in favor of the solutions-oriented Era of Host Defenses. Since we cannot rely on antibiotics as we have in the past, we must now redefine how we approach the bacterium, the person, and, indeed, medicine during this new era. I propose that we describe the way forward—The Era of Host Defenses—as a period in which we marshal our accumulated knowledge in human genetics, biochemistry, physiology, immunology, neuroscience, psychology, and related fields to focus on diagnostics and therapeutics squarely aimed at strengthening the defense and repair systems of the *host*—the person, the individual.

In order to do this, we must recognize the general factors that give rise to strong immune defense, energy, and repair systems. Within this context, we must also realize that each person is unique with regard to her genetic heritage, dietary patterns, lifestyle, psychological tendencies, environmental exposures, and social interactions.

Thus, the Era of Host Defenses also demands that we treat each person as an individual and that we tailor our treatments to the individual. While this requires a fundamental shift in the practice of medicine, medicine has been slowly, if not grudgingly, preparing for this shift for some time. In the Era of Host Defenses, we shift our focus from the microbe to the person. We advance the discipline of personalized medicine as a means to garner robust host defenses, which will permit us to thrive among the microbes and reduce the need for antibiotics.

This does not mean that we ignore the microbe. They are around us, on us, and within us. They permeate all of nature and it is still the microbe's world. It also does not mean that we refrain from appropriate use of antibiotics. They remain a vital tool in our emerging form of medicine. It does mean that our attention to the microbe falls within the context of creating a healthy host—the human-microbe hybrid. We create a healthy host by using our sophisticated knowledge of human biology to build an intelligent system of prevention, treatment, and recovery based on the evidence we have in hand.

Understanding how to create a robust system of immune defense, energy, and repair is the foundation of this new Era of Host Defenses.

Chapter 4

Immune Defense, Energy, and Repair

The immune system is an elaborate network of cells, chemical signals, and physical barriers that keep vigil in our dance of life and death with the microbial world. This sentinel system must continually determine whether the agents it encounters should be designated with "non-danger" or "danger" signals.

The immune system must remember past encounters. It must rise up quickly, though not too quickly. It must remove the potent molecules it produces to destroy bacteria. It must be attentive to false alarms. The barrier systems must allow for the passage of water, nutrients, and vital molecules but prohibit the passage of harmful agents. This system of immune and barrier defenses acts with such intelligence and autonomy that one is tempted to call the system sentient.

As we move forward in our discussion, it is important to understand some fundamental functions of the immune defense system. For the success of our strategies to maintain health in the face of bacterial encounters will depend upon how we attend to the support of these systems.

In this chapter I will go beyond the immune system in describing our defenses. I will repeatedly use the phrase **immune defense, energy, and repair system**. The use of this phrase is appropriate because it recognizes the following:

1. The fundamentals of the **immune system** as it is typically described

2. The heavy dependence of all aspects of human function on an efficient **energy** system, without which we cannot succeed
3. That efficient mechanisms of **repair** must be supported so that we can fully recover from infections, from the treatment associated with infections, and facilitate the repair of all systems that may have been compromised during a microbial encounter

Basic Ideas of Immunity

In this chapter, we are going to take a very quick tour through the immune system. It is not a comprehensive tour, but a journey that will touch on certain points important to building a personalized medicine strategy—a strategy that will help you fortify your immune defense, energy, and repair system.

The key points of this chapter include:

1. The two major branches of the immune system: natural immunity and acquired immunity
2. The importance of balance in the helper lymphocyte system (T-helper)
3. Key components of natural immunity that must be understood in order to make use of the key strategies discussed later

Natural vs. Adaptive Immunity

The most primitive aspect of our immune system is called **natural immunity**. This is our response to invaders in our midst that does not require previous experience. It is nonspecific, in that it does not recognize specific types of bacteria. We share this response with most all our neighboring creatures, from apes to frogs. **Adaptive immunity** is that part of the immune system that builds a response to specific threats, develops a memory, and is then capable of quite rapid response in any future encounter with that same type of microbe. Our natural immu-

■ **Table 4.1. The Two Main Branches of Immunity: Natural and Acquired**

	Natural (Innate, Non-Specific)	**Acquired (Adaptive)**
Anatomical Components	Skin, respiratory tract, gastrointestinal tract	Bone marrow, thymus, mucosal-associated lymphoid tissue, spleen, lymph node
Types of Cells	Neutrophils, monocytes, macrophages, dendritic cells, mast cells, eosinophils, basophils, natural killer cells	B lymphocytes T lymphocytes
Types of Molecules	Interferons Complements Collectin Lysozymes	Immunoglobulins (antibodies; IgA, IgG, IgD, IgM)
Specificity	Innate immunity is not specific in its attack of microbes	Targets specific microbes
Speed of Response	Reacts quickly, within hours	Take days to activate
Immunological Memory	Previous exposure to microbes does not improve function	Previous exposure to microbes significantly improves function and speed of response
Stage of Infection	Acts in the early stage of defenses	Acts in the later stage of defenses
Self-Discrimination	Able to distinguish self from non-self components, but indiscriminate tissue damage can occur	Distinguish self from non-self components, but is imperfect (autoimmunity)

The Two Main Branches of Immunity: Natural and Acquired. Adapted from: Li, P, Yin, YL, Li, D, et al. Amino acids and immune function. Br J Nutr 2007;98:237–52.

nity is quick to act, within hours, whereas adaptive immunity comes more fully into play within a few days.

If we are to thrive in the microbe's world, we must understand those things within our control that positively and negatively affect these two branches of our immune defense, energy, and repair system. Each branch of the immune system is strongly influenced by what we do on a daily basis. This means that an intelligent understanding of the science as we now know it, can form the foundation for a strategic personalized medicine plan.

The Immune System Balancing Act: Th1 and Th2

Our **adaptive** immune system (specific, acquired) is characterized by responses that involve T-cells and B-cells. A great deal of recent attention has been given to specific types of T-cells called T-helpers. They are frequently described at T-helper 1 and T-helper 2 (Th1 and Th2) cells.* T-helper cells usually engage a new infectious organism a few days into an infection, after the innate immune system has been involved.

Th1 cells are involved in cell-mediated immunity. They produce cytokines, such as interferon gamma (INFγ), interleukin-1 (IL-1), and tumor necrosis factor alpha (TNFα). These cytokines stimulate the destruction of harmful microbes by a process called phagocytosis, where cells called macrophages gobble up and eat the microbes. They are essential for controlling **intracellular** (microbes that get inside cells) pathogens like viruses and certain bacteria.

Th2 cells produce a different set of cytokines, namely IL-4, IL-5, IL-9, and IL-13. These provide help for B cells, so they are important for **antibody-mediated immunity**. Antibodies are needed to control harmful microbes that live outside cells and travel through the bloodstream.**

---

*The Th1 and Th2 designation is commonly used in medicine to describe two poles of the T-helper response that are held out as being fairly distinct. It should be noted that emerging research describes an overlap of these two systems and that the Th1 and Th2 designations are not always clear cut, as in some autoimmune diseases, for instance. However, since this concept is widely discussed in medicine, I will continue to make us of it, for there are a wide range of interventions within our control that seem to bring this portion of the immune system back into balance.

**Th17 cells also exist, which protect surfaces (e.g., skin, lining of the intestine) against extracellular bacteria. These are left out for simplicity.

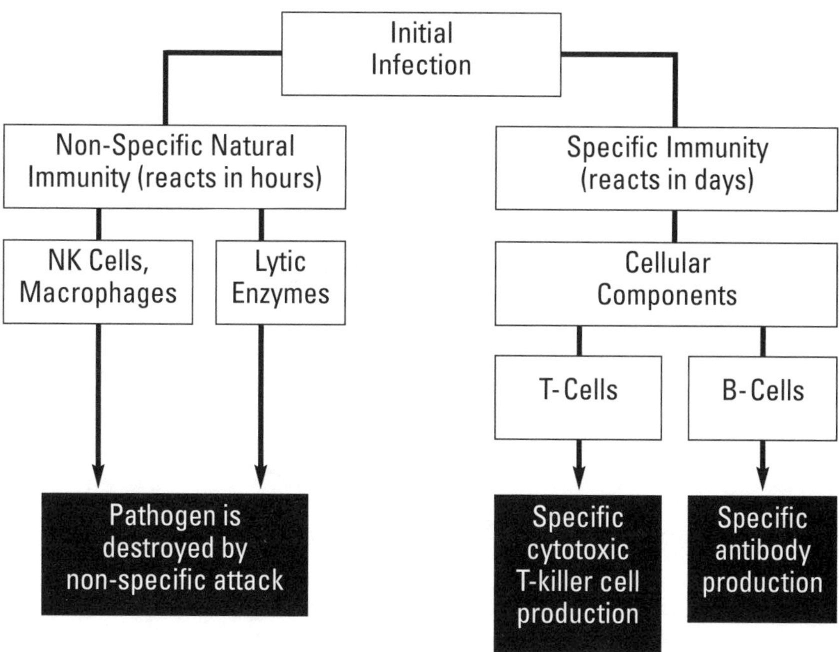

■ **Figure 4.1. Basic Behavior of Natural and Adaptive Immune Systems.** The basic behavior of the natural (nonspecific) immune system and adaptive (specific) immune system. Adapted from: Janeway, C.A. Jr, Travers, P, Walport, MW, Shlomchik, M. Eds. Immunobiology, 5th ed. New York: Garland Publishing, New York, 2001.

The concept of Th1 and Th2 balance in the immune system has gotten a great deal of attention. Though it has limitation and it only describes a portion of the actions of the immune system, it is a useful way to understand three things:

1. Excessive Th1 activity can lead to poor health and altered defense against microbes
2. Excessive Th2 activity can lead to poor health and altered defense against microbes
3. Balance between Th1 and Th2 activity is important in defending against microbes, controlling inflammation, and fostering repair.

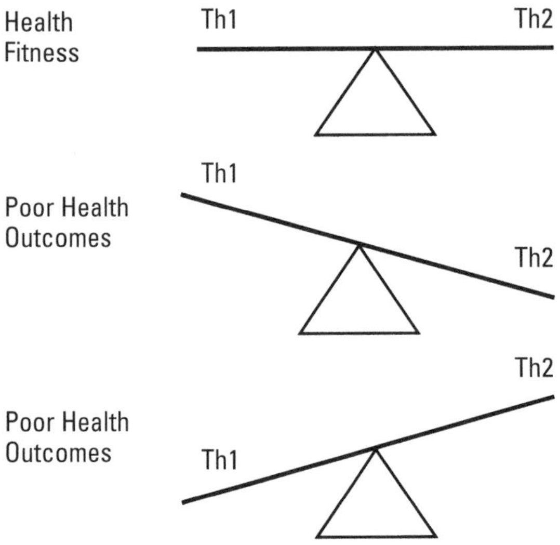

■ **Figure 4.2. Health Outcomes When Immune Proteins (Cytokines) Are Out of Balance.** When the Th1 and Th2 cytokines (immune proteins) are in balance, it is associated with an improved state of health and a balanced defense against microbes. When the Th1 / Th2 balance shifts in either direction, poor health outcomes are more common, such as increased susceptibility to infection and to autoimmune changes. This is an oversimplification, since there can be overlap. But this description is frequently used and it is one helpful way to view the interaction.

As we move forward, I will occasionally raise the issue of Th1 / Th2 balance. This is because there are a wide range of factors, such as sleep, exercise, nutrition, stress, gut bacteria, probiotics, and many other factors within our control that influence the regulation of this part of the immune system.

The Eyes of the Immune System

Our sense of sight, sound, smell, taste, and touch are a means for us to "sample" our surroundings. They relay signals throughout the body and either orchestrate an array of automatic responses or permit us to take conscious actions. Most of what our senses tell us takes place well beneath our conscious awareness. Increasingly, some scientists have begun to view the immune system in a similar light.

Dr. Edwin Blalock has proposed that the immune system is a sensory organ in much the same way as our other five senses.[78] Highlighting the idea of the immune system as a sensory organ, noted immunologist Mark M. Davis has remarked that "Lymphocytes and NK cells can be viewed as cell-sized sensory organs, continuously sampling the internal environment for things that do not belong there or for cellular stress or aberrations. Just as rod cells in the eye can detect even a single photon [of light], cytotoxic T-cells can kill on the advice of only three peptide-MHC ligands."[79]

Scientists have been trying to better understand how the immune system "sees" or "samples" its surroundings. Some scientists looking for the "eyes" of the immune system have proposed that a set of proteins scattered across the surface of white blood cells (and many other cells) just might be these "eyes."

Microbes have all sorts of molecules on their surfaces. Our cells have evolved the tools to recognize the various shapes and sizes of these microbial molecules. The toll-like receptors are among the first tools our cells use to detect these microbial bits.

This might be viewed like a highway toll booth. As you approach the toll stop, the gate is closed. When you throw the correct change into the receptacle, the gate opens. Throw in the wrong change and nothing happens. The toll stop has been designed with a sensing system that recognizes the shape and size of the different coins and only gives the green light and opens the gate when the right combination of shapes and sizes exists.

There are at least a dozen toll-like receptors that help us identify different bacteria. Each one recognizes a different component of a bacterium, such as their DNA, their RNA, and other molecules. While toll receptors alert us to a bacterial presence and activate the immune response, we'll see later how these toll-like receptors can set off false alarms, by "seeing" things in our diet that are not microbial threats. We will also see how bacterial cell wall fragments can ramp up immune function in ways that work to our detriment. This idea of toll-like receptors is important to remember, for it appears that many things within our control might influence false alarm activation of the TLR system.

Barrier Defenses: The Importance of the Gut

While the barriers of our skin, lungs, digestive tract, and other areas form the first line of defense against invading microbes, I am going to focus on the barrier defenses of the intestinal tract, for it is here that a vast, unseen drama is played out every moment of every day. The weakening of our defense, energy, and repair system at this level can have widespread consequences and pose an almost daily threat of which we are typically unaware.

Consider that the mucosal surface of the human digestive tract is about the size of two football fields. Picture a surface this size carpeted with some one hundred to five thousand different types of bacteria all competing for nutrients, food, and a place to attach. This vast surface takes almost one-fourth of the heart's blood supply (while the gut is at rest). According to Dr. Andreas Krack at the Imperial College of London, our helpful gut bacteria help maintain a strong barrier defense in the intestinal tract. This keeps harmful bacteria and bacterial fragments from leaking across our intestinal barrier and gaining access to infect our interior.[80]

This idea of a healthy gut barrier is very important to understand because it links diet, nutrition, lifestyle, psychological stressors, and many other factors that affect our defenses. It may also explain the widespread disruptions in immune defenses that occur with many different types of illness. Of the untold number of bacteria in the human gut, many will die before being eliminated. As they die, their bodies break apart, with fragments scattered throughout the bowel. Much of this dead bacterial debris is eliminated in the stool. However, some of these cell-wall fragments of bacteria (called endotoxins, or LPS) may drift or leak across the gut barrier and make their way into the bloodstream. This is one reason a strong and intact gut barrier defense is so critical.

If the gut barrier defenses weaken (leaky gut), bacterial endotoxin can enter circulation and elicit an immune response, which can have vast repercussions throughout the body. This phenomenon can occur even in conditions that one would expect to have nothing to do with the gut at all. For example, bacterial fragments can leak from the gut into the bloodstream in cases of heart disease, burns, surgery, trauma, and other conditions. If endotoxin enters the blood circulation in people who have severe illness or immune suppression, it can prove lethal. A faulty gut barrier (with leakage of endotoxin) can influence things like bone healing after a fracture, especially if trauma is significant or if surgery is involved.[81] The effects of these bacterial endotoxins are partially driven by the toll-like receptors mentioned above.

Things like stress, alcohol, dietary factors, anti-inflammatory drugs, antibiotics, and other medications can all increase damage to the intestinal lining. We will see throughout this book that the integrity of the gut barrier may be the difference between health and illness (or even survival), and from a wide range of conditions like trauma, heart disease, obesity, diabetes, and more.

Antibiotics and Gut Barrier Disruption

It is important to realize that the process of disrupting the gut barrier can begin very in early in childhood for a variety of reasons. Use of large, single doses or repeated modest doses of antibiotics in childhood often sets the stage for early alterations of gut integrity, which can lead to health problems. It is also important to note that single doses of antibiotics can alter gut bacteria in adulthood, the effects of which can persist for a very long time, in some cases.

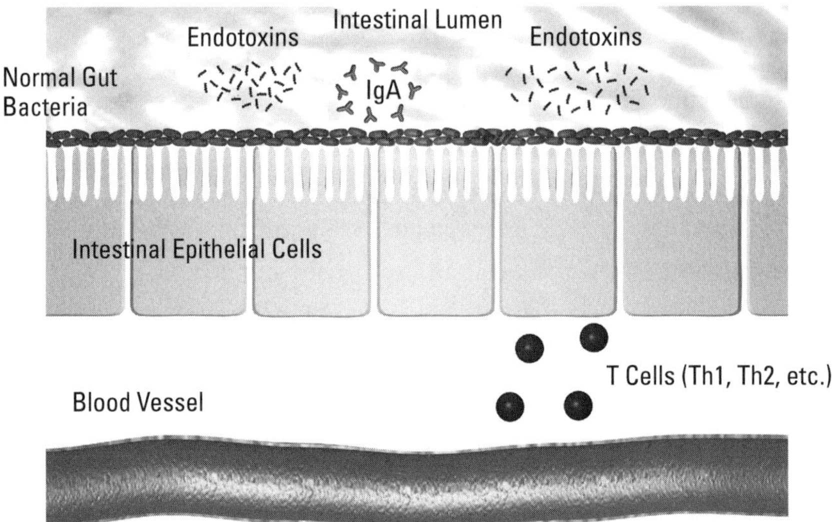

■ **Figure 4.3. The Intestinal Lining (Barrier) and How It Keeps Gut Bacteria from Crossing into the Bloodstream.** A strong intestinal barrier keeps endotoxins and other potentially harmful contents of the gut from leaking into across the barrier and entering the bloodstream.

For instance, one study showed that people who had taken only one course of an antibiotic had significantly lower blood levels of a compound called enterolactone, which persisted for up to sixteen months after the antibiotic was consumed. This was compared to those who were antibiotic-free during the same time period. Enterolactone is formed by the action of gut bacteria on dietary lignans (a form of soluble plant fiber) from foods such as rye. Decreased enterolactone is typically understood to reflect a decrease in gut bacteria that are able to ferment certain dietary fibers.[82] Enterolactone is a helpful byproduct of gut bacteria that has been found to be protective against certain cancers such as breast cancer,[83] as well as against heart disease.[84]

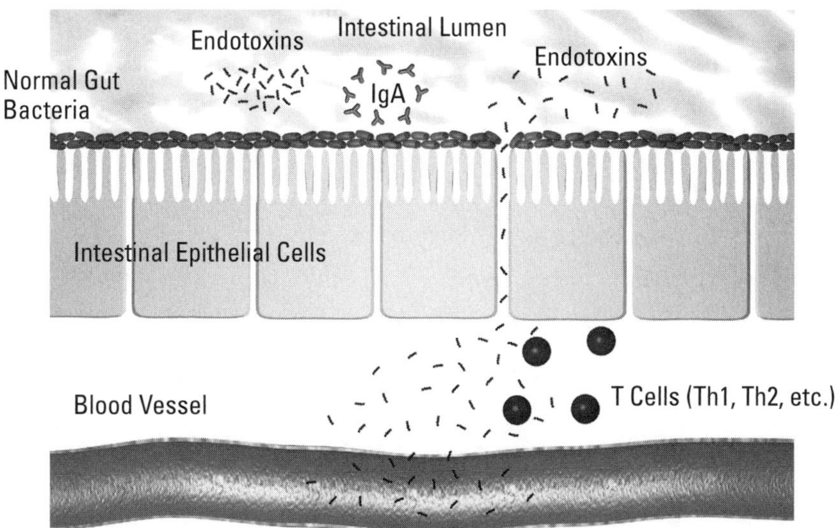

■ **Figure 4.4. How Gut Bacteria Fragments (Endotoxins) Leak into the Bloodstream.** When the intestinal barrier is weakened (the junction between cells is injured), endotoxins and other intestinal molecules can leak across, enter the bloodstream, and elicit a harmful response.

Energy

Defending our bodies amidst so vast a sea of microbes requires a formidable effort, with tremendous energy demands. The process of maintaining and repairing ordinary barrier defenses such the skin, mucous membranes, and gut lining requires an energy-intensive process that takes place well beneath our awareness. When we need to generate a fever, energy must be diverted from ordinary functions like muscle activity to feed the demands of immunity. In fact, *for every 1° Celsius increase in body temperature during fever, a concomitant 7 to 13 percent increase in energy production is required* (which is species-dependent).[85] During infection, the body must activate its production of white blood cells so that it has appropriate forces with which to act against any invader. This process of white blood cell synthesis demands immense quantities of energy.

Immune cells have an ingenious way of conserving energy. T-lymphocytes and memory T-cells can circulate in the bloodstream for long periods in a resting state. They remain in reserve, while the body is free to expend its energy resources on other, more pressing matters, such as writing a report, going to the gym, running a marathon, or giving birth. The T-cells are the lifeguards sitting on a shaded perch, with a careful eye on the water. When the swimmer starts bobbing up and down, crying for help, the quiescent, resting lifeguard springs from his perch, using all the energy of his considerable fitness and expert training. Rushing into sometimes fearsome surf, the lifeguard accelerates his metabolism, surging to the rescue.

When a bacterium plunges into the waters of the body, T-cells are activated by a metabolic switch. The T-cells can ramp up their glucose uptake by a startling twenty times within a mere one hour.[86] These cells may increase their lactate production, a feature of accelerated energy metabolism, by a remarkable forty times. T-cells must increase their numbers. While a single lifeguard can save one swimmer, he surely cannot save one hundred swimmers. The T-cells must replicate to meet the challenge of bacteria that can double their population every twenty minutes.

As impressive as the energy demands of the immune response under challenge are, we must also respect the demands of a resting state. When we go to sleep, our energy use is reduced but we still have what scientists call "house-keeping functions" taking place. We have to be in some functional state while sleeping or we could not repair ourselves or leap out of bed when the baby cries.

Lymphocytes, another type of white blood cell, are no different. They are in a constant state of housekeeping, even while resting. They have to repair the shutters and take out the trash. This requires energy.

Energy requires nutrients. There is no escape from this fundamental law. The immune cells feed on glucose (sugar) in order to make the energy currency ATP. We're usually not short on the raw fuel. However, the cofactors that drive the energy pathways can be limiting. Simple nutrients are needed to drive what we call the citric acid cycle (TCA or Kreb's cycle) and oxidative phosphorylation. Vitamins B1, B2, B3, B6, biotin, coenzyme Q10, iron, magnesium, manganese—these are all cofactors in various steps of the energy process of white blood cells. During a threat, we must also use fatty acids and amino acids to build the nucleotides needed for DNA synthesis in the new white cells.

Seeking to understand these demands on our immunity has turned scientists' attention more fully to how energy might influence our infection susceptibility. In fact, some doctors are now beginning to measure the ATP production of lymphocytes to determine whether lowered energy production may contribute to a patient's poor immunity.

Consider a study in the *Bulletin of Experimental Biology and Medicine.* Fifty-four children and adolescents were selected for study because they had recurrent infections of the upper respiratory tract triggered by bacteria such as *Mycoplasma pneumoniae* and *Chlamydia pneumoniae.* Most had suffered from three to six episodes of acute respiratory tract infections over a one-year period.*

Just as once a rechargeable battery wears down, it cannot run a flashlight until it is recharged, so in our white blood cells, once the charge goes off of ATP (and more remains in the uncharged state as ADP), there is insufficient "charge" for them to efficiently conduct their defensive business. We can now use this measure of "charged" versus "uncharged" ATP to assess energy potential in white blood cells. It

---

*They discovered an average 21 percent decrease in ATP content in lymphocytes during the first two weeks after a respiratory infection in those who were frequently ill. The ratio of ATP to ADP was shifted toward ADP, meaning that once a molecule of ATP was used for energetic purposes, it was not adequately regenerating back to ATP. More of these molecules remained in their ADP state—an unhealthy state.

appeared, from the above study, that children suffering from recurrent illness had deficits in the energy systems of their white blood cells.[87]

So we must pay close attention to the body's energy systems and the molecules (often nutrients) that feed these systems if we wish to maintain robust immunity. One study looked at nutrient supplementation in people with inborn errors of their energy system (called mitochondrial oxidative phosphorylation disorders). In these patients, providing cofactors of the energy system, such as coenzyme Q10, ascorbic acid, vitamin E, riboflavin, thiamine, niacin, vitamin K, and carnitine led to improvements in lymphocyte ATP synthesis.[88] It is believed that if these nutrients can improve lymphocyte ATP in those with genetic disorders it may be supportive in other people, as well.

We can view our energy-immunity requirement by looking at it as a trade-off between vital functions wherein we have a specific amount of metabolic fuel that must be allocated as most needed. This includes locomotion/movement, reproduction, growth, thermogenesis (heat generation), immune function, and cellular maintenance.

Special circumstances have shown us a great deal about how our defenses are dependent upon our energy efficiency.

Pregnancy

It is widely known that pregnancy increases energy demands for expectant mothers. But pregnancy is also associated with suppressed immunity in the mother. The standard hypothesis given for this immune decline is the need to protect the fetus from its mother's aggressive immune defenses. Indeed, there is a clear activation of the innate immune system during pregnancy, with a suppression of the specific immune system (a shift from Th1 to Th2 dominance). However, more recent evidence has doctors convinced that another reason for the immune suppression of pregnancy is the intense energy demands of the growing fetus. Across all animal species, there appears to be a trade-off between energy and immunity. If energy is diverted to one critical function, energy is not fully available to support robust immune defenses.

Some evidence of how strongly pregnancy affects immunity can be found in various infectious outbreaks. Consider the following:

- During the Asian influenza epidemic in New York City (1957), 40 percent of the deaths in those under 50 were pregnant women.[89]
- The incidence of hepatitis in Kashmir was 600 percent higher in pregnant women.[90]
- The odds of developing clinical symptoms of polio were 60 percent higher among pregnant women from 1949 to 1955.[91]

Lactation

The post-pregnancy period associated with lactation is also one of intense energy demands. The mother is simultaneously recovering from the demands of pregnancy and garnering the resources to produce enough milk to grow a young child. It has been estimated that the basal metabolic rate doubles or triples during lactation and that any energy shortages during this time will not support robust immune defenses.[92]

Intense Training

Intensive training regimens like those in the military can take a substantial toll on immunity. For example, men taking part in an extended U.S. Army Rangers training course experience a progressive increase in their rate of infection despite taking large doses of antibiotics.[93] Another study of U.S. military Special Forces trainees showed that during twenty-five weeks of grueling training, the rate of respiratory illness was more than twice the U.S. incidence rate.[94]

Increasing calorie intake may counter some of these effects of declining immunity in extreme conditions. In a study of military special forces, Army Rangers experienced up to a 15.6 percent loss of body mass during two months of intense training. This was associated with a decrease in T-lymphocyte counts and responsiveness. Those who received a 15 percent increase in food intake experienced a greater than 20 percent increase in lymphocyte counts within nine days. This study was undertaken because the Ranger Corps had experienced a high incidence of pneumococcal pneumonia during intense training exercises.[95]

So, it is clear that energy serves immunity and all of the defense and repair functions of the body. We must pay attention to our energy deficits, of which there are many, if we are to walk comfortably in the world of the microbe. Muscle tissue in particular must be considered at the core of building robust energy reserves and capability.

Putting the Muscle in Immunity: How Muscle Mass Fuels Immune Defenses

It is clear that rising to handle a microbial threat can be an energy- and resource-intensive prospect. But from where does this capacity to generate such energy arise? Enter a tissue that has only recently gained recognition as central to immune defenses—skeletal muscle. In fact, it may be the abundance or lack of skeletal muscle that determines much about how we respond to infection or how we defeat microbes over the long haul.

Besides looking at our muscles as the tools to move our bones, we must also see them as reservoirs of metabolic fuels and molecular spare parts. As the energy demands of ramping up immune defenses rise, the demand for fuel rises in concert. The glycogen (a storage form of sugar) that is stored in muscle is depleted rapidly. Luckily, amino acids (the building blocks of protein) that are abundant in muscle are released from muscle proteins and can be used as fuel. In essence, the metabolic demands of infection cause us to break down our own muscle tissue to provide amino acids that fuel the immune defense buildup.

When injury or infection occurs, the body must manufacture new "acute phase" proteins: new white blood cells, natural antimicrobial proteins, immune proteins such as cytokines, immunoglobulins (antibodies), and molecules involved in wound healing. The body must also synthesize antioxidant molecules such as glutathione to attend to the tremendous free-radical stress associated with infection or trauma. All of these require amino acids, which are the building blocks of protein.

With our immune system behaving as a "sixth sense," the activation of all of these processes in the face of a microbial advance takes place well beneath our awareness. Upon activation of our immune surveillance system, the body begins to remove amino acids from the reservoir of structural proteins in muscle. In this way, muscle serves as a bank account to be used in any time of shortage or crisis in the body as a whole. As an infection progresses, we draw down substantial reserves from this muscle storage pool. This is somewhat like burning the furniture to survive a blizzard. You may not be able to go outside to get more wood, so you burn what's in the house to live for another day. In short, we sacrifice our muscle to save ourselves—a fair trade and an elegant system.

The impact of muscle on immunity and recovery is striking. A burn injury (which is associated with a sharply elevated risk to infection) illustrates the dramatic protein needs: The amount of protein needed for the immune activation and cellular repair of a burn to 50 percent of the body is 3 to 4 grams per kilograms of body weight. For a 200-pound (or 90-kilogram) man, that translates into 360 grams of protein daily. For a 120-pound (or 55-kilogram) woman, it translates into a protein requirement of 220 grams per day.[96] This is roughly *four times* the normal amount of our daily requirements, which is very difficult to sustain during an illness, when appetite and activity are low. So, the protein is wisely taken from muscle.

The effect of muscle on survival from critical illness is also impressive. For instance, less than 50 percent of people in intensive care return to work within the first year of discharge. If there is preexisting deficiency of muscle mass before hospitalization, the likelihood of full recovery falls and some people never fully recover from their illness. For example, more than 50 percent of women over 65 who break a hip never walk again.[97] Additionally, survival from severe burn injury has been shown to be lowest in individuals with reduced lean body mass.[98]

Consider that the average muscle mass of young, healthy males ranges from 77 to 110 pounds. In contrast, an elderly woman may have less than 30 pounds of muscle.[99] Looked at another way, muscle accounts for 90 percent of the cross-sectional area in active young men, but only 30 percent in frail older women.[100] Muscle represents about 40 percent of body weight and contains from 50 to 75 percent of all protein in the human body. Remarkably, a mere 10 percent loss of lean body mass is associated with a decline in immune function.[101] From existing research, it is evident that low muscle mass renders one less able to respond to infection, trauma, and disease—especially if it is prolonged or chronic.

It's important to establish appropriate muscle mass for all age groups, since muscle mass declines with age. In fact, loss of muscle mass may be one of the key elements in declining immunity common to aging, as illustrated by a study of 1,017 men that showed declining strength (and lower strength) was the feature most closely linked to survival.[102]

The health effects of physical fitness have been touted for years. Beyond aerobic fitness, we must also direct our attention to muscle mass and muscle strength. It has become evident that a dedicated effort to establish and maintain muscle mass could be central to our long-term insurance against infectious disease. We must include a committed amount of physical activity and protein intake to build the reservoir of muscle-based protein to hold in reserve for times of need. It may be one of our most critical means of establishing a robust immune defense and repair system. The appropriate amounts of protein will be explored later in the chapter on nutrition and immunity.

Muscles Can Recognize Bacteria

One of the remarkable new discoveries about muscle is that it has the capacity to recognize bacteria. It is now clear that muscle cells possess toll-like receptors (TLR), just like those on white blood cells. Once a fragment of the bacterial cell wall (or some other bacterial molecule) docks with the TLR on a muscle cell, a cascade of proteins (cytokines) is released that shuts down muscle protein synthesis. The energy and raw materials typically dedicated to building and preserving muscle are conserved for another purpose—mounting a defense. This reaction is one reason why muscle loss occurs during infection and why muscle wasting occurs during prolonged infection.[103] It also appears that muscle cells behave somewhat like a type of immune cell called an antigen-presenting cell (APC). It is fascinating to think of muscle cells as active participants in the immune defense, energy, and repair system.[104]

Healthy Metabolism

It is clear that efficient energy metabolism and ample protein (muscle) reserves are important to sustain the immune response, the barrier defenses, and the repair process related to infections. In a state of optimum health, one expects that metabolism is at its most efficient and most able to accomplish these response and maintenance functions.

But what happens when metabolism falters, as in a chronic illness? Diabetes is a prime example of such faltering metabolism. Diabetes affects more than 16 million Americans and roughly 250 million people worldwide.Those with diabetes have abnormal white blood cell function, depending upon how poorly controlled their blood sugar. The ability of white blood cells to travel to the site of an infection, adhere to the site, engulf, and destroy bacteria can all be impaired in diabetes.[105] This can translate into more severe disease when microbes are encountered. For instance, people with diabetes were found to be more at risk of complications from pneumonia.[106]

One reason diabetes is so hard on the immune system is that it is linked to such widespread metabolic disturbance. One of these is free radical damage (from oxidative stress). When 21 people with diabetes were given about the amount of sugar in two soft drinks (75 grams of glucose), the free radical products of damaged fatty acids, called isoprostanes, rose by 34 percent in only 90 minutes.* Studies have also shown the converse, that diets *low* in simple sugars *reduce* oxidative stress.[107] Besides damaging fatty acids and cell membranes, free radical stress can cause energy production in the cell to fall, resulting in fatigue and low energy.

These are among the reasons that people with diabetes simply must control the intake of simple carbohydrates in their diets and control their blood sugar. Otherwise, impairment of defense, energy, and repair will most likely follow. People with diabetes who better control their blood glucose have been shown to have improved immune function, improved defense against bacteria, and reduced severity of infections (when infections do occur).[108]

Doctors in the intensive care unit clearly understand the need to maintain healthy metabolism. For years, doctors have given intravenous insulin to ICU patients as a means to prevent infections, since it is well known that controlling blood glucose is central to maintaining a robust immune response.

There are many factors that can affect the efficiency of metabolism, which naturally has an effect on our ability to respond to microbes.

---

*Our cell membranes are made from fatty acids—the same ones found in our diet. Free radicals from many causes can attack the fatty acids, warp their shape, and clip them off their anchoring points in the cell membrane. Isoprostanes are one form of these damaged cell membrane fatty acids. Thus, elevated isoprostanes are both a sign of free radical stress and damaged cell membranes.

Fever as a Defense

There is a long history of doctors using or viewing fever as necessary to our recovery. Then there were more recent periods when fever suppression was in vogue. In our day, fever has generally been viewed as problematic. But amidst that view has been a small chorus of voices arguing the benefits of fever, noting that it is one of the most universal means to combat infection across all animal species. In general, fever is now viewed as an emergency defense that takes over when the specific, or adaptive, immune response has not quickly controlled an infectious agent. Viewed another way, our natural immunity, through such things as fever, must "hold the fort" until specific immunity develops.

This period of rapid elevation of the natural immune defense suppresses the specific immune defenses while the natural immune defense takes over. In doing so, it marshals a tremendous amount of energy, diverting energy from muscles and certain organs not deemed a priority.

Dr. Matthew Kluger has been studying the role of fever in mammals (including humans) and nonmammals for much of his career. While it is beyond the scope of this book to explore the subject in depth, Dr. Kluger's paper published in the *Annals of the New York Academy of Sciences* contains key elements that recognize the importance of fever in survival. His group writes:

> For thousands of years, fever was considered a protective response, and fevers were induced by physicians to combat certain infections. But with the advent of antipyretic drugs, physicians started to reduce fevers, and fever therapy was virtually abandoned. As a result of 1) studies on the evolution of fever, 2) further understanding of just how tightly the process of fever is regulated, and 3) detailed studies on how fever affects host morbidity and mortality, the view of fever as a host defense response has reemerged.

Citing correlational studies, Kluger surmises that "under most conditions, moderate fevers are beneficial in fighting infection, while high fevers are indicators of overwhelming infection and may be maladaptive." Antipyretic studies have shown that use of fever-suppressing agents has *increased illness and death* in many species. Dr. Kluger reviewed one study of patients undergoing colorectal surgery and the effect of hypothermia on surgical wound infection. Those with lower body temperatures had significantly more infections and longer hospital stays than those with a higher body temperature.[109]

It is clear from the fifty studies reviewed by Kluger that fevers that rise too high can be problematic. But the theme that emerges is that fever is an important generalized response to an invading organism that ramps up nonspecific immune defenses until the specific immune defenses can be summoned with sufficient strength to remove the threat.

Kluger is not alone in his caution about fever suppression. A provocative idea has emerged from Anthony Torres at Utah State University regarding the risks of fever suppression. He proposes that the suppression of fever alters the profile of cytokine molecules that influence the brain of a developing fetus or a young child. Doctor Torres suggests that use of fever-suppressing agents such as acetaminophen results in modification of the immunologic development of the brain along with modified gene expression patterns common to autism. His hypothesis specifically states that "The blockage of fever with antipyretics interferes with normal immunological development in the brain leading to neurodevelopmental disorders, such as autism in certain genetically and immunologically disposed individuals." In his paper, he proposes a model to study the controversial hypothesis, but notes that a concerted research effort is needed to definitively say that fever suppression leads to autism.[110]

In dealing with fever, doctors must always balance the severity of the insult, the degree of temperature rise, the appearance of the patient, and the overall strength of the patient's immune response.

Our Natural Antimicrobial Proteins

Our skin, the lining of the digestive tract, and the lining of the lungs form part of the barrier defense network of the immune system. Their role is to form a physical barrier that impedes the advance of any potential microbial threat. The cells of the skin, lungs, and digestive tract (called epithelial cells) are also known to secrete a family of molecules called antimicrobial peptides (AMPs). Selected white blood cells also contain AMPs.[111] Two of the most studied antimicrobial peptides are called cathelicidins and defensins. These peptides (or proteins) directly kill a wide range of microbes including bacteria, fungi, and certain viruses.[112] Researchers are now on an ambitious path to understand how to mimic AMPs in the development of new antimicrobial drugs. Meanwhile, other scientists are trying to better understand how to manipulate or improve the body's own antimicrobial peptide capability.

People with skin conditions, such as atopic dermatitis (who are more susceptible to skin infections) have impaired production of antimicrobial peptides. In the colon, those with defective cathelicidin production are more susceptible to certain bacterial infections. Defensins are also found in high amounts in human breastmilk, which is one of the natural means to protect a nursing child against bacterial disease.[113]

One promising horizon is the manipulation of AMPs through nutrition. For instance, vitamin D3 has been shown to activate the gene promoter for cathelicidin in cells of the skin (keratinocytes) and the immune system (monocytes).[114] The short chain fatty acid *butyrate* was found to activate cathelicidin formation in colon cells.[115] Interestingly, butyrate is formed by certain beneficial gut bacteria in response to dietary oligosaccharides, a kind of complex carbohydrate loved by certain gut bacteria. This would be another example of how gut bacteria might help stimulate the defenses against harmful organisms. Butyrate is also used in supplemental form in colonic disorders. In later chapters, we'll learn about a mind-body practice that appears to increase the natural production of dermicidin, an AMP produced by the sweat glands that protects against skin infection.

Hormones, Infection, and Immunity

Our immune defense and repair system is guided, if not driven, by shifting hormones (and neurotransmitters). Cortisol is one of the most powerful of the immune-suppression hormones, which is why the stress response may take such a toll on immune vigilance. However, cortisol can also be influential in our repair phase, by virtue of its effect on resolvins. Doctors frequently now meausure cortisol at four different time points throughout the day (from 8 a.m. to midnight) in order to determine if disruption of the cortisol cycle might be linked to any state of illness.

Thyroid hormone has a special place in regulation of the immune response. In fact, the natural killer (NK) cell numbers and activity in elderly people have been strongly linked to adequate thyroid hormone levels (T3 and free T4). Thyroid stimulating hormone (TSH) is able to restore the production of the immune protein IL-2. As further evidence for the importance of the thyroid in immunity, lymphocytes even have receptors for thyroid hormones on their surface. Standard approaches to people who suffer from frequent infections or lowered immunity now routinely involve a thyroid hormone panel that includes TSH, T3, T4, antithyroid antibodies, and thyroid peroxidase.

Testosterone is our principal *anabolic* hormone, meaning it is used in building and repairing things. Both males and females require testosterone for this purpose. Testosterone levels change as we age, which is one reason that our immune system weakens with age. Testosterone, estrogen, and sex hormone-binding globulin are widely used to assess imbalances that might be related to compromised defenses.

A testosterone-related hormone called DHEA (dehydroepiendrosterone) is also central to strong immunity, and especially so to recovery and repair. DHEA is another hormone that decreases as we age.[116] Levels of DHEA and the sulfated form of DHEA are routinely measured in blood to assess whether deficiencies in production of this hormone are linked to poor defense, energy, and repair. Vitamin D, a hormonelike vitamin, also now appears to be a requirement for strong defenses.

Another hormone critical to immune defense, energy, and repair is growth hormone (GH).[117] Growth hormone secretion is about 600 mg daily, which peaks at age twenty-five. By age sixty to seventy, growth hormone levels can drop to a meager 15 percent of those peak levels. This can have a pronounced effect on our repair function. Adrenal compounds, such as epinephrine and norepinephrine, form the foundation of our flight-or-fight response to stressors. We'll see later how these molecules of stress shape our immune defenses and how they may even give bacteria the tools to assault us with more vigor. The ability to detect changes in these primary hormones and to use thereapies targeted to our needs will become central in our drive to build strong defenses.

Moving Beyond Antibiotics

With crisis comes opportunity. Our opportunity to devise a new means of living in the microbe's world is clearly upon us. While antibiotics will remain critical to *some* of our encounters with the bacterial world, we should only use them in conjunction with a strategy that takes the necessary steps to strengthen defense, energy, and repair.

This is the fundamental message of the way forward. The path forward will demand that we become more sophisticated in the way that we approach the strengthening of these defenses. If we bring the same level of scientific acumen and energy to this opportunity that we have brought to surgery, emergency medicine, and other fields, I am convinced that an entirely new era of medicine will arise. This new era, the Era of Host Defenses, will ride on the extraordinary discoveries of the past decade. For the average person, some of these strategies can already be translated into steps that can be lived daily, as each of us embark on a personalized journey toward robust immunity.

PART II

How We Can Take Control

Chapter 5

How Nutrients Fuel the Entire System

Without essential nutrients, there can be no efficient immune defense, energy, and repair. Consider that ALL biochemical systems within the human body are dependent upon essential molecules derived from the diet. Essential nutrients (or molecules) are technically defined as **molecules that are necessary for metabolism, but cannot be synthesized by the human body**. This includes eight amino acids, two fatty acids, thirteen vitamins, and twenty one minerals. Our bodies are wholly dependent upon these essential components to make all other molecules. Other nutrients are *conditionally essential,* meaning that we can make them, but under various circumstances (including deficiency of the above) we cannot make enough of them to meet our requirements. (See Appendix C.) Thus, these must also be obtained from the diet.

To be sure, the body is endowed with many redundant systems. For example, we can create energy out of amino acids (protein), fatty acids (fat), or sugars (carbohydrate). If we consume low *quantities* of one, we can generate energy from another (though *quality* surely matters). But even slight deficiencies of micronutrients create widespread disruption. If these deficiencies are too severe, disease ensues. For instance, we cannot methylate our DNA without vitamin B12, folic acid, or choline. Reduce any of these too far and our defense and repair systems suffer. Reduce magnesium levels too far and systemwide failures begin. Reduce vitamin B1 levels too far and energy failures begin. Reduce vitamin C levels too far and barrier defenses begin to fail.

If we reduce the amount of the amino acid tryptophan in the diet, we cannot make the neurotransmitter serotonin. Reduce the amino acid tyrosine or phenylalanine in the diet and we cannot make the neurotransmitter dopamine. Eliminate the vitamin B6 and vitamin C required to convert either of these amino acids into their respective neurotransmitters, and production of both will fail. Our margin for error with essential dietary molecules is small. There are few redundant systems where essential nutrients are concerned.

The body is fully dependent upon essential compounds for the most basic needs. However, add in any unique circumstance and these needs change. Essential nutrient needs can be altered by bacterial infection, viral infection, and parasitic infection. Essential nutrient needs can be altered by heavy exercise, prescription drug use, heavy metal exposure, bowel diseases, chronic illness (like diabetes or cancer), surgery, persistent psychological stressors, or a long list of other influences. Essential nutrient needs can be altered by our genetics.

So, the discussion of nutrition in immune defense, energy, and repair is much more than whether deficiency alters our susceptibility to infection, or whether or not supplements may improve our defenses under certain circumstances. It is without question that nutrients influence immune defense, energy, and repair.

We must really change the question we are asking. The real question is how do we optimize the nutritional status of any given individual in their specific life circumstance, so that we can optimize his or her particular immune defense, energy, and repair system?

This chapter will provide an overview of selected nutrients and their role in aspects of immune defense, energy, and repair. While it is beyond the scope of this book to present an in-depth review, I will use this chapter to explore how nutrients may influence our defensive systems under different circumstances. This begins with a discussion the general role that nutrients may play in illness, followed by a discussion of specific nutrients. (See Appendix C for a more concise description of why nutrients are important.)

As noted in Chapter 4, all functional systems within the human body require energy. All systems require raw materials to build cellular structures and maintain barrier defenses. In essence, all our systems must have sufficient building blocks to make other stuff that we need. These building blocks are derived from the diet. In general, our systems require:

1. Precursors* needed to use as **fuel** (amino acids, sugars, fatty acids)
2. Precursors to serve as **structural** molecules (amino acids, sugars, fatty acids)
3. Precursors to serve as **functional** molecules (amino acids, sugars, fatty acids)
4. **Cofactors** needed to drive the formation of a vast array of structural and functional molecules (magnesium, iron, copper, etc.)
5. **Coenzymes** needed to drive the formation of a vast array of structural and functional molecules (based on vitamins such as thiamin, riboflavin, pyridoxine, etc.)

When we think of nutrition and its effect on our defense, energy, and repair, we must think of our micronutrient needs and our macronutrient needs. Macronutrients occur in the form of protein, carbohydrate, and fat. Micronutrients include minerals, trace elements, and vitamins. We must also consider food factors that do not fit our classical defini-

*A precursor is defined as an item from which something else can be made. A building block is another commonly used term for precursor. Precursor nutrients can be very specific or very general. Certain important molecules can only be made from a single precursor molecule. For instance, thyroid hormone requires the amino acid tyrosine. Thyroid hormone cannot be manufactured from any other amino acid (though we can make tyrosine from phenylalanine). The fatty acids EPA and DHA must be the precursors for repair molecules, such as resolvins, lipoxins, and protectins.

tion of nutrients, yet drive our biology in profound ways. Phytochemicals such as flavones, flavonoids, anthocyanins, and many unrelated families of molecules fall into this category. Salicylates, found in many foods (and in aspirin), can be found circulating in the blood of all people and form a sort of natural anti-inflammatory background defense.

Standard treatment of the subject of nutrition and immunity addresses the classic immune parameters, such as how nutrients affect white blood cell function. In this chapter, we look beyond white blood cells and explore how nutrition affects barrier defenses, energy, repair, and a host of other bodily activities central to successfully living in the microbe's world. Nutritional effects on immunity are vast and profound. They are also complex. It is not always easy to clearly state exactly how a given nutrient affects our defenses. Quite often, a nutrient has opposing effects on immunity depending upon the level of such nutrients. As we will see, iron falls into this category. Also, a single nutrient may stimulate one component of the immune system, while inhibiting another.

Nutrients are the driving force in human biology. They give rise to the structural elements that give us form. They drive the metabolic processes that yield our energy and govern our repair. They are the raw material that fuels every endeavor. Nutrients are an immune system imperative. Thus begins the general question of how nutrients may affect infection susceptibility.

The Influence of Dietary Intake on Infection Susceptibility

There is growing evidence that vitamin and mineral deficiency can lead to diminished immunity and increased infection susceptibility, and that supplementation can boost immunity and build resistance to infection. For instance, in a group of one hundred elderly patients, low blood levels of vitamin E were associated with an increased number of infections.[118] In another study, vitamin E supplementation was shown to increase defenses against a number of infectious agents.[119] These are but two of many studies that have begun to verify the link between nutrition and immunity.

Drs. Paul Newberne and Gail Williams, while at the Massachusetts Institute of Technology, contributed to a book entitled *Nutritional Influences in the Cause of Infectious Disease.* They described four important ways in which nutrition can influence infection. Nutritional deficiency can:[120]

1. Adversely affect the body, which makes it easier for the bacteria or virus to invade
2. Have an adverse effect on the bacteria or virus once it has established itself in the body
3. Increase susceptibility to secondary infection
4. Slow convalescence after infection

Physician and researcher Thomas McKeown spent considerable time investigating the underlying reasons humans become ill. He stated that "the relationship [between man and microorganism] is stable and finely balanced according to the physiological states of the host and parasite; an improvement in nutrition would tip the balance in favor of the former, and a deterioration in favor of the latter."[121] McKeown further stated, "A severe degree of deficiency of almost any of the essential nutrients may have a marked effect on the manner in which the host responds to an infectious agent. The same infection may be mild or even unapparent in a well-nourished host, but virulent and sometimes fatal in one that is malnourished."[122]

A case can also be made that even when antibiotics are used, it is important that nutrients be supplemented as well. A paper in 1997 described a woman suffering from trichomonal vaginitis and low blood levels of zinc who responded to drug treatment *only* after supplements raised her zinc level to normal and four women in whom (vaginal) zinc sulfate lowered the requirement for the drug metronidazole.[123] Another study showed that a zinc-erythromycin solution worked better for acne than erythromycin alone.[124]

The evidence that our nutritional status influences our immune response continues to grow. In one study, people over sixty-five who were given a vitamin and mineral supplement were compared with those given a placebo and followed for one year. The supplement contained nutrients known to effect immune function, but only at levels comparable to the recommended daily allowance (RDA). It was found that those receiving the supplement experienced only half the days of infection as those receiving the placebo.[125]

Further evidence suggests that deficiency of nutrients important to immune function is more common than previously thought. A recent study showed that children in the United States had the lowest blood vitamin E levels of all the industrialized nations. The vitamin E levels of U.S. children was only one-half the level of Japanese children. Dr. Adrian Bendich, the author of this study, pointed out that vitamin E is directly related to the immune response. She also noted that autopsies of children have shown degenerative changes typically associated with aging or old age.[126] This phenomenon is thought to be due to free-radical damage that occurs with the daily exposure to chemical pollutants.

Jeffrey Blumberg, PhD, a senior researcher with the U.S. Department of Agriculture, studied the effects of vitamin C on the activity of white blood cells. He showed that there was a striking relationship between white blood cell activity and vitamin C intake. At 500 mg (almost ten times the RDA) white blood cells were highly active. At 250 mg their activity declined substantially, suggesting that our functional needs for vitamin C are higher than once believed.[127]

Additional evidence can be found in the work of scientists at the University of Alabama, who studied dietary relationships in a condition called bacterial vaginosis* in 1,521 women. Antibiotics are clearly one of the factors that can disrupt the normal flora in the vagina, which can render a woman more susceptible to infection by harmful organisms.

Scientists used a dietary analysis inventory developed and validated by Dr. Gladys Block of the University of California at Berkeley. This inventory is considered among the leading validated tools in dietary studies. The women were divided into one of four groups based on their bacterial vaginosis score (the Nugent score). In this study, 42 percent were classified as having bacterial vaginosis, with 14.9 percent suffering from severe bacterial vaginosis (BV).

The first finding of interest was that dietary fat was associated with both BV and severe BV. In fact, the risk of severe BV was more than twice as high in women with total fat, saturated fat, and monounsaturated fat intakes in the highest one-fourth of fat intake (compared with women in the lowest quartile). Since fatty acids are known modulators of inflammatory status and immune function, it is not surprising that fat showed a strong association with BV. In addition, women with the highest intake of folate, vitamin E, and calcium had a significantly reduced rate of severe BV.[128] We'll see some interesting links between folate and host defenses later in this chapter.

Trace Elements, Burns, and Infection

Infection is one of the greatest complications associated with a major burn and is, in fact, one of the leading causes of death after burns.[129] It is well known that elements such as copper, selenium, and zinc can be depleted in burns, each of which is required in immune function. Reduction of infection through nutrient supplementation in burn cases would represent a significant advance in patient care and would demonstrate the critical role of nutrients in immunity and infection control. A trial

---

*Vaginosis is a condition characterized by abnormal vaginal discharge related to overgrowth of microbes within the vagina.

published in the *American Journal of Clinical Nutrition* examined 21 patients who had received burns on an average of 45 percent of their body. Intravenous copper, selenium, and zinc were given to one group, while a placebo was given by IV to the other group. After thirty days, the number of infections per patient in the placebo group was *twice* that of those in the trace element group. This was represented by a predominant reduction in the rate of respiratory infections. There was also a reduced need for skin grafts in the trace element group.[130]

Skin antioxidant defenses were also improved in those receiving trace elements, which was accompanied by improved wound healing. Specifically, the levels of the powerful antioxidants glutathione and glutathione peroxidase were increased in skin. Though these were increased, skin infections were not reduced by the IV trace elements. The authors suggest that this may have been because, due to the IV nature of the dosing, the lungs may have received priority over the skin for trace elements and, at the low doses used, the skin may have received inadequate concentrations of elements. Another reason may be that the skin has constant exposure to microbes and trace elements may not be enough to overcome such exposure. Nonetheless, these findings suggest a promising role for nutrition in reducing the consequences of infection in serious trauma.

Nutrition in Critical Care and Surgery

According to Karen McCowen and Bruce Bistrian of Harvard University's Beth Israel Hospital, "Despite flaws in many studies, a consistent trend to reduced infectious complications has been seen with immunonutrition, especially in patients undergoing surgery for upper gastrointestinal cancer or trauma." In their important review, they cite the complex literature that has attempted to answer the question of the benefits of nutrition to immunity in critical care patients and the proper form of this nutrient supplementation. Most of the formulas used in these studies have contained various combinations of protein, amino acids (such as arginine and glutamine), omega-3 fatty acids, fat, carbohydrates, and nucleic acids. Two things stand out from their review. One is that the most severely ill patients seemed to benefit little, but that this may be a reflection of the "degree to which the patients receive the assigned feeding." This is related to the second finding that insufficient doses, in general, may be given to critical care patients. Their findings can be summarized as follows:[131]

1. The greatest flaw in most trials has been *underfeeding* of the nutrients being studied, i.e. insufficient amounts of the nutrients were given.
2. Across all studies, there was a trend to a lower rate of infections in those receiving immunonutrition.
3. There was a universal finding of shorter hospital stays in those receiving immunonutrition.
4. There was a universal reduction in complications.
5. Immunonutrition should be delivered early in the illness.

These findings argue that nutrition must take a central role in the management of critical illness and that by such intervention we can reduce infections and reliance upon antibiotics in recovery. This may seem like a statement of the obvious, but it is not the way medicine has been practiced. Attention to immunonutrition has the potential to one day revolutionize critical care medicine.

Diabetes and Chronic Illness

Type 2 diabetes is well known for its effects on immune function and for infections that can be recurring or more difficult to treat. It is also a condition that has very clear negative effects upon immunity, energy metabolism, and repair functions. In a landmark study published in the *New England Journal of Medicine,* doctors divided patients into two groups of eighty people each, one group receiving conventional drug therapy and the other group receiving "multifactorial intervention," also referred to as "intensive therapy," which involved exercise, lifestyle modification, dietary recommendations, and a vitamin and mineral supplement that included[132] vitamin C 250 mg, vitamin E 100 mg (d-alpha-tocopherol), folic acid 400 mcg, and chromium picolinate, 100 mcg.

This study was also noteworthy because it was carried out over the course of almost eight years. Doctors measured the rate of key complications of diabetes including nephropathy (kidney complications), retinopathy (eye complications), cardiovascular events, neuropathy (perhipheral nerve complications), and autonomic neuropathy.*

Those in the supplementation (intensive therapy group) experienced an almost 50 percent reduction in nearly all of the above complications of diabetes (except neuropathy, which was comparable in each group). While the trial lasted almost eight years, favorable outcomes were similar after only four years. This is really quite extraordinary.

While immune parameters, infections, and antibiotic use were not examined in this trial, the study has an important message related to our discussion. As noted, diabetes is a condition of altered immunity, altered energy regulation, and diminished repair capability. The finding that several of the major complications associated with diabetes were reduced by by almost 50 percent with an intensive therapy that included supplementation of nutrients, suggests that nutritional intervention as a component of a chronic illness treatment can have a dramatic impact on energy and repair functions.

The supplementation strategy used in this trial was limited to modest doses of only a small number of key nutrients. It is interesting to speculate on the possible outcomes were a larger number of nutrients

---

*Autonomic neuropathy is not a disease, but a set of symptoms that involve damage to nerves that control digestion, heart rate, blood pressure, bladder function, skin, muscles, internal organs, blood vessels, and many others. Symptoms include, but are not limited to diarrhea, constipation, nausea after eating, heat intolerance, difficulty beginning to urinate, urinary incontinence, and abnormal sweating.

used or where nutrient supplementation was tailored to the individual based on blood analysis of nutrient status.

Healthy People

To address one set of questions about the effect of dietary supplements (vitamins, minerals, etc), Dr. Gladys Block and her colleagues from UC Berkeley studied 278 multiple supplement users, 176 single supplement users, and 602 nonsupplement users. Her group found that the degree of supplement use was linked to more favorable concentrations of disease biomarkers in the blood, such as lower C-reactive protein, homocysteine, lipoprotein cholesterol, and triglycerides. There was also a lower risk of high blood pressure and diabetes. In addition, degree of supplement use was also associated with more favorable (higher) blood levels of nutrients.[133]

It could be argued that those using supplements were more careful in all aspects of their lives, thus accounting for the improved health measures. This is a valid consideration. However, the authors partially address this matter in their statistical analysis, and they state that supplement and nonsupplement users were similar with respect to things like income and socioeconomic status.

Immunonutrition

Scientists will probably some day discover that nearly all nutrients have some direct or indirect role in immune function, especially if we view immunity in terms of energy, defense, recovery, and repair. Some of the more thoroughly understood nutrients are already being used in medicine to prevent infection and to boost immunity during infection. Below is a brief description of selected nutrients and their importance to immunity.

Vitamin A

Vitamin A is typically seen to have the following effects on immune defenses:[134]

- Maintain antibody related immunity
- Maintain cell integrity (barrier defenses in the lungs, skin, and gut)
- Maintain integrity of mucus-secreting cells (which protects barrier membranes)

The role of vitamin A in strong barrier defenses cannot be overstated. Vitamin A helps maintain the cells lining the lungs, skin, intestinal tract, and bladder. These cells are the first barrier of the protective mechanism against infection. In the gut, for instance, vitamin A helps maintain the gap junctions between cells. Strong gap junctions help prevent against leaky gut, and against the penetration of harmful microbes or microbial endotoxins into the bloodstream.[135]

Vitamin A is also necessary for the maintenance of barrier defenses in the lungs, middle ear, and respiratory tract. Among other functions, vitamin A maintains the tiny hairlike cilia in these tissues, which serve to waft microbes and foreign debris out of the tissues.[136]

Vitamin A levels are depleted rapidly during different conditions, including fever, pneumonia, tonsillitis, rheumatic fever, and measles. In one report of children with severe measles, the rate of complications such as pneumonia, croup, and death was cut in half as a result of vitamin A supplementation.[137]

Concerns about vitamin A toxicity are commonly raised, although there are annually only some two hundred reported cases of vitamin A toxicity worldwide.[138] However, there is growing evidence that vitamin A excess can occur in children consuming things like chewable vitamins. Vitamin A excess has also recently been linked to weaknesses in bone density. There seems to be general agreement that vitamin A is vital for immunity, but that doses above the RDI should be restricted to those in whom deficiency has been established through blood testing.

Carotenoids

Professor Marlene Zuk is a biologist at the University of California at Riverside who has spent much of her career studying the behavior of lowly creatures such as parasites, their hosts, the higher mammals, and everything in between.

In her book *Riddled with Life,* she probes the subject of whether the brightly colored beaks and the radiant plumage of male birds, which are so valuable in attracting mates, actually signals to the female that he possesses a robust immune system. She wondered, do the same chemical compounds that render a bird's beak bright yellow or its comb bright red actually have the effect of strengthening the immune system of its bearer? Is the brightly colored bird a better mate because his immune system can withstand the wounds that accompany battle with competitors? Do the bright colors signify that the male will pass on the traits of a robust immune system to its offspring?

To biologists such as Dr. Zuk, this is serious stuff. She and her colleagues discovered that one of the key compounds that renders these colors across animal species is from the family of nutrients called carotenoids—the molecules that color carrots orange, corn yellow, and tomatoes red. They also give fish like salmon and crustaceans like krill their pleasant red color. The effect of carotenoids on animal coloring is so predictable that scientists can observe color changes in birds when the diets are enriched with these molecules.

While carotenoids do brighten things up, they also contribute to strong immune defenses. For one, carotenoids are important free-radical scavengers, mopping up free radicals produced by immune system encounters with invaders. The breadth of Dr. Zuk's work on this subject is compelling. From just a few of the discoveries and observations of her and her colleagues we have learned:[139]

- European blackbirds (which have a bright yellow-orange bill), were injected with a foreign protein that challenges the immune system but does not make the bird ill. In those injected, the carotenoid content of the bills diminished, suggesting that the immune system withdrew carotenoids from the bill in order to bolster immune defenses.

- French workers gave zebra finches carotenoids in their drinking water and tested for changes in immunity and bill color. Both bill color and immune function rose when carotenoid levels were highest. When the immune system was challenged, carotenoid levels in the blood and in the bills was reduced, suggesting, perhaps, that the immune system retrieved carotenoids from tissue stores when needed.
- Dr. Zuk's group measured cell-mediated immunity, humoral immunity, and comb size in jungle chickens. Comb size is one measure of "attractiveness" to females that seems to mirror redness of the comb, but is simple to quantify in the field. Outside the breeding season, males with larger combs had better cell-mediated immunity and humoral immunity than those with smaller combs.
- Dr. Zuk also notes that Egyptian vultures, which are known to consume highly contaminated and infected carcasses, have notoriously robust immune systems. They are adorned with a bright yellow head (rich with carotenoids) to go with their quite ordinary feathers. Evidently, their habit of picking through sheep and cow dung yields a diet rich in carotenoids (as dung was later found to be rich in these nutrients).

Vitamin D and Immunity

Vitamin D is a hormone similar in basic structure to cortisol and testosterone, but it has been classified as a vitamin since its discovery. The potential effect of vitamin D on immunity has long historical roots. For instance, some 90 percent of people infected with the tuberculosis organism (*Mycobacterium tuberculi*) never develop the disease. A link between vitamin D and tuberculosis has been known since the eighteenth century.

Remarkably, cod liver oil (a source of vitamin D) and sunlight (a means for us to produce our own vitamin D) were once among the standard treatments use in TB.[140] In more modern times, it was recognized that immigrants moving from tropical climes to the colder and cloudier United Kingdom experienced up to a tenfold lowering of their vitamin D stores.[141] This may have accounted for the high incidence of non-respiratory manifestations of tuberculosis in people from India who emigrated to the United Kingdom.[142]

It has since been learned that vitamin D is necessary for activation of a key sentinel in cellular immunity called the macrophage (a type of white blood cell).[143] This may account for why people living in the sunnier climate of India showed symptoms of tuberculosis after moving to the United Kingdom. It has been proposed that they may have had a latent infection of tuberculosis, but that their vitamin D levels (once fueled by the sunlight-stimulated conversion of vitamin D in sunny India) were adequate to keep it in check. Once they moved to the UK and their vitamin D levels fell sufficiently, the tubercle bacteria was able to gain ascendance and produce disease.[144]

Such findings have raised interest in vitamin D as an immune-modulating compound, which is now the subject of much current research. The metabolic product of vitamin D is seen as a potent repair and maintenance steroid hormone that targets more than two hundred human genes in a wide variety of tissues.[145] One example of where vitamin D acts is on the gene promoter for the antimicrobial peptide (AMP) cathelicidin in cells of the skin and the immune system (monocytes).

Vitamin D also appears to have a surprising effect on aging of the immune system. Vitamin D concentrations were measured in the blood (serum) of 2,160 women who were part of a cohort of twins. The scientists, based in London, wanted to know how vitamin D status was related to telomere length of white blood cells. Remember that telomeres are sections of DNA that occur at the ends of chromosomes. Shortened telomeres in white blood cells are associated with aging-related disease. Those with higher blood levels of vitamin D were found to have longer telomeres, which would suggest that their immune systems were functionally "younger." According to the authors, this can be roughly translated to mean that those with higher vitamin D levels "had 5 years less telomeric aging." This may suggest that vitamin D supplementation can reduce inflammation and cell deterioration that is associated with aging.[146]

Vitamin D Excess

Because vitamin D is a hormone and because of the profound effects of vitamin D on human physiology, vitamin D excess can be dangerous. Anyone with autoimmune disease should proceed with a blood test for vitamin D before taking vitamin D supplements. Also, supplements and food should be checked carefully for vitamin D content since the cumulative amount of vitamin D from all sources could be higher than is considered safe. This is less of a concern in winter, when vitamin D levels commonly fall (at least in colder, darker climates).

Vitamin E

Vitamin E (tocopherol) exerts an effect on the immune system through its role as an antioxidant. This vitamin protects the fats and cell membranes in the body from oxidation or damage. When vitamin E levels are low, damage to cell membranes easily occurs. Vitamin E also affects immune function by regulating the formation of prostaglandins, the hormonelike substances derived from our dietary fats.

A recent study summarized the dietary vitamin E intake of 8,244 people across all age groups from 1999 to 2000. Using the estimated average requirement (EAR) measure, this study showed that the majority of Americans do not meet the current dietary recommendations of 15 mg alpha-tocopherol per day. The proportion of children below the estimated average requirement was 75 percent for ages 4 to 8 and almost 100 percent for girls aged 14 to 18. Ninety percent of adults have intakes below the EAR level, with low intakes more prevalent in females than in males.[147] This research shows that vitamin E insufficiency is commonplace and that daily supplementation is warranted.

Vitamin E has generally been viewed as having a broad margin of safety. However, there is reason to believe that we should also avoid vitamin E excess. For instance, in one study, providing 300 mg per day of vitamin E for three weeks resulted in depressed bactericidal activity of leukocytes in humans.[148]

Vitamin C

Vitamin C is essential to every cell and there is no question that it is essential to immunity. Vitamin C seems to influence resistance to bacterial and viral infections in two basic ways: by direct inhibition of the virus or bacteria and by stimulating white blood cells' ability to attack bacteria and viruses. One means by which white blood cells destroy bacteria is through a process called phagocytosis, meaning "engulf and destroy." It was demonstrated almost fifty years ago that vitamin C is required for this process. Vitamin C also increases the rate at which white blood cells travel to the site of infection (called chemotaxis).[149]

In a recent study by Susan Ritter and Gailen Marshall, Jr. of the University of Texas Health Science Center, tested the effect of vitamin C on the immune system. Twelve people were supplemented with one gram of vitamin C for two weeks. The scientists then examined the changes in white blood cells and the production of antiviral compounds. They found:

- T-cells produced more interferon gamma, and less interleukin-4 (IL-4) and interleukin-10 (IL-10), shifting the immune system in the direction of Th1 and away from an allergic potential.
- T-cells became more active (though their numbers remained the same).
- The number of natural killer cells increased with vitamin C.

These scientists suggested that one gram (1000 mg) of vitamin C daily may improve the immune response. This is in comparison to the RDI (reference daily intake), which is only 60 mg per day or the DRI (dietary reference intake) of 90 mg per day. These latter references are the levels meant to prevent deficiency diseases like scurvy, but they have nothing to do with optimal health or optimal immune function.

Vitamin C also has a fundamental role in preserving barrier defenses throughout the body via its well-known interaction with an enzyme called prolyl hydroxylase, which helps to assemble large proteins of our connective tissue (the stuff that holds us together). This is why one of the first symptoms of vitamin C deficiency (especially the disease scurvy) is the breakdown of barrier defenses.[150] The connection became clear when the first sign of scurvy in seafarers was the opening up of old wounds that had previously healed, bleeding gums, loose teeth, easy bruising, and a host of other symptoms associated with connective tissue.

Vitamin C is also needed for the synthesis of the nonprotein amino acid carnitine, which helps shuttle fatty acids into mitochondria to be burned as fuel,[151] which is why one of the early symptoms of vitamin C deficit is fatigue and decreased energy. If we put the varied functions of vitamin C together, we can see that it directly affects immune cells (white blood cell activity), barrier defenses, energy (via carnitine), and repair (effects on all of the above).

It has been known for some time that dogs and other animals that make their own vitamin C, increase production ten- to fifteenfold during times of stress or infection. Since humans (and, oddly, guinea pigs) do not make vitamin C, it is necessary for us to get additional vitamin C from food or supplements.

Folic Acid

The major function of folic acid in the human body is the transfer of a humble molecular fragment called a methyl group. Chemically, a methyl group is nearly as simple as it gets—it has one carbon and three hydrogens. But the simplicity of folic acid belies its enormous functional magnitude, for these methyl transfers have far-reaching effects on DNA and cell division. There are few nutrients with such widespread impact.

One study illustrates the potential importance of folate in infection. A study of 2,482 children was conducted to determine the effect of folic acid on lower respiratory infection. Over a four-month period, children in the lowest one-fourth (quartile) of blood folic acid levels had a 44 percent higher incidence of acute lower respiratory tract infections than children in the other three-fourths of folic acid intake.[152]

Immune defense against respiratory and other infections relies upon the ability of immune cells to rapidly multiply and expand their numbers. To do so requires a dramatic increase in DNA synthesis, which requires ample stores of folic acid. Other cells, such as those lining the respiratory tract must also replicate in order to repair themselves in the face of invading microbes. Once again, the rapid cellular reproduction requires substantial folic acid reserves. It has also been shown that the phagocytic and bactericidal ability of white blood cells (neutrophils, for instance) is poor in people with low folate and improves in people in whom folate is replaced.[153]

Many nations have fortified foods with folic acid, so intake has improved. However, folate deficiency remains a problem for certain individuals who do not consume vegetables rich in folate (found in greed leafy vegetables—foliage) or who have a common genetic abnormalities. One specific example is those with a common mutation of the gene known as MTHFR (methylene tetrahydrofolate reductase). Such people have alterations in folate metabolism, which also involves B-12 and riboflavin. One way to be certain of folate status is through plasma or red blood cell analysis for folate.

Iron

We live in conflict with iron in much the same way we live in conflict with fire. We use fire to suit many critical needs, yet fire can destroy nearly any of our creative endeavors.

Iron is essential for proper immune function, with susceptibility to infection as one of the common conditions associated with iron *deficiency.* However, bacteria also need iron to survive. The human body has evolved masterful tactics to shuttle our iron around and keep it from microbes when they threaten.

Scientists have been trying to sort out this immunity/infection/iron conundrum for a long time. It was not uncommon for doctors working with indigenous peoples to prescribe nutrients such as iron and vitamin A, given the poor diets and impoverished living conditions that were common in some populations. Many years ago, New Zealand doctors intended to help Maori babies by giving them injections of iron. Unfortunately, those injected with iron were seven times more likely to suffer from potentially deadly infections, such as meningitis and septicemia (blood poisoning).[154]

Further evidence of the potential effect of iron on infection, at least in infants, arose from sixty-nine cases of infant botulism that occurred in California. When doctors tried to understand the conditions that were associated with babies who died versus those who survived one glaring finding stood out. Babies who were fed iron-supplemented formula were more likely to develop the infection younger. Of the ten babies who died, all had been formula-fed. While it is true that breast milk contains immune modulating proteins and antibodies, the impact of iron on fueling the growth of the *Clostridium botulinum* organism in the small intestine cannot be ruled out.[155]

A noteworthy example of iron fueling infections was on display in a Somali refugee camp in the 1970s, where Dr. John Murray had noticed some paradoxical findings. Somali refugees were exposed to myriad infections, such as brucellosis, tuberculosis, and malaria, yet they seemed unexpectedly protected. At the same time, iron deficiency anemia was prevalent, which would have led one to expect *increased* susceptibility to disease. Dr. Murray decided to conduct a study in which he administered iron supplements to some of the nomads. He was astonished by the results. After iron supplementation, there was a striking surge in the rate of infections in those receiving iron supplements, leading to the conclusion that iron-deficiency anemia might be *protecting* the nomads against a range of life-threatening microbes in their midst.[156] Other studies would seem to support this concern, since data shows that iron supplementation can make some infections, such as malaria and tuberculosis, worse.[157] Scientists working with difficult infections such as tuberculosis have even suggested the use of iron-binding drugs be used (a process called chelation) to lower the body's iron stores.[158]

Determining the relationship between iron, infections, and immunity has grown somewhat confusing. In an effort to better understand the situation and make recommendations, doctors from John's Hopkins University recently examined twenty-six studies of iron supplementation in children in developing countries. While no firm conclusions could be drawn, it appeared that iron supplementation was best used *when iron deficiency was clearly existent.*[159]

How common are iron deficiency and iron excess? In a recent review, 1,016 elderly Americans from the Framingham Heart study were assessed for iron status. Only 3 percent had depleted iron stores. However, 12.9 percent had elevated iron stores, suggesting that iron excess was more problematic than iron deficiency.[160]

Iron *excess* can have the following adverse effects on immunity:[161]

- Decreased antibody-mediated immunity
- Decreased phagocytosis (engulfing and destroying bacteria) by macrophages

- Reduced movement of white blood cells (neutrophils) to the site of infection
- Suppression of one form of natural immunity (complement system)
- Increased rate of infection

It is probably safe to say that iron should not be supplemented on a daily basis (except in bottle-fed babies between six and twelve months) unless it has been established that iron deficiency exists, which can be determined by blood tests described in Chapter 14.

Selenium

Deficiency of selenium results in diminished resistance to bacterial and viral infections, diminished white blood cell activity, reduced antibody production, and reduced ability of T-cells and natural killer cells to destroy pathogenic bacteria. Experimental models have shown that selenium deficiency can affect all components of the immune system, including cellular and humoral immunity. Selenium supplementation in selenium-deficient animals enhances Th1 immune action, improving antiviral, antibacterial, and antifungal defenses.[162] In one study, supplementation with selenium reduced the frequency of upper respiratory infections in children with Down syndrome.[163]

In a recent study of twenty-two healthy adults with low selenium status, scientists wanted to determine whether supplementation with small amounts of selenium led to changes in immune function and in the rates of clearance of a killed form of the polio virus (picornavirus). Subjects were given either 50 mcg/day or 100 mcg/day of selenium for 15 weeks and compared with those taking a placebo. After just six weeks, they were each given an oral form of the polio vaccine. Those receiving selenium cleared the virus from their feces much more quickly than those receiving the placebo. Also, those receiving selenium had a marked increased in cell-mediated immunity (the Th1 response). Those in the selenium groups also mounted an immune response to the polio virus more quickly than those in the placebo group.[164]

The authors of this study suggested that additional "intake of selenium is warranted to optimize immune function," but cautioned that excessive selenium can be harmful. This is an assertion with which most scientists in nutritional medicine would agree. However, it is important to point out the meager selenium intakes in some countries. Current selenium intakes in the UK are only 29 to 39 mcg/day, with a recommended daily intake of 75 mcg/day for men and 60 mcg/day for women.[165] Conditions in the U.S. are not much different, with intakes around 55 mcg/day for both men and women.[166]

Zinc

When it comes to the broader subject of our body defenses, zinc has among the most diverse roles. It is probably the most extensively studied nutrient relative to its role in infection and immunity. A paper published in the *Journal of Infectious Diseases* suggests that an estimated two billion people worldwide are deficient in this trace element.[167] In an important study of zinc's function, zinc was first depleted and then replaced in an attempt to understand how zinc influenced the immune proteins (cytokines) associated with the Th1 and Th2 activity of the immune system (recall from Chapter 4). During the zinc depletion stage, the Th1 cytokines (IL-2 and IFNγ) decreased. When zinc levels were corrected, the Th1 cytokines returned to normal.[168] This would suggest that zinc is critical to maintaining the component necessary for containment of bacterial infection—something numerous studies have found to be true.

Zinc is involved in many DNA-related processes critical to the rapid multiplication of white blood cells that must occur during infection. Zinc is also crucial to cellular repair of tissues that form the barrier defenses against invading microbes, such as the skin, lungs, and lining of the digestive tract. Thus, zinc deficiency can result in poor barrier defenses, which makes microbial invasion and expansion more likely.[169] In fact, zinc supplementation has been shown to strengthen the gut barrier in people with Crohn's disease, who are well-known to have weakened barrier defenses.[170]

Severe zinc deficiency is accompanied by severely depressed immune function and frequent infections. Zinc supplementation has improved resistance to infection in children with Down syndrome.[171] In elderly people, zinc supplementation resulted in improvements in wound healing and resistance to infection.[172] In fact, some believe that immune suppression in the elderly may be due in part to zinc deficiency. Double-blind, placebo-controlled trials of zinc supplementation show that zinc reduces the incidence of acute diarrhea by up to 30 percent.[173] Zinc can also reduce the incidence of acute lower respiratory infection.[175] Twenty-one of thirty-two people with sickle cell disease were found to have zinc deficiency. Zinc supplementation reduced their infection rate by 80 percent.[175]

Zinc, Aging, and Infection

Pneumonia is a growing threat as we age. As our defenses wane, our ability to defend against microbes diminishes. But is our fading ability to defend ourselves a natural part of the aging process—an inevitability? Or is it related to metabolic forces? In one attempt to answer this question, doctors enrolled residents from thirty-three Boston area nursing homes in a study and followed them for one year. Doctors measured blood levels of zinc at the beginning and end of the study, while also giving zinc supplements. They wanted to see how zinc status impacted the rate of pneumonia and, further, its effect on frequency of antibiotic use.

People were categorized as having either low zinc (blood levels less than 70 mcg/dl) or normal zinc (greater than or equal to70 mcg/dl). Each subject received a supplement containing 7 mg of zinc for one year. Other elements were included at 50 percent of the RDA. Compared to those with low zinc concentrations, those with normal zinc levels at the end of the study had:[176]

- A lower overall incidence of pneumonia
- Fewer days of pneumonia in those who developed pneumonia
- Almost 50 percent fewer antibiotic prescriptions
- Fewer days of antibiotic use in those who required antibiotics
- Reduced incidence of death from all causes by 39 percent

This study of almost six hundred people has significant implications because of the widespread nature of zinc deficiency. In one study, dietary intake of zinc was below the RDA in greater than 90 percent of 100 people aged 60 to 89.[177] In another study, 35 percent of elderly people were low in zinc.[178]

The above study also raises an important point that we are urged to bear in mind as we consider the role of nutrition. Subjects in the study were assessed for their **blood levels of zinc,** as opposed to only examination of dietary intake. This and other studies of zinc (and of other nutrients, for that matter) hint that those with low or poor zinc status are more susceptible to infection and that zinc supplementation may be more helpful in those with low blood nutrient levels.

Can Zinc Aggravate Infection?

From a great deal of research, zinc would appear to be a universal solution to bolster immunity. But can zinc have a dark side? Recall that bacteria are masters at using *iron* in order to multiply and spread. To counter this, the human body has developed efficient tools to mop up iron, hide it away, and reduce the availability of iron to bacteria during infection. Zinc may have similar features. At the onset of infection, the blood levels of zinc can decline by 10 to 69 percent, which coincides with an increase in the liver's manufacture of zinc-based immune proteins.[179] This is part of the acute-phase response to infection. Since the body is pulling zinc from the blood, there is some question as to whether elevating zinc during this period can aggravate the infectious process. The answer is not yet clear.

Zinc is generally viewed as an important defense against infections in children. For instance, two studies of children under age two showed that in children with zinc deficiency, zinc supplements reduced the occurrence of severe pneumonia.[180,181] However, studies of hospitalized children given zinc during cases of severe pneumonia have yielded conflicting results.[182]

In an attempt to resolve these conflicts, doctors conducted a new trial of 299 children hospitalized with pneumonia. Some were diagnosed with bacterial pneumonia, while others were classified with non-bacterial pneumonia (viral). Roughly half were given 10 mg of zinc twice a day and the other half a placebo.

Children receiving zinc who were classified as having bacterial pneumonia had significantly longer hospital stays and a slower recovery from severe illness than children receiving the placebo. Children receiving zinc who were classified as having non-bacterial pneumonia had hospital stays similar to those children receiving the placebo. This would suggest that the type of infection (bacterial versus viral) could have an important influence on whether zinc supplementation is appropriate. Previous research with animals has shown that zinc supplementation *at the time of a bacterial challenge* is associated with greater fatality and more serious outcomes.[183] At higher doses, zinc is known to suppress immunity. In one study of 11 men who took 150 mg of zinc twice daily for 6 weeks (almost 8 times the dose in the above study with children), there was a reduction in immune function.[184]

So, does zinc supplementation reduce the incidence of pneumonia in children or does it aggravate pneumonia? There are no clear-cut answers at this time, but there is reason to consider the following:

- Zinc supplementation in children with nonbacterial pneumonia, such as viral pneumonia, appears to be associated with no adverse effects.

- Zinc supplementation *during* acute pneumonia in children with bacterial infection may be associated with worse outcomes and extended hospital stays.
- Zinc *deficiency* is associated with increased susceptibility to infections, such as pneumonia, in children.
- Supplementation (*preventive*) with zinc in children with zinc deficiency appears to reduce the risk to developing infections such as pneumonia.

For practical purposes, it may be wise to avoid zinc supplementation in small children *during* an acute infection thought to be bacterial in origin. For purposes of prevention, it is also important that the zinc status of small children be assessed using blood tests, which provides an accurate measure of zinc status and the correct therapy to raise defenses against infecting organisms.

Magnesium

Magnesium is not widely discussed as a nutrient linked to immunity. But when we expand the discussion to include barrier defenses, energy, and repair magnesium becomes central. This can be illustrated by understanding that magnesium is involved in ALL reactions involving ATP (adenosine triphosphate), the body's energy currency. Magnesium is also involved in six primary steps that we use to convert sugar into energy. In other words, we do not generate energy without magnesium.

As noted elsewhere in this book, diabetes is one condition where impaired defenses are common and magnesium's impact on diabetes is substantial. For example, one study examined 4,637 American adults (age eighteen to thirty) who were free from metabolic syndrome (a prediabetic state) and diabetes. During the next fifteen years, 608 were diagnosed with the metabolic syndrome. For people with the highest magnesium levels, the risk for developing metabolic syndrome was reduced by thirty one percent.[185]

In a different study of obese nondiabetic children and nonobese controls, serum and dietary magnesium were inversely correlated with fasting blood insulin levels.[186] That is, as magnesium levels went lower, insulin levels climbed higher—a dangerous risk to development of diabetes. These discoveries are similar to those of The Women's Health Study and the Atherosclerosis Risk in Communities Study.[187,188] In the Nurse's Health Study, subjects in the highest one-fifth of magnesium intake, had a thirty three percent lower risk of developing type 2 diabetes, than those in the lowest one-fifth of magnesium intake.[189]

Magnesium is important in over three hundred enzyme reactions in the human body. Its impact on diabetes is just one reminder of the capacity for magnesium insufficiency to alter metabolism that affects defenses in significant ways. In our experience of measuring blood magnesium levels in patients, magnesium insufficiency is one of the more common abnormalities we find. This is consistent with the low magnesium intakes reported in many dietary intake studies.

Glutathione

Glutathione (GSH) is a small molecule made from three amino acids: cysteine, glycine, and glutamic acid. Of the amino acids comprising glutathione, cysteine (bearing a sulfur atom) is the most limited by our dietary intake. Glutathione is the most important regulatory antioxidant within cells. In the immune system, it is critical to maintaining control over oxidative stress within white blood cells.

Glutathione is also an important molecule in gut barrier defenses and protection of the gut from toxic molecules encountered through the diet or through ingestion. Glutathione levels in the gut are found to be higher in people consuming higher amounts of fruits and vegetables.[190]

As mentioned in Chapter 4, tremendous efforts are underway to direct the Th1 / Th2 balance of the immune system as a means to regulate immunity in specific diseases. This is a complex task, since manipulation of the immune system with specific cytokines can prove unpredictable.

However, recent evidence suggests that the status of a nutrient indigenous to all cells influences the fate of immune cell populations. More specifically, glutathione reserves are necessary to preserving the balance between Th1 and Th2 activity within the immune system. Specifically, when the white blood cells called macrophages were depleted of their glutathione, they behaved as Th2 cells and they could activate the Th2 path. Macrophages enriched with glutathione led to activation of the immune cells toward Th1 dominance.[191] To simplify, it appears that glutathione may be one important factor within the cell that determines which immune regulatory pathway is dominant within the human body.

During infection and trauma, our antioxidant defenses become depleted. For example, in mice infected with the influenza virus, glutathione levels in blood fell by 45 percent.[192] In patients undergoing abdominal surgery, blood levels of glutathione fell by 10 percent within 24 hours. In skeletal muscle, the levels of glutathione fell a surprising 42 percent during the same postoperative period,[193] which might render a person undergoing a surgical procedure more susceptible to infection.

The importance of antioxidants in times of infection is strongly illustrated by the finding that sepsis (blood infection) is accompanied by a decrease in the total antioxidant capacity of the blood. In one study, the antioxidant capacity normalized over a five-day period in patients who survived. Blood antioxidant status did not normalize in patients who ultimately died from their infection.[194] This finding makes it tempting to conclude that strong antioxidant defenses may protect us from some of the severe consequences of infection and, perhaps, help accelerate recovery.

One compound that has been shown to regenerate glutathione, *N*-acetylcysteine (NAC), may also offer protection. In a separate study of blood infection (sepsis), injection with NAC led to increased blood levels of glutathione, which led to improved respiratory function and fewer days needed in intensive care.[195] In a promising study, NAC has also shortened hospital stays by roughly 60 percent.[196]

Glutathione depletion may also be one reason heavy exercise can lower immunity. When athletes engaged in intense exercise for four weeks, their glutathione levels in blood fell significantly. This resulted in a 30 percent decrease in CD4+ T-cell numbers. Of interest, however, was the fact that supplementation with *N*-acetylcysteine (NAC) prevented the decline in T-cell (white blood cell) numbers.[197]

Taurine

Taurine is another amino acid compound related to glutathione, in that it also contains a sulfur group. We hear little about taurine in the popular literature, but it is the most abundant nitrogenous compound in cells. When the white blood cells called macrophages encounter a harmful bacterium, they activate a "respiratory burst" or "oxidant burst." More simply, they try to bleach the bacterium to death. So we don't bleach ourselves to death in the process, we've got taurine on hand to react with the hypochlorous acid pumped out by our macrophages. The taurine chloramine that is formed in the process also seems to have anti-inflammatory properties of its own. In many species that cannot make taurine (such as cats, who need it from the diet), severe immune suppression occurs when there is no access to this amino acid.

Glutamine

Glutamine is the most abundant of the nonessential amino acids in the human body. While glutamine is found in foods such as meat, poultry, fish, eggs, dairy products, and beans, it can become conditionally essential* during times of infection, trauma, or injury.

According to Dr. Phillip Newsholme of University College in Dublin, glutamine is used at very high rates by cells and tissues important to our immune defense, energy, and repair. Whenever there is an inflam-

*Recall that conditionally essential means that we can make the compound under ordinary circumstances, but that there are certain conditions or circumstances under which we cannot make it or we cannot make enough of it.

matory situation of the sort that occurs during injury or blood infection, the immune system gobbles up glutamine at an accelerated rate. Quite often, the demand for glutamine outstrips the supply, creating a deficiency state of this nutrient. As a result, blood, immunologic tissue and muscle glutamine levels fall.

When our glutamine levels fall too far, the key tissues and organs of our defense and repair system begins to suffer. We essentially enter a "glutamine-deficient" state, where "the immune system is compromised."[198]

Recent studies have shown that during challenge with bacterial endotoxin, the glutamine levels in muscle fall, accompanied by decreased levels of glutamine in the bloodstream.[199] This occurs as the body's immune defenses ramp up to produce more white cells, while activating existing white cells in their attack on microbes.

Glutamine has a most unique role among amino acids. For one, it can be used as a ready source of fuel by white blood cells, much like glucose (sugar) is used as fuel. What is most impressive about glutamine is what appears to occur under stress. During the stress of injury, surgery, trauma, infection, or exertion the stress hormone adrenaline slows the ability of certain white blood cells (neutrophils and monocytes) to produce their bacteria-killing superoxide—a key "bleach-like" molecule. When these white cells are given a source of glutamine, their superoxide production returns to normal. In short, glutamine may circumvent some of the effects that stress has on suppression of immunity.[200] Many doctors now believe that glutamine should be used in gram amounts in any program aimed at immune recovery and repair.

Carnitine and Energy

If you have fatigue and low energy, your energy deficit most likely has some effect on the efficiency of your immune response. This is because fatigue almost always has underlying biochemical influences that also affect white blood cell function, barrier defenses, and repair functions. One nutrient central to our energy metabolism is carnitine.

Carnitine is abundant in our tissues that need to work all the time, like heart muscle and skeletal muscle. In the heart, 60 to 90 percent of the energy comes from burning **fat**. Carnitine helps us shuttle our fatty acids (fats from our diet) into little structures within the cell called mitochondria, where the fats can be burned as fuel. Mitochondria are a bit like tiny furnaces.

You might think of carnitine as the person that carries wood (or in our example, the fat) from the wood pile and puts it into the fireplace to be burned. The carnitine-fatty acid shuttle is how you are able to generate energy from fat in your diet. Too little carnitine, however, and fat is not carried into mitochondria. The fats pile up like so many logs on the wood pile—waiting to be burned. Instead of burning the fat, we store it (usually in the belly, though some within our muscles) As a result, energy production goes down, and fatigue sets in.

We can make our own carnitine—to a point, because there are many things that can interfere with our manufacture of carnitine and, therefore, cause fatigue. As a result, carnitine levels can drop sharply in certain diseases and as we age. (See Appendix C.)

The importance of carnitine supplementation to improving energy was highlighted in a fascinating study of sixty-six people over one hundred years old, who all complained of fatigue after even slight physical activity. They were split into two groups. One group was given two grams of carnitine daily for six months. The other group was given a placebo, or dummy pill. The carnitine-supplemented group experienced the following changes in comparison to the placebo group:[201]

- Improvement in physical fatigue score (-4.10 compared with -1.10)
- Improvement in mental fatigue score (-2.70 compared with 0.30)
- Improvement in fatigue severity score (-23.60 compared with 1.90)
- Improvement in mental state score (MMSE: 4.1 compared with 0.6)
- Reduced total body fat mass (4 pounds compared with 1.3 pounds)

- Increased total body muscle mass (8.4 pounds compared with 1.8 pounds)

This is not an isolated study, meaning that the true effects of carnitine on energy and fatigue are probably quite pronounced and quite real. Another study with eighty-four elderly people receiving two grams of carnitine per day showed the following improvements:[202]

- Physical fatigue: 40 percent improvement (vs. 11% in placebo group)
- Mental fatigue: 45 percent improvement (vs. 8% in placebo group)
- Fat loss: Loss of 6.8 pounds of fat (vs. 1 pound in placebo group)
- Muscle gain: Gain of 4.6 pounds of muscle (vs. 0.5 pounds in placebo group)

These studies are really quite exciting. They emphasize that there are legitimate biochemical tools that can be used to combat symptoms like fatigue as we struggle with health conditions. There are many conditions, such as diabetes, obesity, and cancer, where carnitine has shown similar benefit. There are also many more nutrients, such as magnesium, that fall into the category of substances that benefit energy.

Tryptophan

We all know what it feels like to get sick with a viral or bacterial infection. We lose our appetite, become fatigued, lose interest in things, and withdraw to our quiet spaces. We easily tire with exertion and our sleep is altered. We often become depressed and irritable. In many cases, we become "foggy headed," suffering from short-term difficulties with thinking and mental clarity. For some, this "sickness behavior" seems to persist for long periods after an infection.

But what drives this sickness behavior? One answer appears to lie with the fact that infections can deplete our levels of tryptophan. Tryptophan is an essential amino acid that cannot be manufactured by the human body. We usually get our tryptophan from food sources like eggs, beef, chicken, turkey, lamb, and fish. Most know tryptophan as an amino acid associated with mood disorders, such as depression. Tryptophan is converted to the neurotransmitter serotonin. Tryptophan is also converted to melatonin, associated with sleep and biological rhythms. A whole class of drugs used to treat depression is directed toward manipulation of serotonin activity, while the proposed benefits of melatonin in sleep have been well publicized.

New research has shown that the infection process is often associated with increased activity of an enzyme called IDO (indole dioxygenase). IDO accelerates the conversion of tryptophan into a series of molecules, such as kynurenic acid and quinolinic acid. (These two compounds are problematic in their own right, but I'll leave that for another day.) Of importance here is the finding that, in this rapid conversion of tryptophan to these compounds, tryptophan becomes depleted and unavailable to make things like serotonin and melatonin.

For example, scientists at Innsbruck Medical University studied twenty people with chronic Epstein Barr virus (EBV) infection and compared them with ten healthy people. Epstein Barr virus is also associated with mononucleosis, or "mono." Those with EBV infection had lower blood levels of tryptophan, compared to their healthy cohorts. Of the people with EBV, those with more severe cases had more severe depletion of tryptophan. Scientists believe that some of the energy and mood-related issues associated with the EBV infection could be due to depleted tryptophan levels. Their reasoning goes like this—if there is insufficient tryptophan, the body cannot make enough of the mood-stabilizing compound serotonin, resulting in depression-like symptoms.[203] This phenomenon has also been found in other infections such as chlamydia and malaria, and in diseases of immune activation such as lupus, sarcoidosis, and atopic dermatitis.[204]

We will see in later chapters that things like mood, stress, and coping abilities have a significant impact on immunity and resistance to infectious disease. The phenomenon of depleted serotonin in the face of infection may mean that supplementing the diet with S-hydroxytryptophan, a form of the amino acid tryptophan can become an important solution to prevent adverse psychological changes associated with infection.*

The Surprising Role of Fat and Fatty Acids

The study of fatty acids in immune defense, energy, and repair is wide ranging. There are many scientific papers and books that describe the vital importance of fatty acids, omega-3 fatty acids, omega-6 to omega-3 balance, and the role of saturated fat. Since the entire subject is too broad for this book, only a brief introduction of a few key points will be given here.

Fatty Acids and the Barrier Defenses

To put the importance of fatty acids in perspective, we have to look first at the barriers of the human body since they are the first line of defense against microbes. When they diminish, we become more vulnerable. Consider the total surface area of some of the body structures noted below:

Skin	2 square meters (roughly 2 square yards)
Lungs	100 square meters
Intestines	300 square meters

These vast surfaces are either cloaked in microbes or regularly come into contact with microbes. A highly functioning cell membrane keeps these barriers strong. But what keeps the cell membrane in its highest

---

*Some doctors caution that in very sick individuals, supplementing with tryptophan may spur the production of more quinolinic acid and more kynurenic acid, which could aggravate the neurological state. Given the importance of tryptophan in mood, however, I think an individualized approach to assessing tryptophan status is warranted. This can be done using blood tests, which are described in Chapter 14. For the average person, supplementing with sources of tryptophan and adequate vitamin B6 is probably safe. Many doctors now use 5-hydroxytryptophan.

functional state? First, we have to understand that the cell membranes that comprise these barriers are made of fatty acids, *the* fundamental building blocks. Almost without exception, the amount, ratio, and balance of fatty acids in the diet dictate the integrity of our barrier defenses. Dietary fatty acids also dictate our ability to repair all of our barrier defenses. In some respects, repair of barrier defenses anywhere in the human body is not possible without restoring or maintaining appropriate intake of essential and certain nonessential fatty acids.

To further understand the value of fatty acids, we can look at the surface area of *all* the body's cells. It has been estimated that the total surface area of all our cells is equivalent to about ten football fields. These cells also require fatty acids to maintain the integrity of their membranes. Simply put, the types of fatty acids we consume daily will define the structure of our barrier defenses, the integrity of those defenses, and the ability of those barriers to repair.

*How Unsaturated Fatty Acids Actively Drive Repair**

For many years, it was thought that the process of resolution and repair was a "passive" process. That is, once the acute event (injury, infection, etc.) was over, the body was thought to just slowly work its way back to normal (or not) through some nonspecific process. In science, we frequently run into these roadblocks in our understanding and jokingly insert "... and then a miracle occurs."

Today, we have a new understanding of how this "miracle" of repair occurs. Charles Serhan, MD, of Harvard University has published a summary in the *Annual Review of Immunology* that outlines the critical importance of fatty acids as the foundational molecules in an *active* process of resolving and repairing our tissues after some kind of injury

---

*A detailed discussion of fatty acids written for consumers can be found in *Brain-Building Nutrition: How Dietary Fats and Oils Affect Mental, Physical, and Emotional Intelligence,* Michael A. Schmidt, PhD, North Atlantic Books.

or insult The general term now used is *pro-resolving* mediators, or substances that favor the repair of damaged tissue.

The molecules responsible for this active process of resolution are called lipoxins, resolvins, and defensins. They are derived from EPA, DHA, and arachidonic acid. As his group has described it, once the immunological and inflammatory events associated with the initial phase of dealing with trauma or infection have been brought under control, the cascade of lipoxins, resolvins, and defensins begins to rise, which activates an ongoing series of processes aimed at restoring normality back to our tissues.

These processes are dependent upon the right omega-3 and omega-6 fatty acids. Interestingly, aspirin can play a critical role in formation of one class of these resolving molecules (specifically called aspirin-triggered lipoxins, ATL), which gives a new appreciation for this humble therapy. The role of lipoxins, resolvins, and protectins has spurred efforts to develop drugs that might one day speed the resolution process. These same scientists admit, however, that unsaturated fatty acids (such as those found in fish, krill, flax, and other oils) will always remain central to the inherent capacity of the body for self-resolution.[205]

Beyond resolution and repair functions, fatty acids also appear to be involved in the specific parts of the immune system that helps us "see" bacteria.

Fatty Acids and the Gatekeepers

Recall from Chapter 4 our discussion of the toll-like Receptors (TLR). These are proteins on the cell membrane of white blood cells (also on fat cells, muscle cells, and other cells) that sample the environment looking for the signs that microbes are present. Microbes have all sorts of molecules on their surfaces. Our cells have evolved the tools to recognize the various shapes and sizes of these microbial molecules. The toll-like receptors are one of the first tools our cells use to detect these microbial bits and pieces.

There at least a dozen toll-like receptors that help us identify different bacteria. To expand the toll-booth analogy, some of these toll-like receptors recognize nickels, some recognize quarters, and some recognize dimes. A specific TLR (TLR4) is known to recognize lipopolysaccharide (LPS), one component of the bacterial cell wall. Toll-like receptor 4 excels at identifying the **lipo**- part of these bacterial cell wall fragments. Once a TLR recognizes a bacterium, the white blood cell activates a set of messages that triggers an immune response.

Saturated vs. Unsaturated Fats

Here is where it gets interesting. Lipo- means lipid, or fat. These TLR4 detectors are expert at recognizing the fatty-acid portion of a certain fragment of the bacterial cell wall. (You can think of the fatty-acid portion as a little stick-like molecule made of sixteen to eighteen little carbon fragments.) This got scientists wondering whether the toll receptors might also recognize fatty acids from the diet. Could ordinary dietary fats ramp up or slow down the immune system? Might the toll-like receptors *mistake* dietary fats for bacteria because the molecules "look" the same? Could certain fats, then, trigger shifts in the immune response that upped inflammation at the expense of being able to fight infection? These are fascinating questions.

Several research teams have now used various kinds of fatty acids in different experimental settings to see whether dietary fats activate TLR4 in a manner similar to bacterial cell-wall fragments. They have tested saturated fatty acids such as lauric acid, myristic acid, palmitic acid, and stearic acid, which are the saturated fats found in products such as coconut butter and butter made from cow's milk. Researchers have also tested the polyunsaturated fatty acids EPA and DHA, found in fish oil and krill oil.

Several studies have shown a trend toward saturated fatty acids activating the TLR4 in much the same way as bacterial cell wall fragments (LPS). This is really quite astonishing. Could it be that one means by which saturated fat exerts its adverse effect on us is by fooling the immune system into "thinking" there is a bacterial threat? This could mean that dietary choices could mimic infection-like conditions and evoke a needless (and perhaps harmful) response.

Doctors in the UK recently fed healthy people a high-fat meal to study its affect on endotoxin in the bloodstream. The high-fat meal (about 900 calories) consisted of a cup of tea and 3 slices of toast spread with a total of 50 grams of butter (about one-third of a stick). Endotoxin in the blood increased by an average of 50 percent after a high-fat meal. This is consistent with other human studies that show an increase in inflammation following a high-fat meal and with animal studies showing a two- to three-fold increase in endotoxin after a high-fat meal.[206] Remember, endotoxins are fragments of dead bacteria from the gut that can leak into the bloodstream and activate an immune response—an immune response that is not needed.

In contrast to the effects of a high (saturated) fat meal, new studies have shown that omega-3 fatty acids such as EPA and DHA from fish oil or krill oil may slow the ability of bacterial endotoxin to needlessly activate the inflammatory immune cascade.[207] These findings raise the interesting possibility that long-chain omega-3 fatty acids may help us better regulate our defenses, modulate the effects of certain types of molecules in the diet, and allow us to more successfully thrive in the microbe's world.

But this brings us to one question about fatty acids that has been nagging scientists for years—long-chain fatty acids can suppress immune function at certain doses. Without going into the details of these studies, it is worth pointing out a recent study that has attempted to answer the question of safe levels of omega-3 fatty acids in relation to immunity.

Safe Levels of Omega-3 and Omega-6 Fatty Acids

Doctors recently studied 93 young men and 62 older men who were given low (1.35 gram), medium (2.7 gram), or high (4.05 gram) doses of EPA for 12 weeks and compared them with those given a placebo.

Scientists looked at the activity of two types of white blood cells called mononuclear cells and neutrophils. They wanted to see how the different fatty acid doses affected the ability of the neutrophils to engulf and destroy bacteria, and of the capacity for monocytes to produce the immune proteins called cytokines.

In the young men (age 18 to 42), low, moderate, and high intakes of EPA had no adverse effect on any parameters of immunity in doses of EPA up to 4 grams per day. Men in the older age group (53 to 70) experienced a decline in a neutrophil function called the respiratory burst, which is a process by which white cells essentially bleach a bacterium to death. This occurred in the two higher dose groups, but did not occur in the lower dose of EPA. It should be noted that at the higher doses, EPA can be said to have exerted an anti-inflammatory effect, something for which EPA is well known. It is not clear whether a slight reduction in the respiratory burst is problematic for the immune system in times of infection. No other innate immune functions were altered in the older men at even the highest dose. The authors noted the following about EPA intake and immunity based on their study:

1. Intake of 1.35 grams per day of EPA and 0.3 grams of DHA does not appear to have detrimental effects upon immune function.
2. Older men may handle omega-3 fatty acids differently than younger men.
3. Some immune impairment could occur in older men, but not in younger men at the higher doses of EPA intake (up to 4 grams per day).
4. EPA and DHA intake of 1.65 grams per day is below the dose level required to produce an anti-inflammatory effect in healthy men.

From this study, it would seem that most healthy adults would benefit from the anti-inflammatory effects of EPA by ingesting doses of greater than 2 grams per day and may increase the dose to as high as

4 grams per day (at least for younger men) without any adverse effect on immunity.

In their concluding remarks, the investigators state that "consumption of n-3 PUFAs [Omega-3 fatty acids] could be significantly increased without inducing adverse effects on the innate immune response.[208]

The Need for Protein

In Chapter 4, we explored the importance of muscle mass and strength in supporting our immune defense and repair system. While exercise as a means to build muscle is important, we cannot underestimate the vital role of nutrition, which stands out in its impact. For example, it has been shown that muscle mass and strength can be improved by increased intake of amino acids and that this can occur even in the absence of physical activity. These studies were done with healthy young people on bed rest.[209] We must remember that young people have an inherent advantage over others in the ability to maintain muscle. But it is encouraging to learn of the important role dietary amino acids have in shaping our muscle assets.

Metabolic studies of muscle demonstrate that 15 grams of essential amino acids (those amino acids that our body cannot make) at each meal, within the context of a total protein intake of some 1.5 to 1.8 grams per kilogram of body weight per day, may represent a target level appropriate to maintain appropriate muscle mass and metabolism.[210] This translates into about three ounces of protein for a 130-pound woman.

As noted above, we must also ensure that, as a part of our dietary amino acid complement, we consume adequate amounts of sulfur-bearing amino acids (methionine, cysteine, taurine). These vital sulfur groups permit our complex proteins take their 3-dimensional shapes. They are also essential for the formation of the bridges (called disulfide bridges) that hold the "chains" of our antibodies (immunoglobulins) together. Moreover, sulfur-bearing amino acids such as cysteine are needed to form glutathione, which is central to our antioxidant defenses, detoxification system, and necessary to maintain our Th1 / Th2 immune balance.

While protein is essential, however, excessive protein (especially in the absence of adequate fiber) can lead to production of harmful molecules by gut bacteria. This occurs because dietary substances can shift populations of gut bacteria in certain directions. For instance, it is well known that gut bacteria fed by high protein diets can produce ammonia, amines, indoles, sulfides, phenols, and other potentially harmful compounds. This is why the intake of fibers in amount of greater than twenty grams per day (about two to three tablespoons) is essential to balance out the influence of protein on gut bacteria.

Weight-loss programs often focus on low carbohydrate intake coupled with high protein intake. While the rationale for reducing high-glycemic carbohydrates is sound, it is important that carbohydrate in the form of soluble and insoluble fibers not be reduced. In one study, healthy overweight individuals were fed either a maintenance diet, a high protein, medium carbohydrate diet, or a high protein, low carbohydrate diet.

Those on the low carbohydrate diet experienced a drop in bifidobacteria in the stool as well as a drop in the short chain fatty acid butyrate. Compared to the maintenance diet where butyrate levels were 18 millimoles (mM), the low carbohydrate diet resulted in an average butyrate production of only 4 mM.* Recall that the butyrate produced by our gut bacteria accounts for over 70 percent of the energy used by the cells that line our colon. This drastic reduction in butyrate from the lack of carbohydrate in the diet could quite possibly lead to an energy deficit in the colon cells and eventual disease. The drop in bifidobacteria in

*This study also found a drop in total short chain fatty acids, falling from 114 mM in the maintenance diet condition down to only 56 mM in the high protein, low carbohydrate condition.

this study is also of concern.[211] Stated another way, when gut bacteria are starved of carbodydrates, they do not produce enough butyrate to keep colon cells healthy.

There are a number of conditions in which molecules produced by gut bacteria are thought to contribute to the disease process. Some of these are conditions where the symptoms are predominantly in the intestinal tract, while other symptoms extend far beyond, such as the brain. Recall from Chapter 3, the studies that might link gut bacterial molecules to neurological disease. Thus, while protein is important to maintain healthy defenses, it has to be consumed with an adequate complement of complex fermentable fibers.

Unhealthy Carbs

Carbohydrates can have a significant effect on the tone of our immune system and on the inflammatory state. While this is a lengthy subject, we'll focus briefly on how the glycemic load of the diet can shift our immune proteins in unhealthy directions.

Glycemic Index (GI) is a measure of the degree to which a carbohydrate is likely to raise your blood sugar (glucose) levels. The scale is 0 to 100 (based on either white bread or glucose), with 0 being low and 100 being high. The GI compares equal quantities of carbohydrate and provides a measure of carbohydrate quality but not quantity. Glycemic indices can be misleading because they have been developed using fixed amounts of food that do not accurately reflect what people actually eat.

In 1997, Harvard University scientists introduced the concept of glycemic load (GL). This measure gives a more accurate reflection of the blood sugar effects of a standard portion of food. In short, the GL of a typical serving of food is the product of the *amount* of available carbohydrate in that serving *and* the glycemic index of that food.

In practical terms, the higher the GL of a food, the greater the expected rise in blood glucose and the greater the adverse insulin effects

■ Table 5.1. Glycemic Load of Selected Foods

FOOD	SERVING SIZE (g)	GLYCEMIC LOAD (GL)
DRINKS		
Coca Cola®, average	250	15
Cranberry juice cocktail (Ocean Spray®)	250	24
GRAINS		
White rice, average	150	23
Bagel	35	25
Macaroni, average	180	23
Macaroni and Cheese (Kraft)	180	32
Baked russet potato, average	150	26
FRUIT		
Grapefruit	120	3
Grapes, average	120	8
Orange, average	120	5
Peach, average	120	5
Pear, average	120	4
Apple, average	120	6
NUTS		
Cashews, salted	50	3
Peanuts, average	50	1

of the food. Foods with a GL of 10 or below would be presumed to be less detrimental to health, while those with a GL of 20 and above would have more detrimental affects. Long-term consumption of foods with a high glycemic load appears to be linked to a greater risk to obesity, diabetes, and inflammation. These, in turn, now appear to have negative effects on immune defense, energy, and repair.

Glycemic Load of Common Foods

The table above contains a representative sampling of the glycemic load of some common foods.[212] It immediately becomes clear that foods like potatoes, pasta, bagels, rice, and soft drinks stand out as high glycemic foods. Conversely, fruits and nuts stand out as low glycemic foods.

The affect of high glycemic foods on the production of inflammatory compounds is one reason for concern. For instance, in a recent study published in the *Journal of the American Medical Association,* 244 healthy women were tested to see how their glycemic load (the intake of high or low glycemic foods) affected an immune-inflammation chemical called CRP (C-reactive protein). Women with high glycemic diets had average CRP values of 5.0, while those with low glycemic diets had CRP levels of only 1.6. The highest levels were in women who were overweight.

This is just one piect of evidence showing how a high glycemic load diet can drive our immunological tone toward a state of persistent inflammation. In short, the body behaves somewhat like there is an infection, when no infection is present. It is our high glycemic foods that are driving an alteration in immune function. This can sometimes mean a shift that makes us less able to fight certain types of microbes.

Phytonutrients and Immunity

Molecules derived from a wide range of plants can have beneficial effects on immune defense, energy, and repair. Below is a very brief exploration of selected phytonutrients. It is meant purely as an introduction, as the topic of plant substances and human health is complex.

Quercetin and Polyphenolics

Quercetin belongs to a family of plant-derived molecules called polyphenolics. Quercetin is found concentrated in foods such as onions, apples, grapes, red wine, green tea, and broccoli. Most people in North America get the bulk of their quercetin from onions and apples, roughly 25 to 50 milligrams per day. While there are many polyphenolics worthy of discussion in relation to immunity, the recent work of one scientist has gained attention.

Dr. David Nieman is a professor at Appalachain State University who has been studying the effect of heavy training on immunity and infection for the last two decades. Finding that heavy exertion increases infection susceptibility, Dr. Nieman began studying nutrients in hopes that he might find something to reduce this effect.

Nieman set up his most recent study to be a high-stress condition involving cyclists. Twenty people ingested 1,000 milligrams of quercetin a day for five weeks, while another 20 were given a placebo. The quercetin supplement also contained niacin and vitamin C for improved absorption. After three weeks of preloading with quercetin supplements, the athletes rode a bicycle to the point of exhaustion three hours a day for three days.

His previous research had shown that a grueling task such as this would result in lowered immunity and possible occurrence of opportunistic infections. In this trial, 45 percent of the cyclists taking the placebo reported illness following the extreme exercise, compared with only 5 percent in the quercetin group. This was a double-blind, placebo-controlled study, meaning that neither the participants nor the researchers knew which subjects were receiving the placebo or the quercetin supplement. According to Dr. Nieman, the effects of quercetin did not seem to occur until after the three-day intense exercise period, suggesting that the effects of quercetin on immunity are more pronounced when the body is under stress. More research is underway to determine whether quercetin might influence immunity in healthy, nonstressed individuals.

So, it looks like eating our fair share of apples and onions may, indeed, keep the doctor away.

Cranberries

Cranberries have gained favorable attention for their value in treating urinary tract infections in women. Two studies have been frequently singled out as having promising outcomes. One study was conducted in Canada and involved 150 women who had two or more urinary tract infections in the previous two years. They were divided into groups receiving a combination of cranberry juice, cranberry tablets, placebo juice, or placebo tablets. The study lasted one year. Of those in the placebo group, 32 percent experienced at least one urinary tract infection during the year of study, compared to only 18 percent in the cranberry *tablet* group and 20 percent in the cranberry *juice* group. Thus, the cranberry treatment almost cut the number of infections in half.[213]

A second study that is often cited involves women in a long-term care facility in Boston. Women were given either cranberry juice or a colored drink containing no cranberry products. After one month, there was no difference in the percentage of women who had high bacterial counts in their urine (more than 100,000 colony-forming units/milliliter). However, after one month, the women in the cranberry juice group experienced a consistent decrease in the bacterial and white blood cell counts in their urine. The use of antibiotics for urinary tract infections was cut in half in the cranberry group.[214]

In the most recent and largest study of its kind, 376 men and women in an elderly residence care facility were given a placebo or cranberry juice. The juice contained water, cranberry juice from concentrate (25 percent), sugar, vitamin C, and aspartame as sweetener. The placebo beverage contained no cranberry solids, but contained water, sugar (sucrose), elderberry extract, quinic acid, citric acid, malic acid, vitamin C, and aspartame as sweetener.

A total of 21 patients had at least one urinary tract infection during the 18-day study period—14 in the placebo group and 7 in the cranberry group. Thus, cranberry juice consumption was associated with *half* the incidence of infection. In the cranberry group, there was also a significantly lower rate of *E. coli* infection. *E. coli* is the most common of the bacteria infecting the urinary tract in elderly people. Of all 21 infections, *E. coli* was responsible for 13 of the infections in the placebo group, but only 4 in the cranberry group.

It should be noted that, because the overall incidence of infection in the entire group was small, the study did not reach statistical significance. However, the results are consistent with findings in other studies that cranberry products appear to lower the incidence of urinary tract infection. Also, this trial was conducted for only 18 days, whereas other studies were conducted for one year or more. Long-term use of cranberry products may be needed to achieve maximum results.[215]

Green Tea Extracts

The bacterium *Helicobacter pylori* is known to cause inflammation, oxidative stress, DNA damage, and cell death in cells of the stomach. One way *H. pylori* initiates its damage is by activating the toll-like receptor 4 (TLR4) and triggering inflammation. Scientists in Korea have found that administration of substances found in green tea suppressed the triggering of the toll-like receptor-4. Recall that these are the gatekeepers that are activated by fragments of gut bacteria. It appears that green tea extracts might be one tool to silence or dampen these inflammation triggers. A similar study conducted by an independent group has also shown that a portion of green tea called EGCG might lower the activity of TLR4 when it is exposed to bacterial endotoxins (LPS).[216] These discoveries may mean that one of the mechanisms by which green tea achieves its well-documented effects is through the toll receptor system. It also suggests that green tea could be used as part of a recovery and repair strategy in a variety of circumstances where the effects of gut-based endotoxins are of concern.

Curcumin

Curcumin is a well-known component of the spice turmeric (used in curry powder) and it has been widely studied for its anti-inflammatory and immune-regulating properties. More recently, it has been investigated as yet another plant-derived molecule that could dampen the toll-like receptor 4 and offer protection against the negative effects of bacterial endotoxins. This could mean that curcumin might offer protection against an overactive inflammatory system due to leaky gut. Scientists at the USDA showed that TLR4 is a molecular target of curcumin. They wrote, "These results imply that the activation of TLRs and subsequent immune/inflammatory responses induced by endogenous molecules or chronic infection can be modulated by certain dietary ehydroepiandr we consume daily."[217] In other words, the curcumin found in our humble spice turmeric might be able to help blunt the unhealthy activation of the immune system by bacterial fragments from the gut.

Garlic

Garlic is also known for its positive effects on inflammation and immunity. Some investigators now think that garlic constituents could also be among the phytonutrients that can protect us against gut endotoxins by blocking the toll receptors. Dr. Hyung-Sun Youn and his collaborators found that pretreatment of cells with a garlic extract prevented the activation of the toll-like receptor 4 with endotoxins. They further showed that it appeared to be the sulfur component of the garlic that might be responsible for this blocking effect. More specifically, the sulfur molecules (diallyl disulfide and others) in garlic may link up with the sulfur residues on the toll receptor and prevent endotoxins from sticking to our cell membranes and activating the inflammatory system.[218]

When the garlic data is considered along with the studies on green tea and curcumin, it suggests that these plant constituents (and maybe others) might become part of an overall dietary strategy of using anti-inflammatory herbs to lower the inflammatory risks posed by the harmful components of our gut bacteria.

How Infection Affects Nutritional Status

Not only does nutritional deficiency affect resistance to infection, But infection itself can alter nutritional status. Doctors have known for many years, for example, that conditions such as rheumatoid arthritis, acute tonsillitis, fever, pneumonia, and measles result in inadequate amounts of vitamin A in the tissues. These conditions often lead to depletion of vitamin A, which renders one more susceptible subsequent infections.

An article in the *American Journal of Clinical Nutrition* raised some very interesting points about nutrition and infection. Dr. F. A. Campos and his colleagues found that after an episode of chickenpox, children had inadequate body reserves of vitamin A for three months or longer after the infection.[219] Commenting on this and similar studies of measles, Dr. Thomas R. Frieden of the New York City Department of Health states,

> In developing countries, children who survive measles have increased morbidity [illness] and mortality [death] from respiratory infections and diarrhea for at least 1 year. Since vitamin A deficiency increases the severity of bacterial, viral, and parasitic infections, and is associated with increased diarrheal morbidity and mortality, the decline in total body stores of vitamin A caused by measles may contribute to increased post-measles mortality.[220]

Deficiency of nutrients prior to or as a result of infection has important consequences. As Dr. Frieden's groups showed, children with measles who had low levels of vitamin A were more likely to have fever and to be hospitalized. Other studies have shown that such children are more likely to suffer from pneumonia and diarrhea.

Another group of nutrients adversely influenced by infection is the essential fatty acids. These fats play an important role in regulating inflammation and immune function. Infection by the Epstein-Barr virus, associated with some cases of chronic fatigue syndrome and immune dysfunction, blocks the body's ability to manufacture vital compounds known as prostaglandins (signaling molecules made from fatty acids).

Other viruses are known to do the same. When this blocking occurs, susceptibility to infection by bacteria or reinfection by viruses increases. In people who do not seem to recover from an infection, blood and tissue levels of certain fatty acids (e.g. GLA and EPA) are depressed when compared with those who recover from such infections.[221] When essential fatty acids are given as a supplement, resistance to infection improves markedly.

These studies suggest that infection can cause the loss of nutrients important to immune function. Unless corrected, these deficiencies can render a child or adult susceptible to future viral, bacterial, or parasitic illness. This is not a new discovery. In 1976, researchers discovered that during infection, levels of vitamin C in the blood and tissues fell so low that the mechanisms used by white cells to attack bacteria was impaired.

Food Allergy, Intolerance, and Immunity

Allergy or intolerance to foods is one of the most commonly overlooked contributors to altered immunity and susceptibility to infection. According to James C. Breneman, MD, former chairman of the Food Allergy Committee of the American College of Allergists,

> The incidence of food allergy is greater than the incidence of any other type of illness affecting mankind. By some estimates, 60 percent of the population has unknown food intolerances or allergies. This constitutes a hidden iceberg of food allergy with only a small percentage, roughly 5 percent, of the iceberg showing. The other 95 percent of the food allergy patients go about their suffering unrecognized and untreated.

A classic example is ear infection in children. At the 1991 meeting of the American College of Allergy and Immunology, Dr. T. M. Nsouli presented a study of 104 children with chronic middle ear "infections." Seventy-eight percent of these children tested positive for reactivity to foods. After excluding offending foods from the diet for 11 weeks, 70 of 81 children experienced significant improvement. When offending foods were later

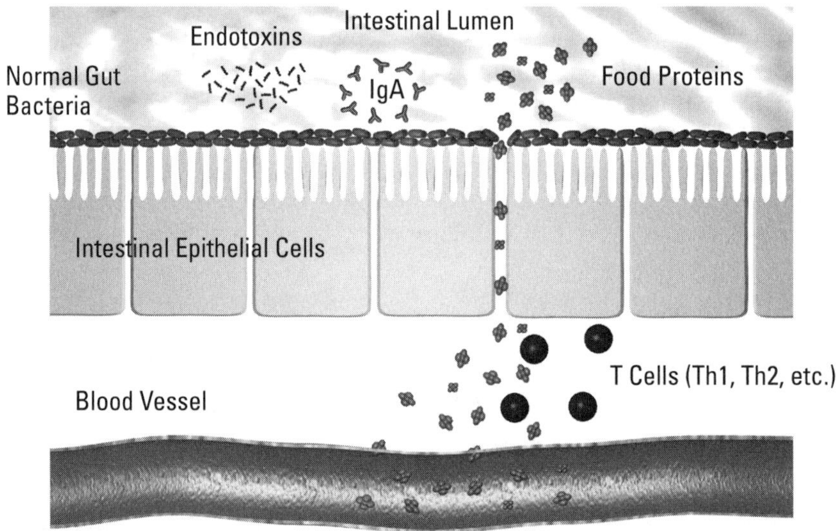

■ **Figure 5.1. How Leaky Gut Allows Food Proteins and Allergens to Pass into the Bloodstream.**

reintroduced—to verify the significance of the food allergy—66 of the 81 children experienced aggravation of their middle ear condition.[222]

Another study compared 56 milk-allergic and 204 non-allergic schoolchildren for their incidence of ear infections. Using the definition of recurrent otitis media as at least 15 episodes of acute earache by the age of ten years, the investigators found that 27 percent of children with cow's milk allergy had recurrent earaches compared with 12 percent of nonallergic children. The number of allergic children who had undergone tonsillectomy or adenoidectomy surgery was 48 percent in the cow's milk-allergic group, compared with 28 percent in the controls.[223]

These sentiments are echoed by Dr. Fred Pullen, an ear, nose, and throat specialist in Miami, Florida. Patients are referred to Dr. Pullen for the sole purpose of having tubes surgically implanted in their eardrums. Before undergoing surgery, however, all patients are first placed on a diet that eliminates dairy products. The result: "three-fourths [of these children] never need tubes."[224]

Intolerance to food may also be evidence of the leaky gut phenomenon. Scientists writing in the journal *Digestive and Liver Diseases* reported on their study of twenty-one people with food allergy and twenty people with food hypersensitivity. Each was tested for "leaky gut," as measured by the lactulose / mannitol test.* Those who reported food allergy or food intolerance had greater evidence of leaky gut. Scientists also found a link between the degree of increased intestinal permeability (leaky gut) and severity of food intolerance symptoms.

Another condition frequently linked to allergy and to weakened barrier defenses is asthma. Thus far, increased gut permeability has been found in one study of adult asthma. A recent study looked at thirty-two children with asthma and compared them with thirty-two children without asthma. Using the lactulose / mannitol ratio to assess permeability, it was found that asthmatic children had significantly increased intestinal permeability.[225]

These studies and others like them do not suggest that allergy or intolerance to food "cause" infection; the issue is much more complex. But one can draw the conclusion that food intolerance may be part of a larger complex of metabolic events wherein host defense and repair have been altered as a result of factors that require deeper investigation. Regardless of the means by which food intolerance and infection susceptibility may be linked, an attention to food allergy testing may be warranted in those with these susceptibilities.

The Most Common Food Allergy Offenders

Although intolerance to almost any food can contribute to or cause sluggish immunity, impaired energy, altered barrier defenses, or diminished repair capability certain offenders are more common than others:

---

*Lactulose is a disaccharide (two sugars) that is poorly absorbed. Mannitol is a simple sugar that is well absorbed. When lactulose appears in the urine, it means that the gut has been excessively permeable to small molecules. A ratio of lactulose to mannitol is used to understand the degree of gut leakiness.

- Dairy products, including milk, butter, cheese, yogurt, cottage cheese, and ice cream
- Wheat, including not only bread and cereal, but anything that contains wheat such as gravies, crackers, and cookies
- Eggs or anything containing eggs
- Corn, or anything containing corn, such as corn flakes
- Soy
- Peanuts and other nuts
- Shellfish
- Sugar
- Yeast

Breast-feeding

Breast-feeding is perhaps the most effective means of preventing not only middle ear infection, but infections of all types in children. In three separate studies, Dr. R. K. Chandra investigated the effect of breast-feeding on the incidence of infection and allergy. He demonstrated that breast-fed infants in India had a lower incidence of otitis media and respiratory infections (as well as diarrhea, dehydration, and pneumonia) than did children who were not breast-fed. In Canada, breast-feeding was again associated with a decrease in the occurrence of otitis media and respiratory infection.[226,227] Dr. Chandra also showed that when newborn siblings of children with allergic disease are exclusively breast-fed for a minimum of six weeks, the number of allergic indicators, including lowered antibodies to cow's milk, are significantly reduced.[228]

The duration of breast-feeding also appears to have an impact on the development of otitis media. Finnish researcher Dr. Ulla Saarinen followed 256 babies, born in the same three months, for one year. Of those breast-fed for more than 6 months, only 6 percent had suffered an attack of otitis by the age of one year, in contrast to 19 percent of bottle-fed infants. Six percent of the children who had prolonged breast-feeding suffered four or more attacks of otitis media between one and three years of age, compared with 26 percent who had early introduction of cow's milk. Dr. Saarinen concluded that early and prolonged breast-feeding exerts a protective effect against otitis media that lasts up to three years.[229]

In another study on the benefits of prolonged breast-feeding, researchers found that breast-feeding protected against the development of otitis media, but that the risk increased four months after breast-feeding was discontinued. Approximately twelve months after breast-feeding was discontinued, the risk of developing otitis media was virtually the same as if the children had never been breast-fed. This led researchers to conclude that "The risk of otitis media depends on the number of months a child is breast-fed and the number of months that pass after breast-feeding is discontinued."[230] It seems to lend further support to the traditional practice in some cultures of mothers breast-feeding their children until they are two to three years old, the age at which children in Western cultures are particularly prone to otitis media.

Breast milk even appears to prevent middle ear problems in children with cleft palate. Most children with cleft palate have difficulty suckling and are usually fed by formula. They suffer inordinately from otitis media, require persistent antibiotic therapy, and often require surgery. Dr. Jack L. Paradise found that when mothers used a breast pump to gather their milk and fed it to their children with cleft palate, the number of episodes of middle ear effusion was significantly reduced. Thirty-two percent of the children given breast milk were free of middle ear fluid at one or more office visits compared with roughly 3 percent of those fed cow's milk or soy formula.[231]

Breast milk is high in an antibody called secretory IgA, something the child does not make in adequate amounts. Secretory IgA is a very important immune protein that protects against infection. Breast milk also contains proteins (called receptor analogues) that protect against attachment of bacteria. When these proteins are present, bacteria may exist in the environment, but their attachment is prevented. The ability of bacteria to attach is strongly associated with their ability to cause illness. Common ear-infecting bacteria such as *H. influenzae* and *S. pneumoniae* can be prevented from attaching by these proteins.[232] A list of natural protective molecules found in human milk can be found in Appendix D.

Infections from Your Food

There is one last issue regarding food and infection that deserves our attention. Intestinal infection by foodborne bacteria is a growing problem in the United States and worldwide. According to a committee of the National Academy of Sciences, one in fifty people in the United States gets sick each year from salmonella or campylobacter.[233] The Centers for Disease Control estimate that foodborne illness strikes roughly 76 million people in the U.S. alone each year.[234]

A study published in 2002 highlights the nature of this crisis. Consumer's Union tested 484 fresh, whole broiler chickens. They found salmonella or campylobacter in about one-half of the samples. Some 34 percent of the salmonella showed some resistance to one or more antibiotics used to treat people. Near 90 percent of the campylobacter tested had resistance to antibiotics.[235]

Most authorities agree that, while foodborne illness can strike anyone, those with weakened immunity or sluggish host defenses are more susceptible.

The Most Common Foodborne Diseases

According to the CDC, the most commonly recognized foodborne infections are those caused by the bacteria campylobacter, salmonella, and E. coli O157:H7, and by a group of viruses called calicivirus, also known as the Norwalk and Norwalk-like viruses.[236]

Campylobacter is a bacterial pathogen that causes fever, diarrhea, and abdominal cramps. It is the most commonly identified bacterial cause of diarrheal illness in the world. These bacteria live in the intestines of healthy birds, and most raw poultry meat has campylobacter on it. Eating undercooked chicken, or other food that has been contaminated with juices dripping from raw chicken is the most frequent source of this infection.

Salmonella is also a bacterium that is widespread in the intestines of birds, reptiles, and mammals. It can spread to humans through a variety of different foods of animal origin. The illness it causes, salmonellosis, typically includes fever, diarrhea, and abdominal cramps. In persons with poor underlying health or weakened immune systems, it can invade the bloodstream and cause life-threatening infections.

***E. coli* O157:H7** is a bacterial pathogen found in cattle and other farm animals. Human illness typically follows consumption of food or water that has been contaminated with microscopic amounts of cow feces. Undercooked hamburger has been one of the most common sources. The illness it causes is often a severe and bloody diarrhea and painful abdominal cramps, without much fever. In 3 percent to 5 percent of cases, a complication called hemolytic uremic syndrome (HUS) can occur several weeks after the initial symptoms. This severe complication includes temporary anemia, profuse bleeding, kidney failure, and sometimes death.

Calicivirus, or **Norwalk-like virus,** is an extremely common cause of foodborne illness, though it is rarely diagnosed because the laboratory test is not widely available. It causes an acute gastrointestinal illness, usually with more vomiting than diarrhea, that resolves within two days. Unlike many foodborne pathogens that have animal reservoirs, it is believed that Norwalk-like viruses spread primarily from one infected person to another. If they have the virus on their hands, infected kitchen workers can contaminate a salad or sandwich as they prepare it. Infected fishermen have contaminated oysters as they harvested them.

Some common diseases are occasionally foodborne, even though they are usually transmitted by other routes. These include infections caused by *Shigella,* hepatitis A, and the parasites *Giardia lamblia* and *Cryptosporidia.* Even strep throats have been transmitted occasionally through food.

In addition to disease caused by direct infection, some foodborne diseases are caused by the presence of a toxin in the food that was produced by a microbe in the food. For example, the bacterium *Staphylococcus aureus* can grow in some foods and produce a toxin that causes intense vomiting. The rare but deadly disease botulism occurs when the bacterium *Clostridium botulinum* grows and produces a powerful paralytic toxin in foods. These toxins can produce illness even if the microbes that produced them are no longer there.

Because we eat so frequently and because we eat so many mass-produced and heavily handled foods, the odds that we will encounter a foodborne illness are fairly high. Strong general immunity, strong barrier defenses, and a healthy and balanced population of gut bacteria are among the most vital elements to our defense, should an exposure to one of these foodborne microbes occur.

Nutrition and Our Defenses

As Dr. Barry Sears is fond of saying, "eating is a hormonal event." We could also add that eating is an event where we shape our inflammatory state and our immunological tone. Our food consists of a complex of nutrients that provide the basic elements of our metabolism. Food consitutents present in excess drive our metabolism in one direction. Elements consumed in inadequate amounts drive our metabolism in another direction. Over time, our bodies will make adaptations, stiving to function in this environment of combined deficiency and excess.

This may seem like an unusual situation, but it is actually more the rule in our modern culture. Excess of carbohydrate triggers adaptations. Inadequate amounts of protein create adaptations. Deficiency of single nutrients causes shifts in our metabolism that alter the normal biochemical behavior.

The growing sophistication of modern biochemistry and genetics has allowed us to peer more deeply into the black box of metabolism, the engine of our immune defense, energy, and repair. From this collective work, it is clear that nutrient imbalance has a powerful influence on how we are able to interact with the microbes around us.

As we move forward to examine the effects of genetics, lifestyle, environment, stress, and other forces on our defenses, we must understand the prominent role of nutrition in shaping our immunity. Many aspects of lifestyle can be improved that will favor strong defenses. But these will only succeed to their full potential if the nutritional building blocks are present to meet the needs of a given situation. This leads us to another class of supplemental agents that are sometimes classified as foods, which we'll explore the next chapter. These are the probiotics.

Chapter 6

How Probiotics Will Change Our Future

We are a human-microbe hybrid cloaked in a blanket of some 1,000 to 5,000 different types of bacteria. An entire field of medicine is emerging that looks to these microbes as both as agents of disease and as agents of healing. Where we once looked to antibiotics to kill harmful microbes, we are now beginning to look toward probiotics to out-compete, destroy, or slow down the harmful microbes. The day may soon arise when we reach not for amoxicillin to treat a sore throat, but for a strain of the helpful *Strep. viridans.* We might one day pull out our spray bottle of *Strep. oralis* to treat an earache. We may even be close to supplying a drink of *Lactobacillus plantarum* or other microbes to modify obesity or diabetes.

Humans have been consuming probiotics for millennia in the form of fermented milk products, fermented vegetable products, and many others. The World Health Organization currently defines probiotics as "live microorganisms that when administered in adequate amounts confer a health benefit on the host."[237] Modern science has now given us the tools to tailor probiotics to specific needs, ushering in a potential revolution in the way we are able to support our defense, energy, and repair capabilities.

When Might Probiotics Help?

Most people are likely familiar with the use of probiotics in support of intestinal health. But it may be surprising to know how much work is being done in applying probiotics to infections of other parts of the body. This is because doctors have come to understand that the organisms that live in our nose, on our skin, in our throats, and elsewhere may be the very things that keep harmful microbes at bay. We might be able to go beyond antibiotics by going toward probiotics in many unexpected instances. Thus, we will consider some of the potential benefits of probiotics applied in unique ways.*

Can Oral Probiotics Reduce Nasal Infections?

As we all know, the nose is home to a wide variety of troublesome microbes. Among them are *Staphylococcus aureus, Steptococcus pneumoniae, Haemophilus influenzae,* and beta-hemolytic streptococci. Reducing nasal bacteria could be helpful for the average person, but especially crucial for someone of lowered immunity, head trauma, or undergoing surgery. This is important because, in 30 percent of wound infections with *Staph aureus,* the patient's nose was the site of origin of the bacteria.[238] In one hospital study, methicillin resistant *Staph aureus* (MRSA) was found in the nasal passage of 46 percent of people hospitalized with liver disease.[239] The findings that nasal bacteria contribute to staph infections is certainly important for patients in critical care, but is also important for any of us who may visit loved ones in such settings.

---

*It is important to understand that studies involving probiotics can have conflicting results. There are many reasons for this, but one fact to bear in mind is that probiotic supplements vary widely in their species, origin, preparation, storage, and other factors. In particular, the probiotic strains that are used in studies are critical. Thus, a negative study using one probiotic may not hold true for another strain of probiotic. On the other hand, a favorable outcome with one probiotic does not mean that another strain would prove equally successful in that condition. Likewise, a particular probiotic successful in one condition may not translate into success in another condition.

In the first study of its kind, doctors in Switzerland studied 209 healthy subjects divided into two groups receiving oral doses of either probiotic cultures or yogurt. The intent was to see if oral probiotics could lower the bacterial count in the nose.

The culture included Lactobacillus GG, Bifidobacterium B420, *Lactobacillus acidophilus* 145, and *Streptococcus thermophilus*. The subjects consumed these cultures for three weeks, which was followed by nasal cultures for the common harmful organisms. Neither the doctors nor the patients were aware of who was receiving which treatment. Harmful bacteria in the nose were reduced by a statistically significant 19 percent. This included the troublesome *Staph aureus* and other gram-positive bacteria. Scientists cannot yet explain the exact mechanism behind this effect, but they speculate that the probiotics somehow modify the immune defenses of the upper respiratory tract. In other words, the gut mucosal immunity and the respiratory immunity may be linked.[240]

Probiotics and Critical Illness

Patients in intensive care units suffer from decreased immunity, breakdown of their intestinal barrier defenses, and increased susceptibility to infection. A trial of twenty-eight critically ill patients was undertaken to see whether ingestion of probiotics would have benefits to patient outcome. Each person in the study received one of three treatments—placebo, probiotics, or probiotics that had been killed by sonication. (With sonication, the bacteria would still be present, but they would not be alive and viable.)

Those receiving the probiotics had significantly larger increases in the immunoglobulins IgA and IgG. Those receiving the probiotics also had reductions in intestinal permeability, which can be translated as improved barrier defenses. This would seemingly be beneficial, since it would reduce the likelihood of harmful microbes traveling across the gut barrier to end up infecting the lymph nodes and blood.[241] Remember from earlier chapters, a leaky gut can permit bacterial endotoxin to cross from the gut into the bloodstream, which can prove serious (if not fatal) to a sick person.

Probiotics and Aging

It is well known that immunity commonly declines with age. With this decline often comes increased susceptibility to opportunistic infections. *Bifidobacterium lactis* is a common probiotic used in clinical studies. The specific strain *Bifidobacterium lactis* HN019 has not been previously shown to influence specific markers of immunity. In this study, doctors enrolled thirty healthy volunteers aged sixty-three to eighty-four. Each was given low-fat milk for one week, followed by one week of the *B. lactis* formula. This was followed by another week of low-fat milk. Immune parameters at each of the three time points were measured and compared.

The probiotic formula was found to affect the following patterns of immunity:

- Increase in the proportion of total helper T-cells ($C4^+$)
- Increase in activated T lymphocytes ($CD25^+$)
- Increase in activated natural killer cells
- Phagocytic activity of monocytes increased
- Phagocytic activity of neutrophils increased
- Tumoricidal activity of natural killer cells increased

The greatest changes in immunity were found in those people whose immune function was lowest at the beginning of the study. The immune system changes ranged from 9 to 82 percent.[242]

Probiotics and Infant Formula

Parents are increasingly using probiotics with their infants and young children as a means to promote health or recover from illness. Use of probiotics has especially been promoted with children who've taken antibiotics for brief or extended periods. A group at John's Hopkins

University School of Medicine conducted a trial in children three to twenty-four months old in an effort to better understand the safety profile of two different doses of probiotics. One hundred and eighteen healthy children received either the probiotic or unsupplemented formula. The probiotic-enriched formula contained a mixture of *Bifidobacterium lactis* and *Streptococcus thermophilus* at two different concentrations.

After an average of 210 days, the probiotic formulas were well accepted. Children on the probiotic formula also experienced less colic and irritability. Of great interest was the finding that these children also experienced a lowered use of antibiotics during the study period than did those not consuming the probiotic.[243]

Probiotics and Ear Infections

Ear infection in children is sometimes characterized by invasion of bacteria, while in other cases inflammation is the predominant feature. When microbes are present, the common infecting bacteria of middle ears in children are *Streptococcus pneumoniae, Haemophilus influenzae,* and *Moraxella catharralis.* Several research groups have wondered whether the work with probiotics, which has been so fruitful in other areas, might be applied to ear infections in children, with the idea that beneficial microbes might take up residence in the ear and prevent harmful ones from taking root.

One novel clinical trial was undertaken with 108 children with recurrent infections between the ages of five months and six years. After a ten-day course of antibiotics, children in the test group were given a nasal spray with strains of *Strep. Mitis, Strep. sanguis,* and *Strep. oralis.* Doctors chose these probiotics based on culture studies showing that these strains could inhibit the growth of the common ear infecting bacteria. The remaining fifty-five children (the placebo group) received a nasal spray consisting only of skim milk.

The portion of children in the placebo group who experienced a recurrence of their ear infections during the three months of the study period was 42 percent. This was in comparison to only 22 percent in the probiotic treatment group.

It should be noted that a follow-up study tested whether antibiotics were needed to first eliminate the harmful microbes in order for the probiotic to work. It appeared from this study that probiotics alone were not sufficient. The probiotics apparently were unable to supplant the harmful strains once the harmful strains had gained a foothold.[244,245] These studies have not yet translated into practical treatments. However, they show the interesting ways in which scientists are viewing the potential merits of probiotics in the treatment of disease.

Whether probiotics given by mouth can reduce the incidence of ear infections in children is unclear. In a recent study, 309 children prone to recurrent acute otitis media (ear infection) were given an oral capsule of lactobacillus, bifidobacterium, and propionibacterium strains for 24 weeks and compared with children given a placebo. The probiotics did not affect the rate of otitis media episodes when compared with the children in the placebo group, though the probiotic group did seem to have a reduction in recurrent respiratory infections.[246] This issue warrants more research, since alpha-streptococci are the most common competing normal bacteria in the upper respiratory tract. A formulation of probiotics similar to the one used in the nasal spray study above may have been more successful in out-competing the harmful organisms in the upper respiratory tract.

It should also be mentioned, however, that many cases of earaches in children are not due to infection but to inflammation, so one might expect conflicting results when studying probiotics in earaches.*

Probiotics, Strep Throat, and Pharyngitis

One of the most common infecting bacteria of the throat and tonsils is called *Streptococcus pyogenes.* In more severe cases, this form of strep

*See: *Childhood Ear Infections,* Michael A. Schmidt, PhD, North Atlantic Books.

can also trigger meningitis, pneumonia, necrotizing fasciitis, arthritis, and septic shock. The pharyngeal area (the throat area) is commonly colonized by another strep called *Strep. viridans,* which secretes substances that are bactericidal or bacteriostatic to *Strep. pyogenes.* Adults seem to harbor more of the protective *Strep. viridans* than do children. This may be one reason that tonsillitis due to strep is more common in children than in adults. These findings have led researchers to experiment with feeding probiotic cultures to people with strep infections of the throat in hopes that recurrence can be reduced.

Two of these studies reflect the promise of this area. In one study giving the alpha-hemolytic strep probiotic ten days after antibiotic therapy, only 2 percent of the patients experienced another episode of infection due to *Strep. pyogenes,* compared with a reinfection rate of 23 percent of the placebo group. In a larger study of 282 people, antibiotic therapy was followed by use of a throat spray that contained the same alpha-strep probiotic. Only 24 percent of the probiotic group became reinfected, compared with 42 percent of those receiving the placebo.[247]

These studies have not as yet been transformed into standard treatments, but the research heralds a new era in medicine where the ecology of the body's natural defenses is considered paramount to any strategy at raising our defenses to the harmful microbes within our midst. Advances in this area will truly take into consideration the human-microbe hybrid, the superorganism.

Probiotics and Eczema

Eczema is an allergic-type disease that commonly runs in families. Doctors interested in the possible role of gut bacteria have wondered if probiotics might have a protective role in families at risk to eczema. Writing in the *Lancet* medical journal, doctors from Finland reported on a study in which they gave the probiotic Lactobacillus GG as a prenatal supplement to pregnant women. These women were known to have at least one first-degree relative (or a partner) with eczema, allergic rhinitis, or asthma. In such women, the likelihood of their offspring developing atopic eczema is high. In addition to the mothers receiving the probiotic, the children were given the same probiotic supplement for a full six months after birth. The frequency of atopic eczema in the probiotic group was only 23 percent, compared with 46 percent in the placebo group.

According to the authors, "Lactobacillus GG was effective in prevention of early atopic disease in children at high risk. Thus, gut microflora might be a hitherto unexplored source of natural immunomodulators and probiotics, for prevention of atopic disease."[248]

Probiotics and Bacterial Vaginosis

Bacterial vaginosis is often treated with antibiotics and it is a condition in which relapse is quite common. A study was conducted to see whether a vaginal antibiotic (clindamycin) combined with vaginal lactobacillus administration might improve the cure rate in one hundred women with vaginosis. These doctors also wanted see how lactobacilli influenced the rate of recurrence, when given repeatedly for three menstrual cycles.

Seventy-six of the women were considered cured. The study found that the treatment combining two different strains of probiotic lactobacilli did not improve the efficacy of the therapy during the first month of treatment. However, after six months, 65 percent of the lactobacilli-treated women were still free of bacterial vaginosis, compared with 46 percent of the placebo-treated women.[249]

Types of Probiotic Organisms Commonly Available

Many strains of probiotics are currently being studied for their potential use as oral and topical therapies. A brief list of some of the most extensively studied is provided below.

■ Table 6.1. Types of Probiotics Available[250]

Genus	Species	Strain
Bacillus	*cereus*	
Bifidobacterium	bifidum	Bb-12
Bifidobacterium	longum	
Bifidobacterium	breve	
Bifidobacterium	infantis	
Bifidobacterium	lactis	HN019
Bifidobacterium	adolescentis	
Enterococcus	feaecalis	
Enterococcus	faecium	
Escherichia	coli	
Lactobacillus	casei	Shirota
Lactobacillus	lactis	
Lactobacillus	plantarum	299v
Lactobacillus	rhamnosus	GR-1, GG (55103), HN110
Lactobacillus	reuteri	RC-14, ATCC 55730
Lactobacillus	johnsonii	LJ-1 (LA-1) NCFB 1748
Saccharomyces	boularidi	
Streptococcus	thermophilus	

Are There Risks with Probiotics?

Probiotics have a long record of safety and an ancient history of use in many cultured foods, so they are clearly safe. But are there cases in which their safety is in question? Perhaps. This is because probiotics *are* live bacteria and they could challenge the weakened defenses of a very sick person, or worse, contribute to sepsis (blood infection).

A review article in the *American Journal of Clinical Nutrition* cited the following circumstances in which probiotic use should be questioned.

The authors suggest that the presence of a single major risk factor or more than one minor risk factor should cause one to proceed with caution in using probiotics.

Major Risk Factors[251]

- Immune compromise, including a debilitated state or malignancy
- Premature infants

Minor Risk Factors

- Central venous catheter
- Impaired intestinal epithelial barrier, e.g. diarrheal illness, intestinal inflammation
- Administration of probiotic by jejunostomy
- Administration of broad-spectrum antibiotics to which probiotic is resistant
- Probiotics with properties of high mucosal adhesion or known pathogenicity
- Cardiac valvular disease (Lactobacillus probiotics only)

Will Probiotics Replace Antibiotics?

Will probiotics replace antibiotics? This is a very interesting question. The fact that it is being asked at all within medical circles heralds a new era in how we approach infection. It is a philosophy that centers on the host, with recognition of our hybrid nature—the superorganism.

Writing in the *Canadian Journal of Infectious Disease and Medical Microbiology,* Dr. Gregor Ried authored a paper entitled "Probiotics to Prevent the Need for and Augment the Use of Antibiotics." He cites three general areas in which probiotics may act as adjuncts to antibiotics:[252]

- Reduce the risk of antibiotic-induced superinfections in the gut and vagina

- Secrete antibacterial substances that lower pathogenic bacterial populations locally and at distant mucosal sites; disrupt biofilms making it easier for antibiotics to function
- Enhance the general mucosal immunity, which in turn aids in the eradication of the organisms at the mucosal site

One could also add to this list the use of probiotics in a preventive manner, so that host defenses can be raised and antibiotic use avoided altogether. Is the idea practical? The simple answer is that probiotics have the potential to replace antibiotics in many circumstances. In other situations, we will likely use them in combination with antibiotics. If we view microbes in their full complexity and humans in our full complexity, it becomes clear that the variations in microbes and uniqueness of each person means that a full complement of tools will be needed to help us navigate this world of the microbe.

Prebiotics

Prebiotics are non-digestible oligosaccharides (complex sugars) that can stimulate the growth of specific or general forms of gut bacteria. There are many forms of prebiotics and many studies on their potential benefits. Here we'll focus on only one, their ability to improve the integrity of the intestinal mucosa by increasing the growth of specific types of gut microbes. One of the best-known forms of prebiotic is called fructooligosaccharide (FOS), found in inulin-containing foods (but there are others, including galactooligosaccharides). FOS has been shown to stimulate bifidobacteria growth in the colon, with its attendant benefits. Some of the foods that contain inulin include artichoke (Jerusalem type preferred), asparagus, banana, unrefined barley, garlic, green beans, honey, leeks, unrefined oats, onions, raisins, soybeans, tomato, sprouted wheat products, and whole grains.

In previous chapters, we explored the process of how cell wall fragments (endotoxins) from certain gut microbes may leak across the gut barrier, enter the bloodstream, and elicit inflammatory changes throughout the body. In Chapter 5, we also discussed how a high-fat diet might further increase the transport of bacterial endotoxins across the gut barrier. A research group in Brussels led by Dr. P. D. Cani has examined whether increasing bifidobacteria numbers in the gut can reduce leaky gut conditions and prevent the translocation of gut bacterial fragments (endotoxins) in rats on a high-fat diet.

In this study, rats fed a high-fat diet had significantly more bacterial endotoxins that leaked from the gut into the bloodstream. Rats that were fed fructooligosaccharide (FOS) along with the high-fat diet had significantly more bifidobacteria in their gut. This was expected, since FOS consistently improves the growth of bifidobacteria. What was of great interest is that feeding FOS *decreased* the amount of bacterial endotoxins that leaked across the gut wall into the bloodstream. In short, the prebiotic FOS slowed the transport of endotoxins from the gut, even under high-fat conditions when endotoxin transport is usually increased. The FOS treatment also improved blood glucose control and reduced the release of inflammatory immune proteins (cytokines).[253]

In humans, FOS intake leads to significant increases in bifidobacteria in the colon.[254] In people with intestinal disorders like Crohn's disease, FOS has raised the level of bifidobacteria and improved symptoms.[255] In a study of elderly people, those in the probiotic (oligosaccharides) group had significantly lower inflammatory markers in the blood, suggesting that the probiotic, even though it was delivered to the gut, had the effect of lowering inflammation elsewhere in the body.[256]

Chapter 7

Genes: We Have More Control than We Think

Some of us have warrior genes. If you carry this warrior gene, it may be what saved your ancestors on the battlefields of the ancient world. The same genes likely also saved them from the bubonic plague during the ominous period of the dark ages of Europe. Had your ancestors not carried this gene, you might not be here reading this book today.

The number of people who carry this gene is staggeringly high, being the most common genetic abnormality found in Caucasians of northern European descent. It is thought that the first mutation arose some seventy generations ago in a single person of Celtic heritage in the British Isles. Today, it is estimated that one in every two hundred people in the United States and Canada has both genes and one in ten is a carrier (possessing one copy of the mutant allele).

The force of the plague was so strong that perhaps as many as two million Americans unknowingly have the double gene mutation, with another 35 to 45 million being silent "carriers" of the single gene mutation. If you are of Irish, Scottish, Norse, or Celtic heritage, you are potentially one of these people. If you actually live in the British Isles, as many as 1 in 4 may be a carrier, with 1 in 64 carrying the double gene mutation. In Australian whites, as many as 14 persons out of 100 is a carrier.

A common notion in genetics is "that which saved your ancestors might kill you today." That phrase is a little drastic, but not entirely untrue. It does make the point that the conditions in which an individual lives strongly shapes who lives and who dies—which genes get passed on to the next generation and which do not. The conditions faced by our ancestors are no longer present, so the gene adaptation that laid the foundation for their survival may no longer serve us. It may, in fact, be to our detriment.

How the Warrior Genes Worked

The warrior gene hypothesis was advanced by Dr. Sharon Moalem in the journal *Medical Hypothesis* in 2002. He expanded his discussion in his book *Survival of the Sickest.* The warrior genes appear to have prevented the bacterium of the bubonic plague, *Yersinia pestis,* from replicating inside white blood cells. It is believed that those who carried this gene were the ones most likely to survive and, therefore, the ones who passed on their genetic heritage in unusually high numbers. Following this logic, if you carry this gene, one of your ancestors likely survived the bubonic plague. Congratulations.

The warrior gene causes its owner to be exceptionally good at conserving iron—so much so that iron builds up over time to levels that have a damaging impact on health. Today, the condition is called hemochromatosis. It is linked to different genes, but the two main ones are known as Hfe mutations C282Y and H63D.

The bubonic plague had a strange set of victims. While many infections claim the young, the old, and the ill (those who were weakened or immune suppressed), the bubonic plague tended to strike those in the prime of life. Healthy males between the ages of twenty and fifty were among those claimed most frequently.

During the bubonic plague, the white blood cells called macrophages likely performed their duty—gobbling up the bacterium called *Yersinia pestis.* Once inside the macrophage, *Yersinia pestis* hijacked the cells' iron reserves and replicated out of control. As the cells were transported to the lymph nodes, the bacteria continued to reproduce, causing swelling of the nodes—the so-called "bubos," from which the bubonic plague derived its name. Once in the lymph nodes, the infection could be distributed almost unimpeded throughout the body.

In Chapter 5, we explored the role of iron in fueling infections. Bacteria need iron and they multiply aggressively in the presence of iron. Also recall that humans have evolved clever strategies to withhold iron from microbes in time of infection. It is one of our crucial defenses. In the two studies cited in Chapter 5, it was clear that iron excess led to an increase in infection incidence and severity.

But, if iron fuels infection, how could hemochromatosis, an iron storage disease, render *protection* against the bubonic plague? First, the normal intestine absorbs one or two milligrams of iron a day from the food we eat. People with hemochromatosis can absorb three or four milligrams a day. That excess iron has to go somewhere, so the body stashes it away in the liver, the joints, the heart, the pancreas, the pituitary gland, the skin, and the bone marrow.

While people with hemochromatosis store iron excessively, one place they do not is in the macrophage (our bug-gobbling white cell). When macrophages of people with the warrior genes encounter a bacterium, there is little iron inside with which to reproduce. With little available iron, the bacteria die out.

Recent studies have perhaps shown why. In one study, the macrophages of people with hemochromatosis were compared to those without hemochromatosis in their ability to kill bacteria in a culture dish. The bacterium used was not the one that causes plague, but another one that replicates inside macrophages, *Mycobacterium tuberculosis* (the cause of tuberculosis). According to scientists at Ohio State University, *M. tuberculosis* in the macrophage of individuals with hereditary hemochromatosis "exhibit a profound defect in their ability to acquire iron. There is also a corresponding decrease in *M. tuberculosis* growth."[257] This has caused doctors like Moalem to suspect that those with hemochromatosis are protected against infection from certain kinds of intracellular bacteria.

While this unusual capacity to withhold iron from *Yersinia pestis* might have protected those exposed to the bubonic plague, it appears now that other iron-loving bacteria pose a special threat to those with hemochromatosis and the so-called warrior genes.

Hemochromatosis and Increased Infection Susceptibility

In the *International Journal of Infectious Diseases,* Dr. Fida Kahn and Melanie Fisher wrote a paper entitled *Association of Hemochromatosis with Infectious Diseases.* In their paper they write, "In the presence of excessive iron, pathogens [harmful bacteria] can much more readily procure iron from molecules of transferrin. In such cases, even microbial strains that are not ordinarily virulent can cause illness. In addition, iron overload compromises the ability of phagocytic cells [white blood cells]. Excess iron decreases chemotactic* response [movement to the infection] and enhances the ability of ingested microorganisms to proliferate within the polymorphonuclear leukocytes (PMN) by lowering bactericidal [bacteria-killing] capacity."[258]

They go on to state one plausible reason for the devastating effect of excess iron on immune cells. They note that "The toxicity of iron for neutrophils [white blood cells] may be due to the formation of excess oxygen radicals, which alter phagocytosis through peroxidation of neutrophil membrane lipids." In other words, iron fuels free radical injury in white blood cells, damaging the cell membranes and diminishing their function.

These scientists make an important summary remark about excess iron in hemochromatosis. They state, "This excess iron burden does not only help the propagation of pathogens, but also plays a sentinel role in modifying the host immune mechanism, specifically by impairment of cell-mediated immune responses."

---

*Chemotaxis refers to the capacity of a white blood cell to migrate or move to a site of infection, injury, or other need.

Iron-Loving Bacteria

There is a long list of bacteria that thrive on iron. This has implications for the person with hemochromatosis and, perhaps more so, for someone who has the genetic mutation but is unaware of it. A person who does not know he has the mutation might suffer from frequent illness or chronic infections without understanding that he might have this fundamental genetic vulnerability. It should also be emphasized that iron stores rise with increasing age and that, over time, the body burden of iron can be significant. This means that susceptibility to infection by this formidable list of bacteria can grow with age, and with the accumulation of more and more iron. In addition, the presence of so much excess iron can even render microbes that are only a minor threat to most people a serious threat to those with hemochromatosis. See Appendix E for infections made worse by iron.

The Alarm System: HLA Genes and Immunity

The hemochromatosis genes are part of an elaborate "alarm system" that accounts for about 50 percent of the impact of genes on immunity. This is called the human leukocytic antigen (HLA) system, which is located on chromosome 6. HLA proteins are created within our cells and then presented on the surface of our cells. Each of us has over 40 genes that code for HLA molecules.

These HLA molecules act as binding sites for foreign proteins that might come from viruses or bacteria. The major function of the HLA system is to alert the T-cell population of the immune system to the presence of a microbe. It is a bit like flipping up the red flag on your mailbox, alerting the postman that there are letters to be picked up. In the case of the HLA system, it hangs a sign out on the cell that says "foreign invader on board." The T-cells, like our mailman, come by to "open the mailbox" and check what's in there. If the T-cell recognizes the protein bound to the HLA molecule as foreign, it activates an immune response. A single one of our cells might contain hundreds of thousands of these HLA-foreign protein complexes. Our T-lymphocytes, which continually circulate through the body, survey our cellular landscape for the presence of these HLA-foreign protein complexes.

The HLA molecular system is divided into two classes, designated I and II. These are recognized by different subtypes of T-cells. The CD8 molecule on the CD8+ T-cell interacts with the class I HLA molecules. The CD4 molecule on the CD4+ T-cell interacts with the class II HLA molecules. Each T-cell is endowed with a structure called a TCR, or T-cell receptor. This allows the T-cell to recognize the foreign protein linked to the HLA molecule on the cell membrane.

HLA genes have the most variation of any genes in humans. These variations are called polymorphisms (single nucleotide polymorphism, or SNPs). This seems to be our adaptation over many, many generations to the vast numbers of infectious agents our ancestors have encountered over the millennia. This wide variation is probably what allows us to be protected against so many and varied forms of infectious bugs.

While the HLA system strengthens our defense against infection, it also increases our risk to autoimmune diseases—when our immune system turns against us. A brief list of autoimmune diseases linked to the HLA system is noted below:

Table 7.1. Diseases Associated with the HLA System[259]

Disease	HLA Antigen
Narcolepsy	HLA-DR2
Ankylosing spondylitis	HLA-B27
Reiter's disease	HLA-B27
Rheumatoid arthritis	HLA-DR4
Hemochromatosis	HLA-A3
Psoriasis	HLA-Cw6
Celiac disease	HLA-DR3
Multiple sclerosis	HLA-DR2

Genes, Mitochondria, and Energy

In Chapter 3, we explored the mitochondrion, the bacteria-like force that drives the energy system within our cells. For decades, scientists have been busy probing the genome and the metabolism of mitochondria to better understand how defects in these tiny organelles contribute to disease. While this subject is well beyond the scope of this book, it is interesting to learn that a mutation in the mitochondrial genome (remember, mitochondria have 37 genes of their own) may actually protect people in times of sepsis, or infection of the blood.

In one study, 150 people with severe sepsis (blood infection) were sent to intensive care for their treatment, wherein they were tested for what is called a **haplogroup**, which is a small set of variations in the mitochondrial DNA that they inherit together. Haplogroup H is the most common type in Europe. It was determined that those with haplogroup H were more than twice as likely to survive their infection as those with other haplotypes. Haplotype H patients were also more likely to experience a higher fever, which we showed in Chapter 4, could be associated with a more robust immune response.[260]

If these findings are confirmed with further research, it may yield a genetic test that allows us to understand which people are most at risk to severe infections or most at risk to severe consequences from particular infections.

Can We Learn Something from Twins?

Scientists discovered decades ago that if you want to tease out aspects of the nature versus nurture argument, find a large group of twins. Though not infallible, this is a powerful way to estimate the strength of environmental influences on whatever feature one is trying to observe. Scientists often compare monozygotic and dizygotic twins. Monozygotic twins derive from the same egg and share 100 percent of their genes. This is why they appear identical. Dizygotic twins derive from two separate eggs and share an average of 50 percent of their genes, which is similar to other siblings. If the results from monozygotic twins and dizygotic twins are similar, environmental influence is strong. If the results from monozygotic twins and dizygotic twins are significantly different, genetics are expected to exert a strong influence.

Not surprisingly, studies of twins have shown a strong genetic effect on susceptibility to infection. In England, doctors recruited 103 monozygotic twins and 186 dizygotic twins to study the effect of genetics on the white blood cell called the T-lymphocyte. Using a "heritability estimate" of the relative contribution of genetics, scientists learned that the ratio of certain T-lymphocytes had a genetic contribution of 65 percent. The contribution of genetics to the absolute T-lymphocyte count was 50 percent.[261]

Doctors have used studies like this to better understand the trends in susceptibility to specific infections. For instance, doctors at the University of Pittsburgh showed that middle ear problems in young children have a strong genetic component, perhaps as high as 74 percent. Other genetic factors could play a role as well. For instance, differences in the HLA system (described below) might account for the susceptibility of some children to infection.[262] Another twin study of middle ear infection showed a high rate of genetic influence, with only about 20 percent ascribed to environmental effects.[263] This was similar to a group of children studied in Norway, where genetic effects explained 62 percent of the variation in recurrent tonsillitis.[264]

It is now becoming clear that our genes have a tremendous effect on our immune defense and repair system—in short, our resistance to and recovery from infection. But the old notion of genes as destiny has given way to a view of genes as powerful architects that are under the influence of a wide array of forces, some of which are under out direct control. As some scientists are fond of saying, "genes load the gun, but environment pulls the trigger."

It is this ability to shape the expression of our genome by our behavior that opens some exciting horizons. If we understand our susceptibility based on our genetic profile and we understand the various forces that may limit or enhance those genetic effects, we suddenly have tools at our disposal that can be used to raise our defenses in our favor.

In order to see where we might have latitude to intervene and mold the influence of our genes on our immunity, we must consider just a sampling of how genes actually do affect immunity.

Inheriting the Stress Response

We have, so far, briefly explored selected ways in which our genetics affects our ability to "cope" with bacteria in our surroundings. It is a kind of stress management at the cellular level. Chapters 10 and 11 will explore the role of psychological stress in immunity and whether our mind influences our defenses against bacterial infection. Since we are on the topic of genes, however, it is worthwhile exploring how genes and heredity might influence our ability to cope with the varied psychological stressors encountered in our lives (since, as we will learn, coping has everything to do with how we respond to the world around us).

Many scientists subscribe to something called *set point* theory. This is based on the notion that our nervous system has a set point around which the ordinary activities fluctuate, akin to the way in which the "set point" of body temperature is kept around 98.6°F. If temperature rises, the body eventually returns to the set point of 98.6°F. If temperature falls, the body eventually returns to the same 98.6°F (or approximately so). The body has many such set points and the variation between individuals is often much greater than the variation in the temperature set point (which is small).

We can return to our twin studies to learn a little about set points and the extent to which these may be influenced by our genes. For example, an ongoing study at the University of Minnesota has been following some 1,491 pairs of twins reared apart in order to learn something about the possible genetic influence on happiness.[265] Based on the Well-Being Scale of the Multidimensional Personality Inventory, about 45 percent of the individual differences in the Well-Being Scale can be attributed to genetic differences in set points. This was determined based on the finding that identical twins, whether reared together or apart, had remarkably similar scores.*

The ten-year follow-up results are even more compelling. Retesting these same people after ten years would allow scientists to determine how stable this set point might be and how much of, in this case, happiness is attributable to genetic influence. In the case of the University of Minnesota twins study, roughly 80 percent of the stability in well-being was attributable to the genetic set point (the remainder would presumably be due to diet, nutrition, stressors, and other influences).

These findings would suggest that, regardless of the negative life events that one might encounter over the course of some years, the individual would generally return to a similar state of happiness. Keep this in mind as we later investigate the role of stress and coping in relation to immune defenses.

The findings on the set point in relation to happiness in twins brings us to another relevant question. Is there a set point, or genetic basis, for depression? As we'll see, depression has a notable effect on one's immune defenses. To answer this question, we can first look to the fascinating work with female twins done by Dr. Kenneth Kendler.[266] He found that 444 identical twin pairs were more alike than 296 fraternal twin pairs—strong indication of a genetic link. Further statistical analysis demonstrated an estimated heritability of depression of about 70 percent. The conclusion, depression is a highly heritable disorder.

---

*While twin studies have been put forth as strong evidence of heritability of psychological traits, various opinions exist in this field. A critical review of this field can be found in *The Gene Illusion* by Jay Joseph.

Another study of female twins looked to examine the effect of genetic predisposition on coping in stressful life events. In this case, the stressors were serious life events like assault, serious illness, divorce, death of a close relative, job loss, or serious illness of a close relative. The odds of depression after a serious life event were 60 percent higher than if no life event had occurred. These scientists concluded that life events were more likely to lead to depression in those women who were genetically predisposed to depression by their genetic heritage.[267] The response to life events that are controllable versus those that are uncontrollable also seems to have a strong heritability factor, especially in response to *controllable* life events.[268]

Moody Genes

So, what are these genes that seem to bend our moods and shape our response to stress? Recent brain imaging studies and genetic analyses have allowed us to peer a little more deeply into this mysterious black box. While the story of these "moody genes" has not been fully written, there is clear evidence that these genes can shape who we are, the response to our environment, and through this, our immune response. For example, the enzyme tryptophan hydroxylase (TPH) helps us form the neurotransmitter serotonin, which has powerful effects on our mood and ability to cope. Variants of the TPH gene strongly influence the development of mood disorders. [269]

Another gene affects our ability to transport serotonin in the brain. The gene codes for a molecule called SERT (serotonin transporter) and there are two main versions. SERT affects how long serotonin hangs around in the synapse. When serotonin lingers too long in between neurons, the symptoms include anxiety, impulsivity, negative thoughts, and even suicidal tendencies. Fearfulness and depression are common in this profile. For those unfortunate enough to inherit a copy of this variant of the gene from each parent, the effects are felt most strongly.[270]

Drugs like Prozac, Zoloft, and others are commonly used to influence the serotonin pathway. Amino acids like tryptophan are used for the same reason.

To keep our neurostransmitter system in balance, we are constantly making and breaking down neurotransmitter substances. Monoamine oxidase (MAO) is an enzyme that helps us break down neurotransmitters such as dopamine and serotonin. Many antidepressant drugs are MAO inhibitors, including Selegiline, Marplan, and Nardil. These drugs are used in some people to help them keep more of the neurotransmitter around longer, so that the benefits of the neurotransmitter can be experienced. Studies have linked the MAO-A gene to a range of difficult psychological profiles. For example, those with low-efficiency MAO-A alleles tend to be more prone to poor impulse control and overreaction to stressful stimuli. Those with low-efficiency MAO-A alleles have been shown to have smaller limbic organs, such as the amygdala and cingulate gyrus, both involved in mood regulation. In fact, the smaller amygdala is partly responsible for the hyper-reactivity in stressful situations.[271]

Another gene that affects our mood and ability to cope is one that codes for the enzyme COMT (short for catechol-O-methyltransferase). COMT helps us break down dopamine and other neurotransmitters, and has an influence on our general intelligence. In the field of psychiatry, people who have variants of the COMT gene are sometimes appropriately dubbed "warrior" or "worrier."[272] (Though this is not related to the "warrior" gene described earlier in this chapter.) The presence of one gene variant is more commonly seen in people with anxiety disorders and obsessive compulsive disorder. Those with certain COMT gene variants do not experience the benefit of soothing opiate-like molecules produced by the brain, which are associated with calming.[273]

Brain-derived neurotrophic factor (BDNF) is a protein that helps survival of neurons and the growth of new synapses. People with one variant of this gene tend to have exceptional memory. The down side is they are prone anxiety, negative moods, and hostility, all of which influence the ability to handle stress.[274] These states are also known the directly affect immunity in negative ways.

Why mention these specific genes, since they are not classic "immune system" genes? As I mentioned briefly and we will explore in later chapters, stress and life events have a tremendous effect on our immune response. Mood disorders like depression have direct effects on immunity. One key feature that protects our immune system from the ravages of stress appears to be our ability to cope. Since our ability to cope is strongly influenced by genes that direct activity in the brain, no discussion of genes and immunity would be complete without also addressing the very powerful influence of genes, the mind, mood, and coping.

But there's more. Outside what we call the genome lies a mysterious domain called the epigenome. Scientists working in this field have not been invited to all the same parties as those working on the human genome project, but it may not be long, for the epigenome shapes our lives in unexpected and dramatic ways.

At the Edges of Our Genes

Just when the Human Genome Project was giving promise to the notion that we would unravel the cause of many diseases, along came **epigenetics**. The epigenome, as it is called, is the component of the genome that takes place "outside of" or "beyond" the basic structure of the gene. The most simple components of the epigenome consists of tiny **methyl** tags and **acetyl** groups that are attached to specific points of the gene. Methyl groups are the tiniest of molecular fragments, consisting of only a single carbon, but their effects are dramatic. These methyl tags can switch the gene on or off depending upon what portion of the gene they are attached to. Likewise with acetyl groups, which are simple two-carbon fragments. Each is a little like putting a padlock on your locker at the gym.

The classic example of the epigenome at work is in cancer. If damaged DNA is allowed to run amok, the result can be the development of abnormal, cancerous cells. Fortunately there are specific genes present in our bodies to repair damaged DNA. However, if the promoter genes for the DNA repair enzymes are excessively methylated, the DNA repair enzymes can be silenced. In other words, you could have just what you need inside the locker, but the padlock is on the door and you can't get anything out. In this case, you can't get at the DNA repair enzymes. Our padlock is like the little methyl tag that hangs on the gene. We have genes that do all sorts of things, but the little methyl groups of the epigenome decide what really gets done.

So, what affects the way in which our genome is methylated (the epigenome)? One important link can be found in diet and nutrition.

The Epigenome and Nutrition

The most fascinating example of how nutrition affects the expression of our genes through the epigenome came with the study of a tiny fellow called the agouti mouse. This little creature, it was discovered over a century ago, contains a gene that produces dramatically different mice depending upon whether the gene is "on" or "off." When switched on, the agouti gene is associated with yellow fur, obesity, diabetes, and cancer. When switched off, the mice become lean, healthy, live long lives, and have a healthy brown coat. In fact, the yellow agouti mice suffer twice the mortality rate as their counterparts with the switched-off gene.

So, what causes the gene to be switched on or off? It is now clear that providing dietary choline switches off the agouti gene. This occurs because the methyl groups found in choline bind to the C-residues (C for cytosine) on strands of the agouti gene and silence the gene. They, in essence, padlock the agouti gene and keep the promoter from getting out of the locker and causing disease (and the yellow fur). In the absence of adequate choline in the diet, the agouti gene is expressed, producing the typical yellow, sickly mice that have become the poster mice for epigenetics.

It is a remarkable thing to see. Withhold dietary choline from these little mice and they turn yellow, grow obese, develop severe disease, and die prematurely. When you enrich their diets in choline, their coat color changes to brown, they become lean, healthy, and live long lives. It was discovered in recent years that if you give choline to an obese agouti mouse mother, her offspring will be born with the genes methylated and they will grow up normal and healthy. This is the power of the epigenome.

Further expanding on nutrients and the epigenome, Dr. Lawrence Harper, a psychologist at the University of California at Davis, suggests that a wide array of personality traits, including temperament and intelligence, may be affected by epigenetic inheritance. He states, "If you have a generation of poor people who suffer from bad nutrition, it may take two or three generations for that population to recover from that hardship and reach its full potential," Harper says. "Because of epigenetic inheritance, it may take several generations to turn around the impact of poverty or war or dislocation on a population."[275]

The Epigenome and Good Parenting

Nutrition is not all that affects the epigenome. The study of twins showed us the astonishing impact of genetics (nature) on our appearance, behavior, and susceptibility to disease. But as the twin research has continued for many decades, the picture is even more fascinating.

In a novel twist, identical twins, with their dramatic similarities, become more different as they age. Some of this divergence has been attributed to epigenetic variations—the effect of nurture or their surroundings. More precisely, younger twins are more alike than older twins and a differing environment (diet, lifestyle, climate, habits, etc.) causes older twins to become more different as they age. This is more pronounced if the twins live in different areas and have different social habits. These different environmental conditions can also cause one twin to have different disease susceptibility compared to the other twin. It is believed that epigenetic effects are, at least in part, at the root of these differences.[276]

The notion that our genetic traits can be influenced after the early imprinting periods of fetal development has given rise to some very exciting prospects. That is, the once cherished notion of DNA as destiny has given way to a view that our postgestational experience can alter the gene expression profile, such that the determinants of our genes is *not* our destiny.

Some of the most interesting work in this area comes from the laboratories of Drs. Michael Meaney and Moshe Szyf at McGill University in Montreal. Meaney has been studying two types of mother rats: those that calmly lick their offspring after birth and those that neglect their newborn pups. He discovered that the rats that were neglected by their mothers grew into adults rats of the sort that scurry about nervously and appear threatened by new environments. In contrast, the pups that were licked by their mothers seemed calm and at ease, by rat standards, at least.

When Meaney's group examined the brain of these rats, the nurtured (licked) rats had better developed hippocampi and lower amounts of the stress hormone cortisol. The hippocampus is a region of the brain associated with memory formation and mood. The licked rats also had a significantly different DNA methylation pattern than the neglected rats.[277] In effect, the nurturing appeared to alter the "switches" that direct the formation of receptors for stress hormones in the rat's brain.

To rule out some unknown genetic effects present between the types of rats, Meaney's group conducted another experiment where the pups were switched at birth. The mother rat who nurtured by licking (we'll call her the "nurturing" mother), was given the pups of the mother who neglected her offspring. The mother rat who neglected her offspring was given the pups of the nurturing mother. This swapping of the offspring was expected to rule out other genetic differences. The result: when the brains of the offspring were examined, the same findings held true. Mothers that nurtured the pups of the "non-nurturing" rats produced pups that were calm, like her own. Non-nurturing mothers that reared the pups of the "nurturing" mother produced pups that were fearful and anxious. Remarkably, nurturing and neglect produced two very different methylation profiles in the genes of the hippocampus, this critical brain region associated with memory and mood.

This work seems to show signs of validation in humans. Meaney has recently examined the brains of adults (using MRI) who were premature babies. Individuals who reported a poor relationship with their mother had hippocampi (on MRI imaging) to be significantly smaller than those reporting a good relationship with their mother. This is not confirmation of the rat study, but it further opens the door into better understanding the way our choices may influence the genome by way of the epigenome.[278]

These findings of the influence of nurturing on the genome are exciting, disturbing, or both, depending upon your perspective. They imply that a lack of early nurturing on the epigenome is almost frightening in its implications. Other studies in this area, however, are showing that modification in adulthood may be possible by providing agents such as the amino acid methionine or certain medications.[279]

The Gene Dimmer Switch

This chapter has briefly touched on the issue of genes that influence immunity, a complex and fascinating field of study. As scientists learn more about the genotypes of susceptibility, our ability to personalize treatment will continue to improve.

But another area of how genes may influence our immune defenses centers on **gene expression**. Simply possessing this or that gene does not write our fate in stone. Genes are continually switched on and switched off, switched up or switched down. They are under the control of complex systems, but they are remarkably responsive to our everyday life. The epigenome is certainly one factor that affects the switching on and off of genes, but there are also factors that can lower or increase the activity of genes—in essence, switching them "up" or "down."

As an example, scientists wanted to see how exercise affected activity of a gene in muscles called lipoprotein lipase. To measure this, they had subjects perform sixty to ninety minutes of exhaustive one-legged knee extensor exercise for five consecutive days, while leaving the other leg dormant. Doctors then biopsied the muscles of each leg to look at the level of expression for the gene coding for lipoprotein lipase (and other genes). There was a significant difference in gene expression between the two legs. In short, exercise up-regulated, or switched higher, the gene coding for this important protein. Another study showed that a single four-hour bout of cycling exercise elicited triggered a five- to more than twentyfold increase in three genes related to metabolism (UCP3, PDK4, and HO-1).[280]

Many such studies have led to the understanding the every thing we do is a potential act of gene regulation. What we eat, the supplements we take, our physical activity, our moods, our lifestyle, and our choices in general, all dictate how our genes are expressed.

It is a fascinating notion that we are driving the expression of our DNA blueprint with the simple choices we make every day. Does eating potato chips switch on the fat, carbohydrate, and insulin genes? Does sitting on the couch switch off our metabolism genes? Does falling in love switch on our neuronal genes? Below is a sampling of our lifestyle choices and their effect on the "switching" of genes.

Effect of Exercise on Gene Expression Related to Immunity

According to scientists at the University of Toronto,

> Every time a bout of exercise is performed, a change in gene expression occurs within the contracting muscle. Over the course of many repeated bouts of exercise (i.e. training), the cumulative effects of these alterations lead to a change in muscle phenotype. One of the most prominent of these adaptations is an increase in mitochondrial content, which confers a greater resistance to muscle fatigue.

With specific reference to the immune system, these selected studies illustrate some effects of exercise on gene expression:

- White blood cells express thousands of genes. After an exhaustive treadmill test (80 percent of maximal oxygen uptake VO2max), 450 genes were up-regulated and 150 genes were down-regulated. The degree of up- or down-regulation was dependent upon how hard the exerciser worked.[281]
- Following two hours of intensive cycling, gene expression for the immune proteins (cytokines) IL-8, IL-10, and IL-1Ra (IL-1 receptor antagonist), is increased in blood leukocytes.[282]
- Cyclists submitted blood samples after two competition stages of 165 km. Gene expression in neutrophils for the antioxidant enzymes catalase, glutathione peroxidase, and superoxide dismutase was increased after exercise.[283]

The literature is full of studies showing how selected choices affect the **expression** of genes that influence our immune response.[284]

Effect of Nutrition on Gene Expression Related to Immunity

Vitamins, minerals, amino acids, fatty acids, carbohydrates, and accessory food factors are well known for their influence on gene expression. In fact, modulation of gene expression is among the primary means by which nutrients exert their effects on us. This is a vast, complex subject, but some brief examples are noted below as they relate to immunity.

- Vitamin D activates the genes for the production of natural antibacterial peptides (called cathelicidin) by skin cells and monocytes (white blood cells).[285]
- Butyric acid (a short-chain fatty acid found as a supplement and produced by gut bacteria) activates the genes that stimulate cells lining the digestive tract to produce natural antibacterial proteins called defensins.[286]
- Vitamin E activates genes associated with the Th1 / Th2 balance in old T-cells (T-lymphocytes).[287]
- Supplementation with EPA-rich fish oil modified over 80 genes in white blood cells of male volunteers over a two month period.[288]
- The flavonoid quercitin, found in onions, apples, tea, and other foods, modified the inflammatory gene expression of peripheral blood monocytes (white blood cells).[289]
- The flavonoid quercitin significantly improved the immune proteins (cytokines) related to the Th-1 and Th-2 balance.[290]
- Zinc deficiency altered the gene expression profile of white blood cells, shifting it in the direction of the pro-inflammatory Th2 profile.[291]

Effect of Stress on Gene Expression Related to Immunity

In later chapters, we'll explore the topic of mood, mind, and infections. But while we're on the topic of genes and immunity, it bears looking at how psychosocial stress acts upon our genes to influence white blood cell behavior. Scientists writing in the *Proceedings of the National Academy of Sciences* summarized their findings on how stress affected peripheral blood monoctyes (PBMCs). PBMCs are vital cells that can transform themselves into macrophages, the workhorse sentinels with a penchant for gobbling up bacteria, viruses, and all manner of cellular debris, alive or dead.

Using human subjects exposed to a brief laboratory stress, 17 of 19 test subjects experienced a rapid activation of the gene transcription factor called NFÎB (nuclear factor kappa B). It was evident from related studies in animals that the stress chemical norepinephrine was a triggering agent for this gene activation. These studies would seem to reveal at least one mechanism by which psychosocial stress alters the expression of genes related to immune function.[292]

Loneliness and Gene Expression Related to Immunity

Doctors have known for centuries that those who are lonely and isolated suffer more disease. Today, physicians observe a trend of increased infections, cardiovascular disease, and higher death rates from various conditions. It seemed reasonable that the immune system was involved, but in what way? For too long, no one seemed to have a clear explanation of how this occurred.

Enter Dr. Steve Cole and his team at UCLA, who studied gene expression in a group of people described as either "high-lonely" or "low-lonely." Using a now-standard tool in genome studies called DNA microarray analysis, Cole's group looked at more than twenty thousand genes to see whether there were differences between the high- and low-loneliness groups.[293]

He found that gene expression was different in 209 sites on the genome of lonely people compared with those not classified as lonely. A large portion of these sites were associated with immune cell and immune protein regulation. Genes associated with a pro-inflammatory state tended to be up-regulated (as though the dimmer switch was left on high), while the anti-inflammatory elements were down-regulated (as though the dimmer switch was turned too low). Some of the gene response elements were centered on appropriate cortisol response. As we've shown, cortisol is an important regulator of immune function.

From this study, it appears that one way in which loneliness may foster increased susceptibility to infections (and all kinds of adverse disease outcomes) is by shifting gene expression toward a profile that favors inflammation at the expense of defense against infectious disease. This is somewhat like the phenomenon of shifting the Th1/Th2 balance toward the more inflammatory state (Th2 dominance).

This is a remarkable breakthrough in our thinking about how a personal and social condition such as loneliness affects us at the genome level. Among the deepest of our human needs is the need for connection with others. In our advancing view of disease prevention and patient care, we must give apt attention to this need for connection.

It has always seemed obvious that the celebration of life that derives from community with others feeds the process of healing and recovery. This "new" biological imperative, that loneliness may foster a shift in our defenses at the gene level or that lack of connection with others shapes the dance of our immunity via the genome, must surely cause us to look to one another in times of need. This conjures images of close-knit societies, where one merely sits at the bedside of another. There is no need for action of any particular sort. It is simply our presence that is needed. It also leads one to the conclusion that having more friends is a pretty good idea.

It is a humbling prospect—that a community might alter the genome of an individual.

How We Control the Fat-Burner Genes

Another way that we control our gene expression is through what we eat. For instance, whenever we make a choice about the fat we consume (and actually consume that fat) we are driving the expression of genes with a widespread impact on metabolism. It is safe to say that if we do not gain control over the type of fat we consume, we lose control over our genes—and thus, our defense, energy, and repair system. In Chapter 8, we'll explore the question of whether being overweight can suppress immunity, activate unfavorable components of the immune system, and increase susceptibility to infection. Not only do fatty acids regulate our immune, inflammatory, and repair system, they greatly influence whether we will store fat in our bellies or burn fat and remain lean.

For example, omega-3 fatty acids up-regulate gene transcription for proteins involved in helping us burn fatty acids as fuel, such as carnitine palmitoyltransferase and acyl-CoA oxidase. At the same time, omega-3 fatty acids down-regulate (dial down) the transcription of genes that code for proteins involved in the manufacture of fat such as fatty acid synthase.[294] In this regard, n-3 fatty acids are being referred to as "fuel partitioners," because of the ways in which they do the following:

- N-3 fatty acids direct fat *away* from triglyceride storage.
- N-3 fatty acids direct fat *toward* fat burning.
- N-3 fatty acids enhance glucose conversion to the storage form called glycogen.
- N-3 fatty acids control the fat-burning capacity by activating the transcription factor PPARα (peroxisome proliferator-activated receptor alpha).[295]

Unsaturated fatty acids control an array of **lipogenic** (fat-making) genes. This means that the right forms of fatty acids can actually limit the amount of fat the body makes for storage. Unsaturated fatty acids also control an array of **lipolytic** (fat-burning) genes. This means that the right forms of fatty acids, such as omega-3 fatty acids can actually accelerate fat *burning.**

So fatty acids increase thermogenesis, decrease body fat deposition, and improve glucose tolerance, which they accomplish, in part, by:

---

*Fat-making (lipogenic) genes controlled by fatty acids include: Hepatic glucokinase, Pyruvate kinase, Pyruvate dehydrogenase, Fatty acid synthase, Adipocyte fatty acid synthase. Fat-burning (lipolytic) genes controlled by fatty acids include: Carnitine palmitoyltransferse, Mitochondrial HMG-CoA synthase, Peroxisomal acyl-CoA oxidase, Fatty acid binding proteins, Fatty acid transporter, UCP-3 (mitochondrial uncoupling protein-3).

- Indirectly reducing aromatase production
- Improving insulin sensitivity
- Upregulating genes that code for proteins that enhance fat burning
- Downregulating genes that code for proteins involved in fat synthesis

Another way that fatty acids can influence fat burning is by indirectly dialing down the aromatase enzyme. Aromatase is the enzyme that helps convert testosterone to estrogen in both men and women. Increased aromatase activity means more testosterone is converted to estradiol (a form of estrogen). This also means that testosterone levels can be lowered. As testosterone levels fall, fat-burning ability falls as well. In fact, as aromatase levels increase, fat cells tend to become more efficient at accumulating fat, which leads to more aromatase.

How Certain Genes May Raise Nutrient Requirements

Bruce Ames, a professor at the Department of Molecular and Cellular Biology at the University of California at Berkeley, is considered one of the most respected scientists in all fields for his work in molecular medicine. Doctor Ames has recognized that there are a large number of genetic mutations that cause certain coenzymes in the body to lose their affinity for their cofactors (which are often vitamins). This renders these cofactors unable to do their jobs of driving metabolism.

For example, one of the most common gene mutations in Caucasians of European descent (occurring in some form in up to 20 percent of the population) is in the enzyme called MTHFR (methylene tetrahydrofolate reductase). This enzyme is critical to what is called the methylation cycle, which transfers carbon fragments from vitamin B12 and folic acid to molecules throughout the body.

■ Table 7.2. A Partial List of Genetic Mutations of Enzymes for Which Nutrient Requirements May Be Increased.

Enzyme	Cofactor	Associated Vitamin Needed in Higher Amounts
MTHFR (methylene tetrahydrofolate reductase)	FAD	Riboflavin (B2)
NADP quinine oxidoreductase	FAD	Riboflavin (B2)
Short-chain acyl-CoA dehydrogenase	FAD	Riboflavin (B2)
Aldehyde dehydrogenase	NAD	Niacin (B3)
Glucose-6-phosphate dehydrogenase	NADP	Nicacin (B3)
Methionine synthase	Ado Cobalamin	Cobalamin (B12)
Folylpolyglutamate carboxypeptidase	Folylpolyglutamates	Folic acid

You may have heard of the more well-known harmful product of this called homocysteine, which is raised when vitamin B12, vitamin B6, and folic acid are low. The MTHFR enzyme is dependent upon a coenzyme hooking up with it. The coenzyme (FAD) formed from vitamin B2, or riboflavin. In people with the MTHFR gene mutation, the "stickiness" of the MTHFR enzyme for riboflavin is reduced by some ten times. It turns out that supplying excessive amounts of riboflavin improves the efficiency of this enzyme and limits the adverse impact in those who carry this common genotype. In short, high-dose vitamins reduce the negative effects of a gene on metabolism.

Citing numerous examples like this, Dr. Ames has taken the general position that very high doses of vitamins that are specific to certain cofactors can be used to *saturate* the coenzyme, which may then influence the enzyme to work more efficiently. Ames argues that this use of high-dose vitamins can reduce the effects of selected genetic defects on health. Put a different way, certain genetic mutations can alter our metabolism merely because our need for certain nutrients is higher than would be obtained by an ordinary diet. In other words, higher levels of nutrients will benefit individuals with certain genotypes. It may even be critical for the health of these people that they receive higher levels of nutrients than normal.

Dr. Ames writes *American Journal of Clinical Nutrition,* "About 50 human genetic diseases due to defective enzymes can be remedied or ameliorated by the administration of high doses of the vitamin component of the corresponding coenzyme, which at least partially restores enzymatic activity."[296] He notes that of the 3,870 enzymes catalogued in the ENZYME database, 860 (22 percent) use a cofactor. Many of these are vitamin-derived coenzymes, as summarized above.

Since the immune defense, energy, and repair system is dependent upon the interaction between genes and nutrients, the importance of what Dr. Ames is saying should not be taken lightly. This is one strong argument in favor of personalized medicine based on laboratory assessment, with the intent to tailor a nutritional strategy to the genotype of the individual.

Shaping our Defense, Energy, and Repair

While we have barely scratched the surface of how our genes influence our susceptibility to infection, it is certain that genes rest at the foundation and hold vast influence over our immunity and capability for repair. It is also true that our genes are not our destiny.

From the very brief discussion on gene expression above, we can only conclude that we are the products of our genes. Yet we are daily shaping our future by our choices via changing the expression of those genes. When we choose chocolate over broccoli, we alter our gene expression. When we choose to watch the movie *Saw* over *The Pink Panther* we are likely changing our gene expression (though I'm not aware that this has been tested). Drinking alcohol, smoking cigarettes, taking drugs, and the varied activities in which people engage, drives the expression of their genes. It must be so.

Our genes form an elaborate system that has helped organize us into our present complexity. They exist in each of us as adaptations by our ancestors. Adaptation to food shortage, cold climates, hot climates, minimal sunlight, abundant sunlight, plague, warfare, and all measure of conditions have forged the genome of each of us. Those who lived with malaria developed a gene adaptation that was protective against infection by the microbe. However, the sickle cell trait that arose does not serve people well who do not live with the threat of malaria today.

What saved us yesterday may kill us tomorrow. What made our grandfather's life survivable under hostile conditions may make ours difficult today. Such is the world of the genome. Such is the marvel of our adaptive capacity. We are living in a world of constantly shifting gene expression, where we modify our gene expression every time we take a vitamin, work out at the club, or drink a glass of wine.

This is, quite obviously, good news and bad news. The good news is that we appear to have a large measure of control over our gene expression—perhaps too much in many cases. The bad news is, we don't yet entirely know all we must do to exert that control. But the day will come when we can answer these questions with greater confidence. Even today, we know how to influence our genes with exercise, nutrition, food, nurturing, community, sleep, medication, and a growing list of activities that can be quite pleasurable.

Chapter 8

How Lifestyle Shapes Our Defenses

Our immune system walks a daily tightrope of vigilance, where there can be no true rest, yet in order to maintain this constant vigil our bodies must be nurtured daily by adequate sleep and rest. Without sufficient rest, our repair systems simply cannot keep up with demands.

It is now evident that one of the most powerful architects of our immune defense, energy, and repair system is sleep. How sleep accomplishes this task of supporting immune vigilance has been a bit murky until recently. A scientific team at the University of Lübeck, led by Tanja Lang, MD, began their investigation into whether sleep might help regulate the Th1 / Th2 balance within the immune system. Recall from Chapter 4 that this balance is important in retaining an immune defense that is vigilant enough to defend against microbes, but not so vigilant that it attacks our own tissues and organs. It is also important because defense against certain microbes clearly require activity of both Th1 and Th2.

In their study, people were subjected to two test conditions. In one, they were permitted to sleep through the night from 11 p.m. to 7 a.m. with lights out. After four weeks had passed, they were subjected to another condition. In this case, they were resting in their beds, but awake from 11 p.m. to 7 a.m. During this time, they watched television, listened to music, and talked to the experimenter, all with normal room light. In each condition, their blood was tested for growth hormone, cortisol, norepinephrine (adrenaline), prolactin, and immune proteins.

Scientists were eager to see whether the sleep condition fostered an immune protein profile that favored the Th1 path. The study first confirmed what had been shown in many previous studies—that sleep supported the production of growth hormone and prolactin.

Next came their immune protein results. Dr. Lang's group stated that, "Nocturnal [nighttime] wakefulness suppressed IL-12^{+} monocyte [white cell] numbers on average to approximately 40 percent of sleep levels and enhanced IL-10^{+} monocyte levels to approximately 170 percent of sleep levels."[297] In other words, the sleep condition favored dominance of the Th1 immune activity, while nighttime wakefulness favored formation of the Th2-dominant condition. They went on to state that "On this clinical background, our data implicate a critical function of sleep for organizing a balanced oscillation in type 1 and type 2 cytokine activity and corroborate the view that sleep supports adaptive immunity."

■ Table 8.1. How Sleep Deprivation Affects Immunity: Th1 and Th2 Balance[298]

	Th1	Th2
Type of Immunity	Cell-mediated	Humoral§
Biochemical Changes	Prolactin ? Growth Hormone ? IL-12^{+} ?	Cortisol ? Norepinephrine ? IL-10^{+} ?
Type of Sleep	Nighttime sleep	Nighttime wakefulness

In the same volume of the *Archives of Internal Medicine,* scientists from ULCA reported on another study looking at gene expression profiles of people subjected to partial sleep deprivation from 11 p.m. to 3 a.m. Sleep deprivation resulted in a threefold elevation of IL-6 and a twofold elevation in TNFα (tumor necrosis factor alpha) messenger RNA. Both are associated with inflammation.

The investigators remarked that "Sleep loss induces a functional alteration of the monocyte pro-inflammatory cytokine response. A modest amount of sleep loss also alters molecular processes that drive cellular immune activation and induce inflammatory cytokines."[299] In short, they showed that moderate sleep deprivation appeared to prime the immune system toward an inflammatory state.

These important studies imply that sleep is necessary for retaining the balance between two key arms of the immune system. They also suggest that sleep deprivation seems to facilitate an inflammatory state. Perhaps one means by which sleep deprivation fuels inflammation is through its stunning effects on the gut.

Can Lack of Sleep Let Gut Bacteria Leak into the Body?

Throughout this book, we've explored the basic premise that integrity of the intestinal barrier protects us from threats posed by harmful components of the gut bacteria. We have also seen how there are many circumstances in which weakness in this gut barrier defense (leaky gut) permits bacterial cell wall fragments (endotoxins) to leak across the gut barrier, enter circulation, and trigger inflammatory immune activation, which can have broad effects on the human body. These effects range from a persistent inflammatory state, to mood disorders, and in people with severe illness, death.

With this understanding, we have to consider the findings in stressed mice. First, there is a fair amount of research showing that when animals are severely stressed, the barrier defenses in their intestinal tract (small intestine, cecum, colon) break down and gut bacteria and bacterial endotoxins can literally "leak" into the bloodstream.

Extending this thinking, scientists from the University of Tennessee College of Medicine wanted to understand to what extent sleep deprivation could trigger this sometimes-fatal migration of bacteria into the bloodstream.[300] In this provocative study, animals were subjected to sleep deprivation over a period of twenty days. Each animal was matched with a paired control that was not sleep deprived, which permitted a direct comparison. At five, ten, fifteen, and twenty days, the rats were tested for bacterial counts in their lymph nodes, bloodstream, and organs.

Ordinarily, when bacteria migrate from the intestine to the interior of the body, they pass first into the lymph nodes, which serve as a launch point for dissemination to the bloodstream and to organs such as liver, kidney, spleen, and lung. In order to count bacteria, scientists use the term **colony-forming units (cfu)**. A colony-forming unit is a measure of living cells, where a colony represents a group of bacterial cells that grow from a single parent cell. The higher the CFUs, the greater the bacterial invasion.

One of the first sites invading bacteria from the colon can be found is in the **mesenteric** lymph nodes—specifically, the lymph nodes associated with the abdominal organs. This, as expected, was the site where migrating bacteria were first detected. By day twenty, the inguinal lymph nodes (comparable to those in the groin in humans) of all the sleep-deprived animals contained from 330 to 40,700 CFUs per gram of tissue. This was compared to only 660 CFU in only one of the control animals.

The cecum is a pouch where the small intestine meets the large intestine. It normally contains an abundance of bacteria, though it contains fewer numbers than those found in the colon. When bacterial populations were cultured after twenty days of sleep deprivation, the gram-negative aerobic bacteria were **thirty-sevenfold higher** in the sleep-deprived rats than in the nonsleep-deprived control animals. The levels of the bacterium *E. coli* in the ileum (the end portion of the small intestine) increased twenty-onefold in sleep-deprived rats after twenty days, compared to controls.

Does Sleep Help Us Contain Our Gut Bacteria?

In the study above, sleep deprivation was associated with weakening of the gut barrier defenses, permitting the passage of whole bacteria into the lymphatic system and into the organs. A growing body of evidence supports this view. According to Dr. Carol Everson at the University of Wisconsin, "In our animal model, impairment of host defenses is chief among sleep deprivation outcomes, as evidenced by *strikingly poor control over indigenous microorganisms** despite an outwardly healthy appearance and robust appetite."[301] [emphasis added]

Citing her view that is based on a series of ongoing studies in rats, Dr. Everson notes that sleep deprivation may lead to a weakening of gut barrier and immune defenses, permitting endotoxins and whole bacteria to enter the body via the gut. This in turn may lead to an activation of one part of the immune system and weakening of another, including the release of inflammatory proteins and generation of a general proinflammatory state.

If these conclusions by Dr. Everson and colleagues hold true, it represents a remarkable advance in our understanding of factors that may strengthen or weaken our host defenses. It could represent a vastly underutilized tool in our effort to reduce antibiotic use and to stand strong in the world of the microbe.

To understand the implications, it is useful to think of the gut barrier as a dike that holds back the microbe-laden waters of the GI tract. Our system of defense is organized to keep these bacteria on other side of the dike. We do this by strong cell-to-cell junctions, a mucus layer, a water layer, immune cells, antibodies, and a range of other protections. Dr. Everson's studies suggest that sleep deprivation weakens the dike until it is breached, allowing contaminated waters to rush to the other side—to the interior of our body. Once the whole microbes or endotoxins

---

*Indigenous microbes refers to bacteria that reside on and in the body. In this case, it refers to microbes that reside within the gut. Please note that obesity has been included in the lifestyle chapter because obesity often emerges because of lifestyle (diet, physical activity, stress) and that obesity is responsive to lifestyle intervention. In placing obesity here, it does not diminish the influence of things like genetics, environmental factors, infection, and other elements that are less within our control.

break through the dike, however small the numbers, our systemic immune system must engage to protect us.

From Dr. Everson's work it appears that as sleep deprivation weakens the dike, microbes and microbial fragments seep into the body, pressing our immune system into action. In this scenario, prolonged sleep deprivation and the endotoxin load might be the source of ongoing stress that drives the immune system toward excessive activation on the one hand and weakened capability to respond to true infections on the other.

Collectively, these and other studies on sleep show that sleep is one of the most fundamentally essential components needed to maintain strong immune defenses, efficient energy production, and appropriate recovery and repair functions.

The Essentials of Exercise

Exercise is another of the very powerful tools we have to stimulate immune function and resist the microbes around us. An article published in the *International Journal of Sports Medicine* is one of many papers that illustrates the effect exercise can have on infections. In this study, only 45 minutes of brisk walking per day was shown to lower the incidence of upper respiratory symptoms, cut the duration of illness in half and increase natural killer-cell activity in people prone to upper respiratory tract infections.[302]

In one of the longest and most recent studies of its kind, doctors at the Fred Hutchinson Cancer Center in Seattle set out to assess whether modest exercise influenced immunity. A total of 115 overweight, postmenopausal Seattle-area women were enrolled. The women were randomly assigned to one of two groups. One group exercised 45 minutes a day, five days a week, for one year. The other group merely stretched 45 minutes a day, five days a week, for one year. Over the twelve-month study period, those in the stretcher group experienced twice as many

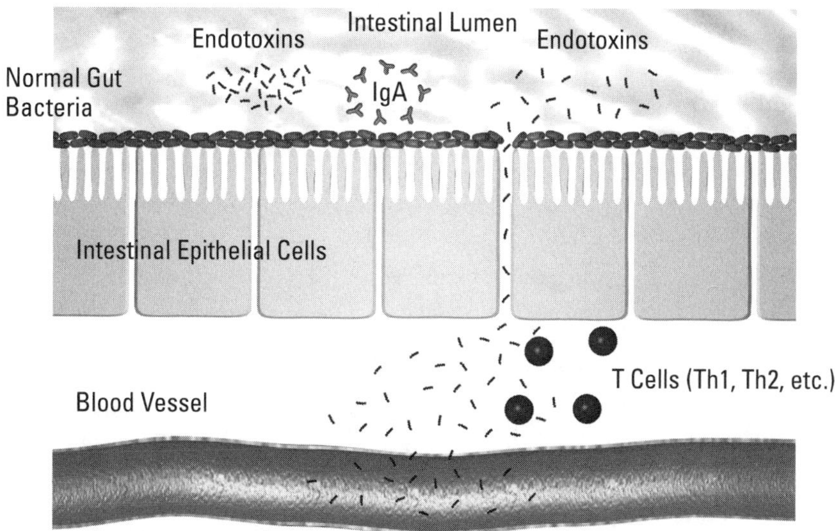

■ **Figure 8.1. How Sleep Deprivation or Heavy Exercise May Allow Gut Bacteria Fragments (Endotoxins) to Leak into the Bloodstream.**

colds. Other studies have shown that moderate exercise may strengthen immunity by increasing lymphocyte numbers.[303]

The Risks of Extreme Training

While the benefits of exercise on immunity continue to become apparent, highly strenuous training can temporarily weaken immune function. When researchers at Loma Linda University studied runners of the Los Angeles Marathon, they found immune function to be depressed for several hours. According to Dr. David Nieman, "Those who train more than 60 miles a week double their odds of getting sick, compared with a runner training less than 20 miles a week."[304]

Runners of a Cape Town, South Africa marathon, had twice the incidence of upper respiratory infections in the two weeks following the race of non-runners. Runners with the fastest times suffered from more infections than runners with slower times.[305] A follow-up study at study at the University of Cape Town showed that the best marathon runners experienced a profound drop in white blood cell counts in the day immediately following a race. Scientists at the U of Queensland in Australia have observed that antibody levels in saliva (sIgA) fall by as much as 70 percent after just 2 hours of cycling at a racing pace.[306]

Evidence of the effects of extreme training on immunity is highlighted by the plight of two of Great Britain's most noted distance runners, Sebastian Coe and Diane Edwards. Both runners have had to drop out of international competition after contracting a rare protozoan infection called toxoplasmosis. Usually carried by cats and generally benign in humans, toxoplasmosis typically afflicts only those who suffer from suppressed immunity.

Extreme Training and Gut Bacteria

Whenever we exercise, blood supply is diverted *away* from the gut to our hard-working muscles, to the lungs, and elsewhere. There is now evidence that heavy exercise can weaken the gut barrier in some athletes and permit gut bacteria to migrate across a leaky gut.[307] In one study, Danish scientists examined 89 exhausted runners from a marathon. Eighty-one percent of these exhausted runners had levels of endotoxin above the limit of 0.1 nanograms per milliliter. Recall that endotoxin is made up of tiny fragments of bacterial cell walls. The presence of endotoxins in the blood of runners indicates that gut bacteria or fragments of gut bacteria likely passed into the bloodstream of these stressed runners.[308] Another study examining blood from athletes after a long-distance triathalon showed that 68 percent had evidence of endotoxin.[309]

As it becomes clearer that heavy exertion can impair immunity, energy, and barrier defenses, in the future we will no longer look with surprise when a well-trained athlete succumbs to infection. We should instead anticipate that the well-trained (often highly stressed) athlete is among those who might actually be at greater risk of infection. Special care should be taken to avoid overtraining, ensure optimum nutrition, optimum sleep, and other means of supporting immune defense, energy, and repair.

How Exercise May Regulate Immune Overactivity

While *heavy* exercise appears to stress the body so gut bacteria can pass, moderate exercise may have an opposing effect. In fact, there is now evidence that moderate exercise can actually dampen the toll-like receptors that we've discussed previously. In some exercise studies, the number of toll-like receptors on cells has been shown to go down and the ability to trigger inflammatory immune activation is reduced. This may be one of the ways that exercise reduces inflammation and dampens the inflammation common in aging.[310]

Can Being Overweight Weaken Immunity?

Chapter 3 explored the question of whether or not antibiotics could make us fat by virtue of their effect on gut bacteria. A separate question relating to being overweight is, can increased body fat disrupt our immune defense, energy, and repair system?*

Dr. Salomon Amar at Boston University has been studying the immune response of obese and lean mice for many years. In one experiment, his group exposed mice to a gum-infecting bacterium called *P. gingivalis* by tying a string coated with the bacterium around the molars of the mice. The obese mice had a more sluggish immune response to the gum infection, which was also accompanied by infection of the entire body (determined by elevated bacterial counts in the mice and bone loss). Important immune-signaling molecules were also lowered

---

*Please note that obesity has been included in the lifestyle chapter because obesity often emerges because of lifestyle (diet, physical activity, stress) and obesity is responsive to lifestyle intervention. In placing obesity here, it does not diminish the influence of things like genetics, environmental factors, infection, and other elements that are less within our control.

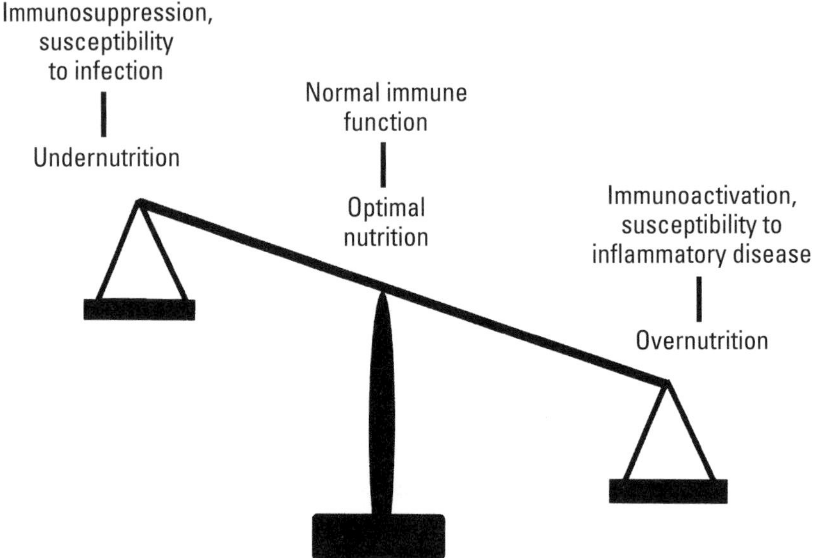

■ **Figure 8.2. How Undernutrition and Overnutrition Create Immune Imbalance.** Undernutrition (insufficiency of selected nutrients) is well known to decrease immune defense, energy, and repair. However, overnutrition (excessive caloric intake), as found in people who are overweight or overtly obese, may shift the immune system toward an inflammatory profile that is also associated with lowered defenses against microbes. Adapted from: Wellen, KE, Hotamisligil, GS. Inflammation, stress, and diabetes. J Clin Invest 2005;115(5):1111–19.

in the obese mice when compared with the lean mice. This study seemed to support the idea obese mice had lowered immunity when compared to lean mice.[311]

In the human population, increased body weight seems to be linked to altered immune function in children. For instance, in a study of obese children between the ages of six and eighteen, those with the highest percentage body fat and body mass index (BMI) had higher numbers of white blood cells. Included in the elevated white blood cells were neutrophils, monocytes, total T-lymphocytes, and helper T-cells. While elevated white blood cells might seem like a good thing, elevated white blood cell numbers indicate a persistent inflammatory state. These findings suggest that obesity is related to persistent low-grade inflammation.[312]

Another study with overweight children also found that obesity was linked with a low-grade inflammatory state. These researchers wanted to further see how exercise affected immunity in the overweight kids. Exercise lowered some immune cell populations (monocytes) and raised others, again suggesting the presence of an adverse immune response.[313]

Belly Fat and Confused Immunity?

Doctors have long been puzzled as to why overweight people have so many inflammatory molecules floating around in their blood. Recently they have begun to tease out the identity of some of the hidden cells burrowed into the fat mass. It now turns out that buried within the belly fat and subcutaneous fat of overweight people are cells of the immune system clean-up crew—the macrophage.

Recall that the word macrophage means "big eater" in Greek. Macrophages are phagocytes. Their role is to engulf and then digest (phagocytize) bacteria and cellular debris. Macrophages also produce signaling molecules that stimulate other immune cells to respond to invading microbes. By virtue of this, macrophages are involved in nonspecific defenses (innate immunity) and specific defenses (cell-mediated immunity).

Fat cells recruit macrophages by sending out signals that call these white blood cells to fat stores like belly fat. As fat stores grow larger, the signals get louder, and more macrophages are recruited. Because of this, the actual number of macrophages in belly fat is correlated to the body mass index (BMI).[314] The greater the body mass, the greater the number of macrophages. Once in their fatty new home, the macrophages seem to adopt a new personality. It is like these cells have moved into a new neighborhood and bought guns. Macrophages in belly fat go from being anti-inflammatory cells to becoming agents that fuel inflammation, weaken defenses against microbes, and degrade health.

Why are macrophages drawn to our belly fat (and other fat stores)? Recent studies suggest that they are drawn there to clean up dead and dying fat cells. The theory is that as fat cells get too large and too filled with fat, they can no longer sustain themselves and begin to die. The macrophages, then, move in for at least two possible reasons. First, macrophages are well known to gather up fat from other cells (such as the fat inside blood vessels). Macrophages may be drawn to belly fat tissue simply to remove the excess fat. Second, macrophages could be moving to fat stores to clean up dead fat cells. They could even be there to help "execute" dying fat cells.[315]

In this view, obesity may be a condition where belly fat is filled with dying fat cells and our white blood cells rush to the site to clean things up. While there, the macrophages pump out inflammatory cytokines that activate other aspects of the immune system. Unfortunately, this persistent state of inflammation causes a shift away from strong cellular defenses, which can impair our ability to fight against bacteria.

Losing weight can be one way to shift the inflammatory macrophages back to a native state that better serves our overall defense objectives. For example, in one study, 29 obese people were fed a very low calorie diet, which resulted in weight loss. After 28 days on the low calorie diet, inflammatory genes were quieted and inflammatory protein production was reduced in fat cells and in macrophages.[316] This fits with the recognition that the macrophages of lean people tend to be anti-inflammatory, while those of obese people tend to be pro-inflammatory.

A further way to understand the effect of obesity on immune function would be to measure immune function of severely obese people after radical weight loss. This was done by doctors at Washington University School of Medicine, who looked at the release of immune proteins in extremely obese people undergoing gastric bypass surgery. After the subjects lost nearly 30 percent of their body weight, their depressed immune response (measured as reduction in a protein called MCP-1) had returned to that comparable to a group of lean subjects used for comparison.[317] MCP-1 is a protein that recruits macrophages, so reduction in this protein with weight loss is important.

Overweight and Leaky Gut

Another group of scientists wanted to find out whether the system that recognizes bacteria (the toll-like receptors) could be activated by dietary fat and trigger an inflammatory activation much like bacteria do. As noted in Chapter 5, scientists found that the saturated fats stearic, palmitic, and (to a lesser degree) lauric acid can act through these receptors (TLR4) on fat cells, muscle cells, and white blood cells (macrophages) to "induce inflammatory signaling."[318] This might also be how saturated fat alters the insulin response. In short, too much saturated fat may "fool" the body into thinking a bacterium is present, which triggers an inflammatory response. This in turns alters insulin and contributes to the accumulation of body fat.

These results suggest a likely interplay between the obese or overweight condition, gut bacterial endotoxins, dietary fat, and a persistent inflammatory state. With the finding of these studies and others like them, reducing body weight may be of critical importance in bringing the immune defense and repair system back to a state of balance. Conversely, it also means that being overweight may make sustaining robust immune defense and repair more difficult due to the persistent inflammatory load that shifts the immune system toward an inflammatory state.

Diabetes, Leaky Gut, and Altered Immunity

Obesity and diabetes have much in common, since many people with diabetes are overweight. But people with diabetes have unique disruptions to their immune regulatory system. Doctors at the University of Warwick Medical School in England studied obese nondiabetic people and compared them to obese people with type 2 diabetes in order to tease out the effect of diabetes from the effect of obesity.

One of the key features they measured was the presence of bacterial endotoxins (LPS) in the blood of individuals from each group. In people with type 2 diabetes, the level of endotoxin circulating in the blood was found to be 76 percent higher, on average, than that of the people in the obese group.

The authors made an interesting observation on why the endotoxin levels may be so high in diabetes and why it might be associated with inflammation (immune disruption). They wrote,

> The innate immune system . . . may have been a means of first-line defense from bacterial and fungal organisms that breach the barrier of the skin and the GI mucosa, potentially causing deleterious systemic effects. However, this reaction could have become disadvantageous in those with increasing adiposity (increasing body fat). The protective inflammatory effects are therefore exaggerated by the sheer volume of adipose tissue (belly fat) that accompanies obesity.

They also went on to note that increased intestinal permeability is common in diabetes, creating conditions whereby gut bacterial endotoxins might drift across the gut barrier to elicit inflammatory immune responses.[319]

In essence, they seem to be suggesting that diabetes in obese individuals is linked to a leaky gut condition, which permits bacterial endotoxins to drift across the gut barrier. As these endotoxins circulate, they come in contact with cell receptors (on white blood cells and on fat cells) that activate inflammation within the immune system. Because the fat cells are so numerous in obesity and diabetes, the endotoxins have vastly more cells on which to bind, so there are more cells triggering immune hyperactivation. This may, in part, explain why diabetes and obesity are linked with disrupted immunity, weakened defenses, and heightened inflammation.

Light and the Immune Response

The average person in our Western world spends less than one hour daily outdoors. We sleep in darkness, awaken indoors to artificial light, drive to work in a car, toil for eight hours under artificial fluorescent light, complete our work, drive home, eat dinner indoors, and go to bed. Depending on the day of the week or the season, we may get a few hours outdoors. But generally, we're short on natural light.

In contrast, our predecessors of a hundred years ago spent the bulk of their day outdoors. Artificial light had nowhere near the impact it does today. There is now evidence that the absence of light experienced by most of us exacts a measurable toll on our mood, behavior, productivity, and general level of health.

In some people, absence of adequate sunlight leads to development of a condition called seasonal affective disorder, or SAD. This condition is characterized by lethargy, fatigue, depression, insomnia, and irritability. It is most pronounced during the winter months—especially in northern climates where it has been called "cabin fever." Sufferers show dramatic improvements with daily exposure to full-spectrum light. These people have found by trial and error that a winter week in Florida, Arizona, or the Caribbean dramatically improves their outlook on life.

SAD is not the only condition that responds to sunlight. Scientists have known for decades that treatment of jaundiced babies with blue light results in a rapid elimination of excess bilirubin from the body (full-spectrum lights work even better).

Light is as vital to our health as vitamins and minerals. In fact, the manufacture of vitamin D is actually dependent upon adequate exposure to ultraviolet light from the sun. We are only beginning to discover the many bodily processes that are dependent upon daily exposure to natural light. Whether light actually enhances immune function or increases resistance to disease is another question. However, recent reports suggest that light plays a role in these vital functions as well.

German researcher Dr. Fritz Hollwich discovered that when subjects sat under standard cool-white fluorescent lights, the levels of ACTH and cortisol (stress hormones) rose to levels comparable to those found in people under stress. In contrast, those sitting under full-spectrum light experienced no such rise in stress hormones. High levels of these hormones are known to have an adverse effect upon immune function. In view of this research, German hospitals are no longer allowed to use cool-white fluorescent bulbs.[320]

A recent study found that switching from cool-white fluorescent lights to full-spectrum lights reduced the number of workplace absences due to illness. Based on this and other evidence, some doctors suggest that full-spectrum light boosts immune function much like natural sunlight.

Studies in Germany and Russia suggest that providing adequate ultraviolet light can be useful in managing infectious diseases in schools and in the workplace.[321,322,323] In one study conducted in the 1940s, modifying environmental factors such as lighting in the classroom of school children resulted in a 43.3 percent reduction in the incidence of chronic infections.[324]

Washing Up

In the face of untold organisms, some of which are uniquely harmful, it is humbling to realize that something as mundane as hand washing is still among the most powerful tools to prevent microbial illness. As mentioned previously, there are still some 76 million illnesses due to foodborne microbes in the United States each year. Some of this illness can be eliminated by hand washing. Transmission of infections within hospitals, nursing homes, schools, and other care facilities can also be dramatically reduced by simple hand washing.

Hand washing might be dull, but it actually does work. Consider the findings of four representative studies summarized below:

- 769 elementary school children were studied for the effects of hand-washing on respiratory illness. Half used an alcohol-free, instant hand sanitizer containing surfactants, allantoin, and benzalkonium chloride. After 5 weeks, students using the active product were 33 percent less likely to have been absent because of illness when compared with the placebo group.[325]
- 430 students were recruited from 4 residence halls during the fall semester at the University of Colorado at Boulder. Alcohol gel hand-sanitizer dispensers were installed in every room, bathroom, and dining hall. Reductions in upper respiratory-illness symptoms in the hand washing group were as high as 40 percent. Total improvement in illness rate was 20 percent. The product group had 43 percent less missed school and work days.[326]
- Military recruits had 43 percent reduction in outpatient visits for respiratory illness after initiation of a hand washing program over a three-year period.[327]
- Diarrheal illness in children over 2 years of age was reduced by 66 percent when children and caregivers carefully followed a hand washing program.[328]

Below is a list of circumstances where hand washing is likely to be important in reducing the spread of illness-causing microbes.[329]

- After using the toilet
- After changing a diaper—wash the diaper-wearer's hands, too
- After touching animals or animal waste
- Before and after preparing food, especially before and immediately after handling raw meat, poultry, or fish
- Before eating
- After blowing your nose
- After coughing or sneezing into your hands
- Before and after treating wounds or cuts
- Before and after touching a sick or injured person

- After handling garbage
- Before inserting or removing contact lenses
- When using public restrooms, such as those in airports, train stations, bus stations, and restaurants

According to the CDC, washing with soap and water alone is sufficient for most uses.

Many scientists concerned about antibiotic-resistant bacteria are concerned about the widespread presence of triclocarban (and its cousin, triclosan) in common handwashing products. This is discussed in following chapters.

Where There's Smoke There's . . . Illness

Information about the adverse health effects of cigarette smoke is nothing new. We know those who smoke are more likely to develop heart disease, lung cancer, and a variety of other ills. The negative effects of secondhand smoke are receiving more attention lately. In fact, the EPA has recently listed secondhand cigarette smoke as a carcinogen (cancer-causing agent).

Beyond its ability to cause cancer, second-hand smoke serves as a respiratory irritant that can contribute to recurrent ear, bronchial, and sinus infections. Kids who live in homes with smokers have up to a fourfold greater risk of developing middle ear infections than kids who live in homes without smokers. Hospitalization for respiratory illness is also higher among those who live in homes with smokers.

Cigarette smoke causes excessive amounts of vitamin C to be eliminated from the body and increases the need for other nutrients such as vitamin E and beta-carotene. In a recent study, only one-third of smokers consumed enough vitamin C to meet the very conservative RDA. Moreover, the smokers required over twice as much vitamin C daily to achieve the same amount of vitamin C in the blood as nonsmokers.[330]

The Search for Meaningful Touch

The skin is the largest sense organ in the body. Stimulation of the skin of the entire body is an important component of maintaining healthy contact with our external world and fostering health in our internal world. Unfortunately, many of us have become touch-starved.

When premature babies were massaged three times per day, they gained 28 percent more weight over a ten-day period than did babies who were not massaged. They were also less easily startled and smiled more often. In a study at Duke University, researchers showed that massage increased levels of certain digestive hormones, allowing babies to more efficiently absorb nutrients from their food. Massage also lowers anxiety in children.[331]

Appropriate touch benefits growth, development, and immune function. In a series of experiments, those animals given frequent touch utilized food better, developed more rapidly, learned more efficiently, and showed greater emotional stability in stressful situations. Remarkably, when confronted with stressful stimuli, the output of stress hormones was considerably lower in animals that received frequent touch than in those receiving less touch.[332]

When animals are touched or handled extensively in infancy, as adults they show more efficiently developed immune systems than animals that have received less tactile stimulation. They suffer fewer infections and have a lower mortality rate than their lesser-touched counterparts.[333]

In subtle but profound ways, touch even influences our perception of people and events. Robert Tisserand reports on a study conducted at Purdue University in 1986. As students left the library after checking out books, they were asked questions regarding their opinion of the library and whether the librarian smiled at them. The library assistant treated everyone the same way, except that every other student was lightly touched on the hand as their library card was handed back to them. Those who were touched formed a more positive view of the library than those who were not and often thought that the assistant had smiled at them, even though she had not.[334]

Noise Pollution

Unwanted noise is well known to create stress and contribute to a variety of physiological ills. Noise pollution can cause these problems alone, but is more apt to cause problems if one perceives to have little or no control over the source of the noise or the noise level.

In Chapter 11, we discuss the impact of emotions, perception, coping, and stress on immune function. Noise can have an insidious effect upon how we interpret and respond to events around us. For example, in a report published in *Psychology Today,* a researcher with a cast on one arm carried an armload of books and papers down the sidewalk and dropped them as another pedestrian approached. The researcher would then helplessly attempt to gather up the books. Nearby, another researcher was operating a power lawn mower. When the lawn mower was on, only 15 percent of the passersby stopped to help pick up the books. In contrast, when the mower was silent, 80 percent stopped to lend a hand.[335]

Turning Up the Heat

In Chapter 4, we explored the importance of fever in fighting infection. Fever is an elevation in body temperature that is controlled internally. This is in contrast to hyperthermia, which is an elevation of body temperature that is generated externally. However, hyperthermia as a means to promote health has been a part of human activity for millennia.

Perhaps one of today's most overlooked hygienic practices for improving health is the use of saunas and steambaths. These have been used by people from many cultures for centuries. Virtually all of the Indians of North America used steambaths. According to anthropologist Jack Weatherford,

> The widespread and persistent use of the steambaths and of the water baths by the Indians paralleled the practices of ancient Mediterranean cultures, but stood in sharp contrast to the practice of the Europeans who arrived in the New World. *The bathing probably served to reduce disease among the Indians prior to the European arrival and thereby partly accounted for the general freedom from epidemic diseases. The destruction of the lodges by the Europeans and their denunciation of frequent bathing quite probably contributed to the rapid spread of Old World epidemics among the natives of North America.*[336] [emphasis added]

Steambaths and saunas are also a well-known component of the Finnish repertoire of healthy living. The Finnish people have long contended that weekly saunas are an essential part of preventing disease and living a long life. They also serve as a kind of social encounter in which families and friends gather to share stories, laugh, and play.

But is there a scientific basis to these beliefs about the benefits of saunas and steambaths? Perhaps. German researchers have studied twenty-two kindergarten children who partook of a weekly sauna and compared them with a control group who took no saunas. The children were followed for eighteen months and a careful record was made of their incidence of ear infections, colds, and other upper respiratory problems. Children who took no saunas suffered from *twice* the number of sick days as their steamier counterparts. The conclusion: children who sauna regularly have an improved resistance to infections.[337]

This chapter merely scratches the surface of lifestyle influences on immune defense, energy, and repair. Unlike many environmental stressors, lifestyle factors are well within our control. A growing body of research has shown that lifestyle affects almost all aspects of health and disease.

Chapter 9

Environmental Threats to Robust Immunity

A handful of scientists from Colorado State University have been scavenging ponds, streams, pastures, and all manner of terrestrial sites. They are DNA hunters. Environmental engineer Amy Pruden and her group are part of an international forensic effort to understand the risks and extent of DNA pollution.

They have been probing these sites in search of naked DNA—DNA that has escaped its host microbe and is found freely in the environment. Many of these naked genes actually code for resistance to antibiotics. Once these naked, antibiotic-resistance genes are loose in the environment, they are theoretically free to interact with all kinds of microbes, transmitting antibiotic-resistance genes to a new host. Scientists are unsure of how severe this problem is, but they have confirmed that naked DNA can bind to things like clay in stream sediment and persist in the environment. This represents one of the newly discovered environmental threats that are certain to change how we view our interaction with our microbial surroundings. And there are others.

Antibiotic Drugs in Our Environment

Discovery of naked, antibiotic-resistant DNA in the environment begs a simple question: How did it get there? While we cannot be certain, it is becoming clear that a related contaminant may be at least partially to

Table 9.1. Antibiotic Drugs Found in U.S. Waterways

Carbodox	Chlortetracycline	Ciprofloxacin
Doxycycline	Enrofloxacin	Erythromycin-H2O
Lincomycin	Norfloxacin	Oxytetracycline
Roxithromycin	Sarafloxacin	Sulfachloropyridazine
Sulfadimethoxine	Sulfadimethoxine	Sulfamerazine
Sulfamethazine	Sulfamethizole	Sulfamethoxazole
Sulfathiazole	Tetracycline	Trimethoprim
Tylosin	Virginiamycin	

blame. For many years, scientists have quietly been aware that the antibiotics we use in the home, the hospital, and the farm end up being flushed down the toilet or washed down the drain. Most antibiotics used in medicine and animal care are not absorbed from the intestinal tract into the body. So, most just pass on through out into the environment.

In addition, most antibiotics are not biochemically converted or broken down. In fact, 85 to 95 percent of antibiotics used remain in their basic molecular form once they hit the environment. What if they end up in our water supply? This concern has led to some disturbing findings.

Studies by the U.S. Geological Survey have found the nation's waterways awash in a vast number of prescription drugs. Additional studies by Johns Hopkins University have found some thirty different types of antibiotics in these waterways.[338] Since the concentrations vary, the health effects from these amounts are currently unclear. If, as we've discussed earlier, our repertoire of antibiotics is dwindling and there are few new antibiotic drugs in development, then we must take seriously the findings of additional antibiotic exposure through environmental sources. Table 9.1 contains a brief summary of antibiotics detected in U.S. waterways.

Triclosan in the Environment

A special note should be made about triclocarban (triclosan), an antibacterial additive. Currently, triclocarban is widely used (some one million pounds annually) in many antibacterial soaps and cleaning products. Its use is expanding as more companies perceive an advantage to marketing their products as antibacterial. This, of course, plays on legitimate concerns about emerging and virulent infections. A tragic irony is that recognition of the issue of emerging infections is driving well-meaning people to use antibacterial products where they are not needed—furthering the problem of antibiotic resistance. A list of common products that contain triclosan is noted below:[339]

- Hand soap
- Dishwashing products
- Laundry detergents and softeners
- Plastics (e.g., toys, cutting boards)
- Toothpaste
- Deodorants and antiperspirants
- Cosmetics
- Hair conditioners
- Impregnated sponges
- Pesticides (as an inert ingredient)

Many scientists concerned about antibiotic resistant bacteria are concerned about the widespread presence of triclocarban in the environment and the possible effect of this triclocarban further expanding antibiotic resistance.

The John's Hopkins study noted above found that triclocarban (a cousin of triclosan) was present in 60 percent of the U.S. water sources tested. This means that triclocarban was the fifth most commonly found contaminant among the ninety-six pharmaceuticals, personal care products, and wastewater contaminants tested.

And this triclosan is finding its way into human bodies. In a Swedish study of thirty-six nursing mothers, triclosan was found in the mothers' blood and breastmilk. A close examination of personal care products found that nine of the women used toothpaste, deodorant, or soap containing triclosan. Triclosan levels were higher in the women using personal care products, but it was detected in all women, suggesting an environmental source. Triclosan levels were higher in blood than in breastmilk, though levels in breastmilk were still significant.[340]

What's in That Dirt?

It is more clear than ever that this is the microbe's world. Scoop up a handful of dirt and you would be holding a sample of the most crafty living things on the planet. We have known for decades that all manner of bugs live in the soil. In fact, the bugs in the soil are often to our benefit, as they help prime our immune systems. Most of these are nonthreatening organisms, but our immune systems still must do some work at recognition. You might say that when you send your little ones out to play in the dirt, you're also sending them out for a little immune system practice. Chalk one up for our friends the soil bugs.

But soil bugs have also been found to possess an astonishing set of talents, which have only recently become clear to us.

Bugs That Eat Antibiotics for Breakfast

In Chapter 1, we learned about soil bacteria that eat antibiotics for breakfast.[341] To more fully appreciate this, we'll look a bit more closely at the work of a team of Harvard scientists led by Dr. George Church, who recently gathered soil from eleven different sites, ranging from manure-fed cornfields to a pristine forest. They were initially looking for bacteria that might be used to convert agricultural waste into biofuels—a noble effort, indeed. In their investigation, however, they were astonished to find that every soil sample tested contained microbes that could *digest* antibiotics. Not only did the bacteria digest antibiotics, they could actually use the antibiotics as a carbon source—a basic source of fuel to survive. The microbes tested came from eleven different orders of bacteria. Included were human disease-causing microbes such as *E. coli*

0157:H7 and *Shigella flexneri,* well known for invading the human gut and causing disease.

According to Dr. Church, some of the soil microbes could tolerate antibiotics at more than fifty times the concentration used to establish a bacterium as resistant. He stated, "Almost all the drugs that we consider as our mainline defense against bacterial infections are at risk from bacteria that not only resist the drugs but eat them for breakfast."[342] Those antibiotics tested are foundations of our antibiotic arsenal, including:

Table 9.2. Antibiotics that Resistant Bacteria Could Use as a Food Source

D-cycloserine	Amikacin	Gentamycin
Kanamycin	Sisomycine	Chloramphenicol
Thiamphenicol	Carbenicillin	Penicillin-G
Vancomycin	Ciproflaxin	Levoflaxin
Mafenide	Sulfamethizole	Sulfisoxazole
Trimethoprim		

Not all antibiotic-resistant or antibiotic-eating soil bacteria got that way because of *our* antibiotics. While we must be held accountable for overusing antibiotics in medicine, animal husbandry, and spraying fruit trees, soil bugs have been busy figuring out how to defend themselves for eons.

The Gene Collectors

Bacteria are the consummate collectors and traders. But they don't trade antiques, baseball cards, or fine art. They collect genes. Scientists have long puzzled over the immense capacity of bacteria to develop resistance to antibiotics they had not previously encountered. How was this possible? Clearly the process of evolving the capacity to do so through mutations in their own DNA would just take far too long; impossible to do in the short time bacteria were developing resistance.

It then became clear that bacteria were swapping genes with other bacteria that already had the genes for resistance.

It is a little like borrowing the antivirus software from your neighbor's computer. You know you're unprotected from the bugs floating all over the Internet. Writing your own anti-virus software is too complex and going to the store will take too long, so you pop next door to get your neighbor's copy. You walk home with the disk, insert it into your computer, download the program, and your computer is suddenly protected against a range of viruses—just like your neighbor. You avoided the laborious and perhaps impossible task of having to write the new software yourself.

Bacteria take these genes for resistance to antibiotics from their neighbors, insert them into their own DNA, and *voila,* they now have the software, if you will, and they are now resistant to a new class of antibiotic drugs.

This passing of genes for antibiotic resistance is an endless process taking place constantly in the invisible microbial world. Their ability to rapidly transfer these resistance capacities back and forth means that they will likely always remain more than one step ahead of our efforts to defeat them.

How Did Bacteria Get So Good at Gene Collecting?

Of course, the above scenario of swapping genes is deliberately simplified. While conceptually accurate, the real story of the means by which bacteria transfer these genes is of bewildering complexity and is only beginning to be understood by scientists. Basically, we know they are swapping these genes, but a full understanding of "how" is elusive.

There are two main schools of thought on our gene-collecting bacteria. First, many soil-based bacteria are actually antibiotic *producers.* That is, these bacteria manufacture their own antibiotic compounds in order to fend off rival microbes in their surroundings. Since the antibiotic-producers do not want to succumb to the antibiotics they manufacture to kill off their neighbors, they have developed protective means (resistance genes) in order to remain unharmed. It is a brilliant and necessary survival strategy.

Besides having to protect against their own antibiotic compounds, bacteria in the soil have another arch nemesis.

Living in a Plant World

If you're a soil bacterium not living in a desert, there's a pretty good chance you live around plants. Plants are quite vulnerable, as they sit there waiting for just about anything to land on them, attack them, or eat them. So most plants have developed a formidable arsenal of chemical agents to ward off all manner of pests. Bacteria that live around these plants and their antipest arsenal must develop their own defenses against the plant defenses. In many cases, this means that the bacterial genome has crafted a series of "resistance genes" to protect the bacterium. It just so happens that the plant-derived molecules against which the bacterial genes have afforded protection have a lot in common with certain antibiotics in use today. Thus, the toxic products of plant defense have pressured the soil microbes to develop antibiotic-resistance genes as a side-effect.

Living in a Heavy Metal World

Another way that bacteria develop resistance genes is by living in areas contaminated by heavy metals such as lead, mercury, cadmium, copper, or arsenic. This is how resistance to erythromycin occurs in the bacterium *S. maltophilia.*[343] It has become clear that one means by which microbes eliminate heavy metals is through the use of *efflux pumps*—a fancy word for something akin to a water pump in the basement that pumps out water during a heavy flood. Microbes use efflux pumps to get rid of heavy metals. They have also learned how to adapt these heavy-metal pumps to get rid of antibiotics—they just pump them out.

A Not-So Healthy Lawn

Beyond metals in the soil, other contaminants of modern life may contribute to development of antibiotic-resistant bacteria. A report published in *Infectious Disease News* noted that spraying lawns with chemical fungicides and bacteriocides increases bacterial resistance. The authors recognized that treated lawns harbor bacteria that are resistant to multiple drugs, that lawn chemicals can increase the number and amount of drug-resistant bacteria in the environment, and that they could cause serious problems in the treatment of life-threatening bacterial infections.

Heavy Metals and Immunity

We now know that heavy metals can trigger the development of antibiotic resistance in bacteria, rendering us less able to treat certain infections when they occur. But heavy metals can also reduce our ability to defeat microbes by lowering our immune defense and repair system directly or indirectly.

Exposure to lead, mercury, cadmium, aluminum, nickel, arsenic, and other metals can occur in infancy, childhood, or adulthood. Metals can cause problems when present individually in high amounts. When more than one metal is present, which is often the case, even low levels can be damaging. This is because of a synergistic effect and the total toxic load.

A recent study on prenatal exposure to heavy metals shows just how dramatic this effect can be. Amniotic fluid was taken from 92 pregnant women and tested for the presence of seven heavy metals—cadmium, chromium, cobalt, lead, mercury, nickel, and silver. A prenatal toxic risk score was assigned based on the presence and amount of the different heavy metals detected. This score was then correlated with the health of the children at age three. The researchers found that children with higher toxic risk scores *in utero* suffered from more infectious disease and allergies at age three than did children with low toxic risk scores. Listed in the category of infections were coughs, fever, sore throat, congestion, diarrhea, vomiting, ear infection, and constipation. The authors of this paper wrote, "The toxic risk score predicted the total number of illnesses and the number of infectious illnesses."[344]

In a study of blood lead and immunity in 193 children, nine months to six years old, blood lead levels were correlated with a *decreased* antibody response to diphtheria and rubella vaccination.[345] This essentially means that lead exposure lowered the immune response.

The effect of lead exposure on immunity in adults has also been examined. In one study, scientists looked at immune competence in thirty-nine workers who were exposed to lead on the job. These were compared with thirty workers with no apparent occupational exposure. The average blood lead concentration was 42.9 micrograms per deciliter in the exposed workers, compared to 19.5 micrograms per deciliter in the nonexposed group.* In the lead-exposed group, the concentrations of the following immune components were found to be significantly depressed:[346]

- Serum immunoglobulins IgG, IgM (two main antibodies)
- Complement component proteins C3 and C4 (part of natural immunity)
- Chemotaxis of neutrophils (the ability of this white blood cell to migrate to the site of invading microbes)

Also of interest, C-reactive protein (CRP) was significantly higher in the high lead group. CRP is an immune protein associated with an inflammatory state and has long-term detrimental affects on health.

Another study looked at lead exposure, testing blood lead levels in people working in occupations, such as car battery shop workers, car painters, welders of car radiators and exhausts, and printing office workers between the ages of 15 and 70 years. Elevated blood lead was associated with depressed immunoglobulins, especially in the IgG antibodies.[347]

---

*Note that 19.5 micrograms per deciliter is still considered above the safe threshold.

Beyond being severely toxic to the nervous system, mercury may also have a negative impact on immunity. In one effort to study mercury's effects on immunity, a multicenter study was performed on 117 workers exposed to very low doses of inorganic mercury and 172 subjects from the general population of the same geographical area with environmental exposure to mercury from dental amalgams and dietary fish intake. In the mercury-exposed workers, lower interleukin-8 (IL-8) was discovered, which may be associated with depressed immunity.[348]

Mercury Fillings and Antibiotic Resistance

Recently, a new controversy has emerged surrounding the potential health hazards of mercury fillings, suggesting that mercury from dental fillings can bring about changes in bacteria that cause them to be resistant to antibiotics. This would be consistent with what's been found when soil bacteria are exposed to mercury. In a paper presented at the Annual Meeting of the American Society for Microbiology, Dr. A. O. Summers and colleagues reported on their study in which mercury fillings were placed in the mouths of monkeys. Various types of bacteria that live in the mouth and intestines were tested for resistance to antibiotics before and after placement of the fillings.

After installation of the fillings, investigators found a dramatic increase in bacterial resistance to multiple antibiotics including tetracycline, ampicillin, streptomycin, chloramphenicol, and sulfadiazine. After five months, the mercury amalgam fillings were replaced by composite resin fillings that contained no mercury and the proportion of antibiotic-resistant bacteria declined. The researchers concluded that, "Constant exposure to Hg [mercury] arising from dental amalgams constitutes continuous selective pressure for the maintenance of multiply resistant bacteria in both oral and fecal flora of primates."[349] In other words, the fillings favored development of bacteria resistant to some of the most commonly used antibiotics in the medical arsenal.

Recent efforts to confirm these findings have left us with an unclear picture. In a laboratory biofilm study, 71 percent of mercury-resistant bacteria were resistant to a wide range of antibiotics, with resistance to tetracycline being most common.[350] In another study, dental plaque and saliva samples from sixteen children without mercury amalgam restorations were screened for bacteria resistant to mercury or to one of the antibiotics before and one month after placement of mercury fillings. Mercury amalgams appeared *not* to trigger greater resistance to mercury, penicillin, ampicillin, erythromycin, or tetracycline.[351] In a follow-up study using a control group, bacteria from the mouths of forty-one children mercury amalgam fillings and forty-two children without these fillings were tested for resistance to mercury and to antibiotics. Antibiotic-resistant bacteria were common in both groups, suggesting that there was no greater prevalence in those with mercury amalgams.[352]

Heavy Metal Sources

The presence of lead, mercury, cadmium, aluminum and other metals can take a considerable toll on our immune systems. When metals are identified and removed from the body, major improvements in well-being typically follow. Below is a list of the most important heavy metals, their sources, and nutrients that are protective.

Mercury

Sources of mercury in the environment include dental amalgams (fillings that are mixtures of mercury, silver, and other metals), saltwater fish, some freshwater fish, shellfish, plastics, latex paint, selected vaccines, organomercurial pesticides with fungicides, grains and seeds treated with methyl mercury or mercury chloride, and chlorine bleaches.

Nutrients that protect against mercury exposure include selenium, vitamin C, vitamin E, pectin, and the amino acids cysteine, cystine, and methionine.

Lead

Common sources of lead include drinking water, lead dust from paint used in old homes, atmospheric pollution, leaded gasoline (some countries), lead-glazed pottery, wine, and "tin cans" soldered with lead-containing solder. In some countries, canned tuna is a major source of lead in children.

Nutrients that antagonize and protect against lead exposure include calcium, vitamin C, vitamin E, B-complex, pectin, and the amino acids cystine, cysteine, and methionine.

Cadmium

Sources of cadmium include cigarette smoke, shellfish and other seafood, teas, paints, welding pigments, drinking water, galvanized pipes, batteries, auto exhaust, and industrial smoke and waste. The processing of whole grains such as wheat into white flour strips off the zinc, a natural antagonist of cadmium, and leaves the cadmium to be sold to consumers.

Nutrients that protect against cadmium include zinc, vitamin C, selenium, and to a limited extent, calcium.

Aluminum

Sources of aluminum include aluminum-containing antacids, aluminum-containing baking powder, aluminum antiperspirants, aluminum pots and pans, soft water, and aluminum foil. Aluminum is not efficiently absorbed into humans.

Nutrients that protect against aluminum exposure include vitamin C, magnesium and calcium.

Arsenic

Sources of arsenic include drinking water, tobacco smoke, smog, pesticides, caulks, glues, and building materials that contain fungicides, beer, table salt, colored chalk, and household laundry products.

Nutrients that protect against arsenic include selenium and vitamin C.

Indoor Air Pollutants: Can Buildings Make Us Sick?

Three main factors have given rise to an increase in illness and complaints related to buildings. First, there has been a shift to more energy-efficient buildings. This has limited the amount of fresh air that circulates through homes, offices, and schools. Second, there has been a dramatic increase in the use of synthetic building materials and furnishings (though this has changed in some areas). Many of these materials are made from petrochemicals that slowly release vapors over time (a process called outgassing). These vapors are known carcinogens and respiratory irritants. Finally, the proliferation of air-conditioned buildings has led to more bacterial and mold-related illness among people working in such places.

Offices with air conditioning typically produce the greatest number of complaints among office workers. According to an article in the *American Journal of Public Health,* air-conditioned buildings are "consistently associated with increased prevalence of work-related headache, lethargy, and upper respiratory / mucous membrane symptoms."[353]

Next on the list of symptom producers are *new* homes and offices. Several years ago, and with great irony, workers at the office of the EPA (Environmental Protection Agency) were forced to move out of their new headquarters because of a flood of complaints of headache, nausea, burning eyes, fatigue, and irritability. The culprits, formaldehyde and other volatile substances, were being released from building materials and paper supplies such as file folders. This certainly brought the issue of indoor air pollution to the fore.

Mold in the Home: A Hidden Hazard

Mold is something we usually associate with those dark spots lurking inside the shower curtain or perhaps that cheese that has spent too long in the refrigerator. Whatever the source, mold is an insidious culprit that can permeate the home and be a constant source of immune system stress. For some, the constant presence of mold in the home so heavily taxes the immune system on a daily basis that they easily succumb to opportunistic germs. Researchers in Canada reported that respiratory symptoms such as bronchitis and cough were much more common in homes where there was dampness or mold. Of the 15,000 homes studied, 32.4 percent reported mold, 21.4 percent reported flooding and 14.1 percent reported moisture from other causes.[354]

It should be noted that the sensitivity to mold varies considerably between individuals. However, recall the studies from Chapter 3 showing increased allergy or sensitivity in those who had received antibiotics. Those with a history of extensive antibiotic use, hospitalization, use of immunosuppressive drugs (for cancer, organ transplant, or other reasons), chronic airway disease, or genetic immunosuppressive disorders should pay careful attention to mold as a potential problem.

Pesticides in Our Food

Exposure to a variety of pesticides through fruits and vegetables has raised concern because of the frequency with which these foods are consumed. As government and medical organizations stress the consumption of more fruits and vegetables, there must be awareness of the added exposure to agricultural chemicals that comes with conventional produce. The effects of these chemicals on immune defense, energy, and repair are very complex. Most toxicology studies do not examine cocktails of multiple chemicals, but it is well understood that these compounds at trace levels pose some risk and that their intake should be limited as stringently as possible.

■ Table 9.3. Most Heavily Contaminated Fruits and Vegetables in U.S. Food Supply

Food	Score
Peaches (N. America)	4,848
Peaches (Chile)	471
Winter squash (U.S.A.)	1,706
Apples (U.S.A.)	550
Pears (U.S.A.)	435
Pears (Mexico)	415
Spinach (U.S.A.)	349
Spinach (Mexico)	256
Grapes (U.S.A.)	228
Grapes (Chile)	339
Celery (U.S.A.)	255
Green beans (U.S.A.)	222

Pesticides used on fruits and vegetables generally include:

- antimicrobials to control bacteria
- fungicides to control mold and fungus
- herbicides to control weeds
- insecticides to control insects
- rodenticides to control rodents

As with all issues related to immunity, those for whom extra caution must be taken are children, pregnant or nursing mothers, the elderly, those who are immunocompromised, and those in general poor health.

Foods with the Greatest Degree of Contamination

The USDA recently undertook a collaborative study examining the pesticide content of a wide variety of foods. In their analysis, produce was scored based on the following (where each sample represented about five pounds of food):

- How many samples contained pesticides
- The average amount of each pesticide
- The toxicity of particular pesticides found in the food

A score over one hundred was deemed a cause for concern. Contrary to what has been suspected, many of the most heavily contaminated fruits and vegetables were grown in the U.S.[355]

Organic Fruits and Vegetables Significantly Better

The USDA study discussed above also compared the pesticide levels in organic vs. commercial foods (done in collaboration with the Consumers Union and the Organic Materials Research Institute). The combined efforts of the three groups studied more than 94,000 food samples from more than 20 different crops. In this study, organic food was found to be dramatically lower in pesticide residues.[356] For instance:

- 73 percent of conventionally grown foods had at least one pesticide residue, while only 23 percent of organically grown samples of the same crops had any residues.
- More than 90 percent of the USDA's samples of conventionally grown apples, peaches, pears, strawberries, and celery had residues.
- Conventionally grown crops were six times as likely as organic to contain multiple pesticide residues.
- Consumer's Union tests found pesticide residues in 79 percent of conventionally grown samples and 27 percent of organically grown samples.

As noted, the effect of exposure to multiple pesticides in trace amounts over time is complex, but there at least two important considerations to bear in mind. In Chapter 3, I discussed the drug-metabolizing enzymes called cytochrome P450 (CYP450). This is the system that

■ Table 9.4. Percentage of Samples Testing Positive for One or More Pesticide Residues*

Data Set	Organic Samples	Conventional Samples
PDP	23%	73%
DPR	6.5%	31%
CU	27%	79%

■ Table 9.5. Percentages of Samples Testing Positive for Multiple Pesticide Residues

Data Set	Organic Samples	Conventional Samples
PDP	7%	46%
DPR	1%	12%
CU	6%	44%

detoxifies drugs entering the human body and the same system that detoxifies chemicals we encounter through our food. Constant exposure to chemicals through our food places this system under a constant state of demand. Also, some chemicals and drugs have complex effects on this detoxication system; some can block it and some can activate it. In other words, drugs can impair our ability to detoxify chemicals and vice versa.

Second, removal of chemicals in the body is a biochemical process about which we know a great deal (though by no means everything). We will see below how ongoing exposures can deplete nutrients needed for defense and repair as well as those needed for the detoxication process itself.

*PDP=USDA Pesticide Data Program; DPR=California Department of Pesticide Regulation; CU=Consumer's Union

Environmental Toxins and Immunity

There is increasing concern that exposure to chemicals can have a negative effect on immune function. One effect may be immune activation, meaning the immune system becomes hypervigilant and attacks the body's own tissues. Another effect may be immune suppression, in which infection and tumor-fighting ability is compromised.

With recent reports suggesting that exposure to chemicals is more prevalent than previously thought, the issue of chemical exposure and immune function is becoming more urgent. For instance, the EPA published results of a study in which they analyzed the urine of 7,000 Americans for the presence of toxic chemical residue. Chemicals such as pentachloraphenol, a wood preservative, were found in 71 percent of those tested. The subjects of this study were not people who worked in chemical plants or those who lived near landfills; they were selected at random from all walks of life.[357]

According to William Rea, MD, author of *Chemical Sensitivity,* some toxic chemicals, such as pentachloraphenol and hexachlorobenzene, will suppress the ability of white blood cells to engulf and destroy bacteria. Hexachlorobenzene and PCB (polychlorinated biphenyl) have been found in 51 percent of the chemically sensitive patients studied by Dr. Rea. These and other chemicals reduce resistance to infection in mice by 20 to 30 percent.[358]

Dr. Rea has also observed that patients with recurrent respiratory tract infection, recurrent vaginal infection, and some children with recurrent middle ear infection have decreased resistance to infection because of chemical exposure. When the chemical load is reduced, recurrent infections cease; when reexposure occurs, reinfection follows. Dr. Rea also found that the greater numbers and higher levels of organochlorine pesticides in the body corresponded to lower levels of T-cells in the immune system.

In another study, ninety women referred for endocrine abnormality were tested for chemicals such as pentachloraphenol and lindane.

Twenty-two were found to have elevated levels of one or both compounds. Of these, 71 percent had immune system abnormalities. When the source of toxic exposure was removed, symptoms improved in twelve out of twelve women. Only two of twelve cases where chemical exposure was not reduced showed improvement.[359]

A group of 289 people who worked at a computer manufacturing plant were evaluated for chemical exposure and immune function. Phthalic anhydride, formaldehyde, isocyanate, trimellitic anhydride, and aliphatic and aromatic hydrocarbons were among the chemicals to which they were exposed. A significant adverse effect on immune function was found based on many different measurements of immune health. Some individuals experienced a decline in immune function, while others experienced an autoimmune response wherein the immune system attacks the body's own tissue.[360]

Competitive swimmers suffer inordinately from asthma. They also become more susceptible to infection as the season progresses. In one study, 92 percent of 251 competitive swimmers had symptoms of respiratory distress. Roughly three-fourths of those with asthma were diagnosed *after* taking up swimming. One important contributor is continued exposure to chloride from swimming pools. Chloride is a powerful oxidant that interacts with lung tissue, leading to inflammation and mucus formation. Chloroform, a byproduct of chlorination, is present in indoor swimming pools due to the use of sodium hypochlorite. In a study of 127 people, researchers compared the level of chloroform in the blood of people who swam every day, a few days a week, and those who were merely in the pool area. Those who swam most frequently during the week had higher blood levels of chloroform.[361]

Children, Toxins, and Immunity

Doctors at Harvard University and the University of California at Berkeley have been taking a serious look at environmental exposure and how it affects childhood immunity. In their analyses, they have examined a wide range of immune system proteins in relation to levels of toxic substances found in the blood of pregnant women, umbilical cord blood, and the urine and blood of children.

For example, one study looked at immune function in children living in an environmentally "clean" area compared with an area polluted from power plants and coal-home heating. Children living in the polluted area had significantly more ear infections, respiratory infections, gastrointestinal infections, and pneumonia.[362] In other studies, children living in agricultural environments where chemicals are used have been found to have alterations in their immune parameters, such as in the Th1 / Th2 ratio.

The authors of one study wrote, "Th2 was higher in children with mothers who performed agricultural fieldwork or had other agricultural workers living in the household. The presence of a gas stove in the home was also strongly associated with higher Th2."[363] Recall that the Th1 / Th2 balance is critical in establishing an immune response that supports a balance between healthy defenses against microbes and preventing unhealthy responses that tend toward allergy or intolerance.

According Berkeley and Harvard scientists Duramad, Tager, and Holland, a growing body of research has linked environmental chemical exposure to alterations of the immune response in children. A brief summary of reports is adapted from their review below:[364]

It is difficult to comprehend the number of chemicals to which we are exposed. We do not routinely have our blood tested for chemicals, so there is little personal experience with our individual chemical burden. But the reality is that most of us are exposed on a daily basis, though to varying degrees. The National Academy of Sciences reports that an average American consumes roughly 40 milligrams of pesticides (DDT, DDE, DDD, etc.) each year in food alone and carries about 100 milligrams permanently in his or her body fat.

A simple example of how environmental chemicals pass through

■ Table 9.6. Immune Measures in Toxicology Studies of Children

Environmental Toxicant	Immune Parameters Measured
Volatile organic compounds; Napthalene, benzene, thrichloroethylene	Inteferon gamma, IL-4[v]
Environmental tobacco smoke	Nasopharyngeal aspirate for IL-13[vi]
Arsenic	Granulocyte macrophage colony stimulating factor[vii]
Mercury	Cord blood immune cell subsets[viii]
Polychlorinated biphenyls	Cell counts (CD4)[ix]
Organophosphates	Interferon gamma and IL-4
Organochlorines	Cord blood immune cells (IL-10, TNF?)
Hexachlorobenzene	Cell counts, IL-2 cytokine

Adapted from: Duramad, P, Tager, IB, Holland, NT. Cytokines and other immunological biomarkers in children's environmental health studies. Toxicol Let 2007;172:48–59.

the human body is found in cigarette smoke. Cotinine is a by-product of nicotine that is eliminated in the urine of smokers and people exposed to cigarette smoke. Only 8 percent of infants in nonsmoking households show elevated levels of this chemical. In homes where one or both parents smoke, 96 percent of infants show elevated levels. Children of smoking parents suffer from more frequent respiratory infections, asthma, and hospitalization than do other children. The chemicals found in cigarette smoke are known to contribute to this.[365]

One group of doctors analyzed the blood of two hundred people reporting sensitivity to chemicals for sixteen different synthetic compounds. An average of 3.4 chemical compounds was found per individual. The most common included hexachlorobenzene, heptachlorepoxide, and members of the DDT family—dieldrin, beta-BHC, and endosulfan-1.[366]

Weather and Climate

In the United States alone, some 1.68 million people are hospitalized each year and an average of 41,400 die annually from influenza. In northern climates, influenza viruses circulate from November to March. In the southern hemisphere, the trend is reversed, with the season ranging from May to September.[367]

While theories abound as to why such seasonal variations occur, a recent study on humidity and temperature has gained attention. Anice Lowen and her team at Mount Sinai School of Medicine in New York have performed a series of twenty replicated experiments with guinea pigs in which the only condition varied were temperature and humidity. Guinea pigs were then exposed to varying temperature and humidity.

Five different relative humidity conditions were used: 20%, 35%, 50%, 65%, and 80%. Various temperature conditions were varied along with relative humidity. The temperature conditions included: 5°C, 20°C, and 30°C (41°F, 68°F, and 86°F respectively). After exposing the guinea pigs to influenza virus under numerous combined conditions, it became clear that low temperature (5°C) and low relative humidity (20–35%) were the optimum conditions for viral transmission.

The research team suggested that if these findings apply to humans, influenza virus transmission could be reduced by "simply maintaining room air at warm temperatures (>68°F) and either intermediate (50%) or high (80%) relative humidity."

The Electromagnetic Sea

As our society becomes more reliant upon electrical appliances and instruments, our exposure increases to what was once thought harmless forms of energy. Whenever an electrical motor is operated or electricity travels through a wire, an electromagnetic field is produced. Depending on certain factors such as amperage, wattage, frequency, wavelength, and so on, the field can be projected great distances. For instance, the field from overhead power lines can project hundreds of feet into nearby homes. Radio waves and microwaves are projected nearly everywhere from towers high atop tall buildings. Exposure to both high-frequency and low-frequency electromagnetic waves is inescapable.

There is considerable debate over whether electromagnetic fields have an adverse effect on immune function. But a growing number of researchers are beginning to uncover a link that raises serious questions about how we will be able to manage immune system illness in the future. According to Robert O. Becker, MD, "Impaired immune response has been found at many frequencies. Several groups of Soviet researchers have found a decline in the efficiency of white blood cells in rats and guinea pigs after the animals had been exposed to radio waves and microwaves." Reporting on the work of one researcher, Becker writes ". . . the most dramatic effect on immune response has been produce by ELF [extremely low frequency] fields. Yuri N. Udintsev found that the concentration of bacteria needed to kill mice in such an environment was only one-fifth that needed without the field."[368]

Becker also reports on the work of Yu N. Achkasova of the Crimean Medical Institute in Simferopol. Becker writes,

> In 1978 they reported the results of exposing thirteen standard strains of bacteria—including anthrax, typhus, pneumonia, and staphylococcus—to electric and magnetic fields. After accounting for magnetic storms, ionospheric flux, passage of the interplanetary magnetic-field boundaries, and other variables, they found clear evidence that an electric field only slightly stronger than earth's background stimulated growth of all bacteria and increased their resistance to antibiotics.... Every field tested had an effect, even after one four-hour exposure. In many cases, longer exposure produced *permanent* changes in bacterial metabolism.[369]

It may be that with our technology we are altering the way in which our immune systems function *and* the virulence of organisms that live on this planet. It also suggests that we may need to look to our environment to answer some of our more puzzling medical questions.

Pollutants and Nutrient Depletion

One effect of exposure to chemicals in our environment is the loss or destruction of nutrients in our bodies. Loss of nutrients may render us susceptible to harm by subsequent exposure to these and other chemicals in the future. For example, vitamin B6 is essential for the enzymes that detoxify the toxic substance toluene. Yet, B6 can be antagonized by exposure to this and other toxic substances, making the job of detoxication* much more difficult. Moreover, nutrients antagonized by toxic exposure, such as vitamins A and C and the mineral zinc, are critical to optimum function of the immune system. Consider only a few examples cited in a chapter entitled "Environmental Medicine" published in *The Kellogg Report* by Joseph Beasley, MD:[370]

- Workers handling pesticides suffer from severe disruption of vitamin A.
- Exposure to even low levels of PCBs cuts the vitamin A stored in the liver of animals by 50 percent.
- Deficiency of vitamin E worsens the ill effects of nitrogen dioxide from smog.
- More than 20 cigarettes per day lowers blood levels of vitamin C by 40 percent.

Nutrients have also been used to protect against pollutants and to treat exposure. For example:

- Zinc reduces liver damage by the chemical solvent carbon tetrachloride.

*The term detoxication is usually used to describe the body's own mechanism for handling toxic substances. It refers to a therapeutic process used to rid the body of toxins.

- Selenium and vitamin E protect against lung damage by ozone.
- In workers exposed to toxic fluorine, vitamin C enabled the body to excrete the toxin more rapidly.

Toxic Compounds and Glutathione Depletion

A final note should be considered in regard to how toxins might influence nutritional status and immune function. It begins with understanding how the body rids itself of chemicals. Many chemicals go through two distinct phases of processing by the human body in preparation for elimination. Phase I is by the cytochrome P450 system. The first step in processing many drugs, it also processes many molecules to which we are exposed through a toxic environment.

The next step for elimination is called Phase II (conjugation). In this step, the body binds the toxin with molecules (often nutrient molecules) such as glutathione, the amino acid taurine, the amino acid cysteine, the amino acid glycine, and others. When this occurs, the toxic molecule becomes more soluble in the bloodstream and is shuttled to the kidneys for elimination.

This process, by necessity, also removes the nutrient molecule. Thus, for every toxic molecule removed by this means, one nutrient molecule is also removed. (This is somewhat oversimplified, but still accurate.) It is easy to see how toxic exposure can deplete the body of key nutrients. As a toxin is removed, a nutrient is removed, so if the body is not regularly replacing these nutrients, insufficiency ensues, followed by deficiency.

One of the key nutrients that participates in these detoxication reactions is glutathione. Glutathione is critical for immunity, critical for energy, critical for barrier defenses, and critical for repair. Glutathione is required for removal of many heavy metals and toxic volatile compounds. In so doing, glutathione molecules are removed and depleted as they carry out the toxic molecules to which they bind.

Chemicals have the capacity to affect almost any aspect of our system of immune defense, energy, and repair. Since most doctors do not test for environmental chemicals or their byproducts in patients, this issue is almost never addressed. Though it is more commonly done in people who work in occupations where there is known chemical exposure, it is rarely done with people who might have background exposures from their daily lives. There are several straightforward means to assess chemical exposure using laboratory methods. Some of these methods are discussed in Chapter 14.

Chapter 10

Mood, Mind, Stress, and Infections

If we are to become masters of our ability to thrive in this world of the microbe, we must understand the ways in which stress shapes our immune defense, energy, and repair systems. Psychiatrist Stephen Locke describes stress as "the perception of individuals that their life circumstances have exceeded their capacity to cope."[371] Noted personality researcher H. J. Eysenck points out that we must distinguish between "stress" and "strain" much as an engineer or a physicist would. Stress is the outside force brought to bear upon the individual. Strain is our reaction to the outside force.[372] Dr. Hans Selye, who is credited with bringing the concept of stress to public attention, gave this definition: "Stress is the nonspecific response of the body to any demand made upon it."[373] Selye realized that some stress was necessary for survival. He made a distinction between pleasurable or "eustress" and painful or "dis-stress."

During the past several decades, scientists have learned that stress can have a profound effect on immune function and susceptibility to disorders ranging from infectious disease to arthritis to cancer.

Stress, Life Events, and Infections

Infectious disease expert Dr. Tohru Ishegami observed at the turn of the century that the principal factor determining whether tuberculosis patients would survive or succumb to this infectious disease was their emotional state. He realized that stressful life events took a toll on patients suffering from tuberculosis (TB). Stress seemed to be predictive of who became sick and who did not become sick. It also seemed to explain why reasonably healthy individuals became seriously ill. Dr. Ishegami commented on the factors that influence susceptibility to TB. He stated, "The personal history usually reveals failure in business, lack of harmony in the family, or jealousy of some sort. Nervous individuals are especially prone to attacks of this type, and the prognosis is generally bad." He continued, "Again, in chronic cases, patients may go on apparently well until some misfortune happens. This immediately alters the course of the disease."[374]

This "novel" concept, that stress and life events might influence the course of infectious disease, was published in 1919. Since Dr. Ishegami's time, the germ theory of disease and antibiotic treatments dominated the medical scene. Little attention was given to the psychosocial aspects of infection. Only since about 1980 have we seen the emergence of a concerted effort to understand infection from this perspective.

Dr. W. Thomas Boyce and his colleagues raised several important questions regarding infections in children. They wrote,

> Despite major advances in the microbiology of respiratory disease, why and how a child becomes ill remain poorly understood. In over half of respiratory illnesses, complete cultures fail to yield an etiologic [infectious or causative] agent. Conversely, 30 percent of a school-age population can harbor group A *Streptococci* without developing symptoms, three-quarters of preschool children infected with *Mycoplasma pneumoniae* remain asymptomatic, and as many as 42 percent of upper respiratory tract cultures from well children yield pneumococci.[375]

Dr. Boyce and his colleagues at the University of North Carolina at Chapel Hill believed that stressful events in the life of children played a role in why some children became sick while others exposed to the same infectious germs did not. They also theorized that having well-established routines such as waking, bathing, eating, napping, and playing at the same time each day would be protective against the adversity of stressful events.

They sought to test their hypothesis through a carefully designed study. Each child was scored on a "Life Events" test that looked at the relative degree of stress brought about by difficult life changes such as death of a grandparent, parental divorce, a move to a new city, and so on. (These were based on the original work by Holmes and Rahe, who developed the Social Readjustment Rating Scale.) Each child was then observed daily for signs of respiratory illness. In addition, nasopharyngeal cultures were taken to determine whether viruses or bacteria were present.

After factoring out all variables such as age, sex, race, income, and family size, the researchers found that "life change scores were significantly and independently predictive of the average *duration* of illness." Then a surprising finding emerged. High life change (or life event) scores *coupled with* rigid family routines were together related to the *severity* of illness. According to Boyce, "It appears that illnesses became more severe as the magnitude of life change and the strength of family routines jointly increased." Dr. Boyce was surprised to learn that routine helped to increase rather than decrease susceptibility to severe illness. The researchers concluded that:

- Life change was the strongest single predictor of how long a child stayed ill.
- Major life change in the setting of a highly ritualized family appeared to predispose to greater illness severity.
- Scores for life change and family routines had no noticeable influence on the growth of harmful bacteria or viruses from the respiratory tract in either health or disease.

While life changes and routine affected duration and severity of illness, they did not affect the presence of germs in the respiratory tract. In other words, bacteria and viruses were present in both high-stress and low-stress children, but the high-stress children suffered from more prolonged and severe illness.

This finding is similar to that of an earlier study in which sixteen families were followed for one year. Every three weeks each family member had a physical exam that included a throat culture for streptococcal bacteria. Family members also kept diaries documenting events that occurred during the one-year test period.

At the end of one year, researchers reviewed the data to determine whether there was an association between stressful life events and illness. They discovered that:

- Stress was four times more likely to precede an infection than to follow an infection.
- When throat cultures revealed a streptococcal infection, one-half of those under high stress became ill.
- Of the low-stress individuals with a positive strep culture, only one-fifth became ill.
- One out of four outbreaks of illness followed some form of family crisis.[376]

Scientists at the University of Rochester have looked at how family stress impacts the immunity of children. In this study, they examined parental psychiatric health, including symptoms of stress, anxiety, and depression. The total number of illnesses in the children was directly related the emotional distress reported by the parents. Immune activation in the children was also linked to stress in the parents.[377]

A study organized by investigators from the University of California at San Francisco Department of Medicine and Pediatrics was conducted on 236 three- to five-year-olds attending San Francisco child care centers. The researchers found that children who responded to challenging developmental tasks or familial stress with elevated blood pressure were more likely to develop childhood respiratory disease.[378]

In one of the largest studies of its kind, physicians from England and

Scotland studied 640 middle-aged and 582 elderly people to measure how stressful life events effected the mucosal antibody secretory IgA (sIgA). Recall that sIgA is a general antibody produced at the surface of the respiratory and digestive tract as a first line of defense against invading microbes.[379]

No one has gone so far as to say stress causes infections. But as the above studies show, stress and life events indeed have a significant impact on susceptibility to infection. Dr. Hans Selye offered this observation in 1978. He wrote, "If a microbe is in or around us all the time and yet causes no disease until we are exposed to stress, what is the 'cause' of our illness, the microbe or the stress? I think both are and equally so. In most instances the disease is due . . . to the inadequacy of our reactions against the germ."[380]

Stress and the Common Cold

The most universal affliction of humans—the common cold—also appears to be influenced by stress. When individuals were exposed to one of five common cold viruses, 90 percent of those under high stress became infected compared with only 74 percent of those under low stress. Of those in the low-stress group, only 27 percent actually became ill, in contrast to 47 percent of those in the high stress group, suggesting that stress nearly doubles the likelihood of becoming ill when exposed to a cold virus.[381]

Dr. Sheldon Cohen and his associates in the Department of Psychology at Carnegie Mellon University observed that the stress-infection connection occurred among three very different viruses (rhinovirus, coronovirus, and respiratory syncytial virus), leading them to conclude ". . . stress is associated with the suppression of a general resistance process in the host, leaving persons susceptible to multiple infectious agents . . . stress is associated with the suppression of many different immune processes, with similar results."[382]

Abuse and Illness

We are only beginning to understand the many ways in which humans are affected by abuse. One adverse effect of abuse seems to be an increase in susceptibility to disease. Tamerra P. Moeller and Gloria A. Bachmann of the University of Medicine and Dentistry of New Jersey measured the effects of childhood abuse on the rate of illness in women. Their findings showed that 53 percent of the women reported suffering one or more kinds of abuse as children (physical, emotional, or sexual). The women reporting abuse were more likely to report symptoms such as fatigue, insomnia, and headaches. They also reported more illness and required more hospitalization than did those not reporting a history of childhood abuse.[383]

Violent crimes such as rape may also cause adaptive changes to the immune system. When fifteen women reporting rape were compared with sixteen women who had no history of rape, there were notable differences in immune system function. Those reporting rape had higher cytotoxic T-cells, lower B-lymphocyte counts, decreased lymphocyte proliferation, and higher levels of pro-inflammatory immune proteins. These are signs of activation of the innate immune system and some suppression of adaptive immunity. In essence, there was a shift in the Th1 / Th2 balance.

Stress, Care-Giving, and Immunity

We have long known that the stress of caring for a loved one who has a protracted illness or medical condition can have a decidedly negative effect on the caregiver. But recent evidence of the effect of caregiving on immunity calls us to give greater attention to those who care for others. Scientists at the University of California, San Francisco (UCSF), set out to measure a set of features of immune cells (which are also present in other cells) called telomeres in fifty-eight women who were biological mothers of either a healthy child or a chronically ill child.

Telomeres are complex structures at the ends of chromosomes that protect the chromosome from degradation and foster completion of DNA replication at the chromosome ends. Shortening of telomeres is commonly associated with cellular aging. Each cell is capable of only a finite number of cell division cycles. After so many cycles of cell division, telomeric DNA has been depleted and cellular division can no longer take place. In the UCSF study, those caring for sick children had shorter telomeric DNA in their immune cells, suggesting that their immune cells had aged excessively.[384] There was also a striking 48 percent reduction in telomerase activity in the caregivers. Telomerase is an enzyme that is protective against excessive telomere shortening. In addition, markers of oxidative stress (isoprostane to vitamin E ratio) was much higher in the caregivers. Thus, caregivers had shorter telomeres, lower telomerase activity, and greater oxidative stress. We might say that there nerves were frayed and so were their chromosomes.

Some scientists have urged that we be careful as we interpret such studies, since measuring telomeres in complex cell populations like white blood cells can be tricky. However, a rare condition involving telomere shortening should give us pause. A condition called dyskeratosis congenita is associated with a 50 percent deficiency in telomerase RNA gene dosage. The individuals suffer from bone marrow failure and increased vulnerability to infection.[385] Also, people with early heart attacks had white blood cell telomere lengths that were similar to those of a person almost eleven years older.[386] This is about the level of increased cellular aging found in the caregiving mothers above.

Stress and Vaccine Success

If stress has an effect on our immune system, one way to test this effect would be to see whether people developed an appropriate level of antibodies in response to a vaccine while they were under stress. When a person receives a vaccine, the goal is that their immune system produces sufficient antibodies from the stimulation of the vaccine so that their immune system can defeat the real virus/bacteria should it come along in the future.

It is well known that elderly people have diminished immune systems and that they respond in less vigorous ways to vaccines in general. Their immune systems do not produce as many antibodies against the targeted microbe if they are under stress when the vaccine is given. This weakened response can last for many months.

The question is, do young healthy people under stress also have a reduced antibody production to vaccines? To answer this question, doctors at Carnegie-Mellon University in Pittsburgh, Pennsylvania enrolled eighty-three first-year college students with an average age of about eighteen years. Students were asked to report on their stress levels in a diary. Each person was given a vaccine containing the following viruses: New Caledonia, Panama, Victoria, and Yamanashi. The students were followed for four months, with doctors monitoring their blood for antibodies, saliva for cortisol, and diaries for stress profiles.

Those reporting the highest cumulative stress produced antibodies to the New Caledonia virus at a much slower rate than the lower stress group. Those reporting high stress also demonstrated lower antibody levels at the four-month period. The conclusion was that high stress did have an effect of lowering the antibody response to this one virus in young, healthy people. As for the other viruses in the vaccine, stress did not seem to have an effect on antibody response. However, it should be noted that not all students received the full complement of vaccine; only 65 percent and 35 percent received the Victoria and Yamanashi components of the vaccine.

This study then raised an interesting question. Can we determine why stress negatively affected the immune response to these vaccines? The simple guess would be cortisol. But in this study, causality was not that clear. What emerged from the analysis was that stress was linked with reduced quantity of sleep. But did stress *cause* the poor sleep or did poor sleep lead to more stressful days? I'll spare you the arduous statistical calculations and summarize by saying that it appears that stress and sleep work in both directions. Sleep affects stress and stress affects sleep. Scientists call this a feed-forward relationship, in which one begets the other; each promotes the other.[387]

Stressed-Out Students

Students in high school and college are commonly under persistent stress. When stress is coupled with the high expectations of self, parent, or other pressure, the effects on immunity can be pronounced.

Research conducted at Yale University by Stanislav Kasl and his colleagues lends support to this view. They looked at the enrollment and medical records of West Point cadets. Contained in the record was information about family history and background, including personal and parental expectations. The investigators were particularly interested in laboratory tests for Epstein-Barr virus, the cause of infectious mononucleosis. They wondered why some cadets infected with the virus became ill while others seemed unaffected.

The answer appeared to lie in the psychosocial record. Kasl found that the cadets who became ill shared three common features: The fathers were described as "overachievers;" the cadets were strongly committed to a military career; and the cadets were performing poorly academically. The combined effect of poor performance and high expectations seemed to increase the likelihood of succumbing to infection. Surprisingly, as academic rank went down, the severity of the infection went up.[388]

In conversations I've had with high school and college administrators, students who either take on too much or who perform below expectations often suffer tremendous stress, some of which results in physical symptoms. Many of these symptoms are gastrointestinal in nature. Some students are known to develop recurrent infections and even fevers of unknown origins. One way that persistent stress in students (or anyone) may impact health is by altering intestinal permeability.

Stress and Gut Barrier Defenses

As we've seen, increased leakiness of the gut permits transport of gut microbes or gut bacterial cell wall fragments, which can trigger an adverse immune response. Ongoing studies suggest that stress is another factor that can upset the barrier defenses of the intestines, leading to leaky gut.

In a study of rats, it was shown that one hour of stress per day led to migration of bacteria from the gut through the intestinal barrier defenses. Of particular interest in this study was the finding that the number of one type of white blood cell (called a mast cell) tripled in the portion of the small intestine known as the ileum, which suggests that a strong immune response accompanies the migration of these bacteria.[389]

A group at McMaster University in Ontario, Canada studied the affect of early psychological trauma on gut barrier function. They separated young rat pups from their mothers for three hours per day, for two weeks before weaning. In this study, maternal separation led to behavioral changes along with disruption of gut barrier function. The rats also had higher levels of the stress hormone cortisol. Of great interest was the finding that feeding the probiotics *L. rhamnosus* and *L. helveticus* "prevented the long term effects of maternal separation."[390]

In one of the more interesting studies of its kind, scientists wondered how a water-immersion stress would affect rats and whether a probiotic supplement might reduce the effects of this stress. In this study, rats were placed in a water-filled vessel and forced to float on a block of wood, while avoiding the water for one hour daily for ten days. Their response to this water avoidance test was compared with a control group. Another group of rats was fed a probiotic culture of *Lactobacillus rhamnosus* and *Lactobacillus helveticus* for seven days prior to the study and for the full ten days of the study.

It is known from previous studies that water avoidance stress facilitates the migration of harmful gut bacteria through the gut and into the lymph nodes. The scientists conducting this study wanted to learn whether the probiotics could reduce this occurrence. Consistent with other studies, 70 percent of the rats in the stress group had movement of gut bacteria into the lymph nodes (mesenteric lymph nodes). As predicted, no bacteria were found in the lymph nodes of the unstressed control group. In the rats pretreated with probiotic bacteria, migration of gut bacteria to the lymph nodes was prevented. Probiotics also prevented the other gut bacteria from adhering to the cells that line the intestines.

These findings confirm previous work that water avoidance stress in animals leads to migration of gut bacteria into the lymph nodes. This implies that stress harms the barrier defenses in the gut, permitting gut microbes to end up inside the body, which becomes a substantial challenge to the immune system. The study also showed that probiotics might mitigate or reduce the effects of stress on the gut barrier defenses.[391]

Studies have looked at stress and gut bacteria in humans as well. In one study, there was a 20 to 30 percent increase of *Bacteroides fragilis* in the guts of people responding to anger or fearful situations.[392] Studies have found that an immune protein known as secretory immunoglobulin A (sIgA), an immune protein that protects the gut mucosa, is depressed in college students during or shortly after taking exams. The fact that sIgA is lowered during stress may be one reason that gut defenses diminish during stress.[393] Another reason for weakening gut defense and bacterial overgrowth during stress may be related to the stress compounds epinephrine and norepinephrine (adrenaline compounds) that are produced during stress.

Can Stress Make Bacteria More Dangerous?

When we are under stress, levels of stress compounds such as norepinephrine increase in our bodies. These levels also increase in the intestinal tract, which is part of a network that accounts for almost 50 percent of the adrenaline produced in the entire body (the mesenteric organs).[394] New research suggests that norepinephrine can stimulate the growth of a range of harmful bacteria in the gut. In one study, for example, the common gut-infecting bacteria *Campylobacter jejuni* was found to be more invasive in the presence of norepinephrine.[395]

At the University of Texas Southwestern Medical Center, Dr. Vanessa Sperandio has been studying the harmful forms of *E. coli* that can infect our gut. Among these is the notorious *E. coli* O157:H7, which is known to cause severe kidney damage and even death. It is most well known for contaminating improperly cooked hamburger and causes illness in over seventy thousand people in the U.S. each year. Her group found that epinephrine helps to alert this form of *E. coli* that it is in the intestinal tract, which seems to trigger the *E. coli* to activate its virulence (harm-causing) genes.[396]

Another bacterium that can have severe effects on us is called *Pseudomonas aeruginosa*. In fact, this microbe has been found to prove fatal in some 40 percent of hospitalized patients who contract the infection. It appears that *P. aeruginosa* is another bacterium that is good at using the stress hormones epinephrine and norepinephrine to get a foothold in our intestines. The stress molecules are used by the bacteria to switch on their virulence genes, compete with our beneficial gut bacteria, and exact a severe toll on the body.[397]

It is a compelling thought that our own stress chemicals give the harmful organisms around us the advantage they need. On a positive note, this may mean that controlling the stress response or blocking the release of our stress compounds could be a means by which we strengthen our defenses against harmful microbes.

Stress and the Cortisol Response

Scientists have known of the adverse effects of excess cortisol on health for decades. Our understanding of the details of cortisol's adverse effects on the immune system continues to grow. Without going into great depth on the effects of cortisol on immunity, it does bear mentioning its effect on the Th1/Th2 balance. Recall that these two "poles" of the adaptive immune response are based on the T-helper lymphocyte profile. When the ratio is skewed, it can raise susceptibility to acute and chronic infections, as well as to allergy and autoimmune disease. There is now evidence that cortisol can cause selective suppression of the Th1-cellular immunity axis and forge a shift toward the Th2-dominated humoral immunity.

As noted by Dr. Ilia Elenkov at the National Institute of Mental Health in Bethesda, Maryland, "A major factor governing outcome of infectious diseases is the selection of Th1- versus Th2-predominant adaptive responses during and after the initial invasion of the host [the person]."* Dr. Elenkov also notes that epinephrine and norepinephrine, (which are also produced under stress, as mentioned above) cause a shift toward the Th2 pole of immunity. Dr. Elenkov states that "the Th2 shift may have a profound effect on the susceptibility of the organism to an infection, and/or may influence its course. Thus, stress has a substantial effect on the defense system where cellular immunity mechanisms have a primary role."[398]

But immunity shifted toward Th2 is not the only potential problem. In people with an underactive (or hypoactive) stress responses, the balance can tip toward Th1-dominance, which is seen in such autoimmune conditions like type I diabetes, multiple sclerosis, rheumatoid arthritis, and autoimmune thyroid disease.[399]

---

*This refers to the initial invasion of the person by a bacterium, for instance.

How Leaky Gut May Alter Mood and Energy

While the effects of stress on fostering conditions of a leaky gut have been documented, there is also now evidence that mood disorders like depression may be triggered or aggravated by leaky gut and by gut bacteria. To explain why, it bears repeating a concept we've explored previously. When the integrity of the intestinal mucosa (lining) is breached or compromised, it permits the passage of LPS (lipopolysaccharides) endotoxins, which are fragments from the outer membrane of the cell walls of dead gram-negative bacteria that live in the gut. Once inside the bloodstream, these LPS endotoxins provoke an inflammatory immune reaction that can have systemwide effects on the body and, in this case, influence the brain.

Dr. Michael Maes of Belgium and his colleagues at Vanderbilt University wanted to understand the role that leaky gut and LPS endotoxins might have in major depression. To do this, they measured blood levels of antibodies against LPS endotoxins of six different kinds of gram-negative gut bacteria. Remember, antibodies are Y-shaped proteins that the immune system produces *en mass* when harmful microbes and fragments of microbes breach our boundaries. If people with depression had more antibodies against the cell wall fragments of these gut bacteria, it would mean that the gut was leaky enough to permit passage of these fragments into the bloodstream, and might imply that depression was related in some way (or perhaps in some people) to leaky gut.

Dr. Maes' group found that the levels of IgA and IgM antibodies against the gut-derived bacterial fragments were "significantly greater in patients with major depressive disorder than in normal volunteers." The symptoms reported by those with depression included fatigue, autonomic and gastro-intestinal symptoms, and a subjective feeling of infection. Dr. Maes went on to remark,

> The results show that intestinal mucosal dysfunction characterized by an increased translocation of gram-negative bacteria (leaky gut) plays a

> role in the inflammatory pathophysiology of depression. It is suggested that the increased LPS translocation may mount an immune response and thus IRS [inflammatory response system] activation in some patients with major depressive disorder (MDD) and may induce specific "sickness behaviour" symptoms. It is suggested that patients with MDD should be checked for leaky gut by means of the IgM and IgA panel used in the present study and accordingly should be treated for leaky gut.[400]

Another study looked at leaky gut and chronic fatigue symptoms. Using the same method of measuring IgA and IgM antibodies against gut-derived bacterial cell wall fragments, Dr. Maes' group studied patients with symptoms including irritable bowel, muscular tension, fatigue, concentration difficulties, and failing memory. Their assessment also included the FibroFatigue Scale.

They found that blood values "for serum IgA against the LPS endotoxins of enterobacteria are significantly greater in patients with chronic fatigue syndrome than in normal volunteers and patients with partial chronic fatigue syndrome. Serum IgA levels were significantly correlated to the severity of illness."

In summary, they wrote "The results show that enterobacteria [gut bacteria] are involved in the etiology [cause] of chronic fatigue syndrome and that an increased gut (intestinal) permeability has caused an immune response to the LPS endotoxins of gram-negative enterobacteria."[401]

It is really quite fascinating to consider that leaky gut and migrating gut bacterial fragments might contribute to depression and to symptoms of fatigue. It certainly fits with the growing research on how bacterial cell wall fragments passing through a leaky gut can alter the systemic immune response and even complicate things like surgery and heart failure. All findings of this type point us toward evaluating gut integrity in disorders that have previously been thought to have little association with the gut—at least according to our old paradigms.

But if the leaky gut is involved in depression or chronic fatigue, we should expect an improvement in these conditions if the leaky gut condition is repaired. Dr. Maes and his group recently reported on their work with a thirteen-year-old girl with chronic fatigue. She was found to have high blood levels of IgM antibodies against endotoxins (LPS) of certain gut bacteria along with other signs of immune activation and inflammation. She was treated with specific antioxidants and a diet aimed at repairing the leaky gut. She was also given intravenous immunoglobulins. The result: the passage of intestinal LPS into her bloodstream was reduced, which lead to "a complete remission of the CFS symptoms."[402]

How Infection May Alter Mood

The findings of Dr. Maes' group on the effect of gut bacterial fragments on mood is compelling because it fits with a phenomenon long known to doctors as "sickness behavior." It is widely known that when the body is fighting infection, it engages in a range of behaviors such as decreased appetite, fatigue, altered sleep, irritability, depressed mood, and loss of mental clarity. It is now known that some of these behaviors are driven by immune proteins like cytokines.

What has become increasingly clear is that "sickness behaviors" can carry over for long periods of time, long after some infections have seemingly resolved. These behaviors would manifest in the form of altered mood and include symptoms like fatigue, social withdrawal, loss of appetite, and anxiety. In other words, the carryover from an infection episode can affect mood long after the infection. More precisely, past or current infections may alter mood in a manner that affects our ability to cope with stressful stimuli.

We explored one possible reason for a kind of persistent sickness behavior in Chapter 5, where I noted the amino acid tryptophan can be depleted with some infections. When tryptophan is low we cannot make adequate adequate amounts of the neurotransmitter serotonin, which has a powerful effect on mood. Also, the immune proteins called cytokines can remain altered or elevated in the body for long periods. Past infections can also leave the Th1 / Th2 balance of the immune system altered, which may have lasting effects. This is of particular concern in people with digestive disorders, autoimmune disorders, obesity, diabetes, and other conditions with heightened or inflammatory immune activation.

Stress and the Immune System

It was not long ago that doctors believed the immune system operated completely independent of all other body systems. As research began to support a link between mind and immunity, however, it became evident that thoughts, feelings, and images have a direct impact upon immune function. But how?

Many researchers were stunned by the discovery that the immune system is "hard wired" to the nervous system. Nerve fibers of the autonomic nervous system—our automatic pilot—branch directly into the tissue of the lymph nodes, spleen, bone marrow, and thymus gland. They are in *direct communication* with pools of white blood cells. Moreover, white blood cells have been shown to possess receptors on their surfaces for neurochemicals such as adrenaline and noradrenaline.

Scientists once believed that these neurochemicals acted *only* on nerves, That they were the messengers that carried information from nerve cell to nerve cell. With the remarkable finding of a direct neurochemical link between the nervous and immune systems came profound implications for our understanding of health and disease. Mind and immunity are connected. The brain and immune system are engaged in constant dialogue. The immune system increasingly seems to act like a "wandering nervous system" that is inextricably linked to our state of mind.

This brings us back to the concept of the immune system as a sensory organ, much like the eyes. Does the immune system "see" microbes and alert the host defense network? As noted immunologist Dr. Mark Davis reflects,

> Lymphocytes and NK [natural killer] cells can be viewed as cell-sized sensory organs, continuously sampling the internal environment for things that do not belong there or for cellular stress or aberrations. Just as rod cells in the eye can detect even a single photon [of light], cytotoxic T-cells can kill on the advice of only three peptide-MHC ligands.[403]

So, if stressors affect our defenses via the interplay of our immune and nervous systems, we should be able to take conscious action to modify this interaction. Indeed, this is where a range of human attributes and strategies bring control of immunity within our reach.

Chapter 11

Coping Strategies That Make Us Strong

We have a tremendous amount of control over how stress affects our defenses and, ultimately, our lives. This is the inspiring truth hidden within the rather gloomy research on stress and immunity.

Stressors are most certainly an inevitable part of life. But many features of our personality, habits, coping strategies, and outlook will shape the way in which stressors ultimately affect our immune defense, energy, and repair. In one respect, how we choose to translate the events in our lives will have a profound influence on whether stress depletes our defenses.

In this chapter, we'll explore some of the human traits that seem to allow us to thrive and even grow in the face of difficult times. We'll also examine a handful of intriguing findings that not only seem to support robust immunity, but that also make life more enjoyable. It appears celebrating life could be the road toward strong defenses.

Perception and Control

How we look at things and how we translate events for ourselves have powerful effects on our physiology. More precisely, our *perception* may be one of the most critical determinants of how we respond to stress. For instance, while deer probably fear cougars, people seem to fear public speaking. In fact, in surveys of what people say they fear most, public speaking is always listed at the top (well ahead of fear of heights and even death). Someone unaccustomed to public speaking may begin to develop anxiety attacks months in advance of the speaking date. As the date approaches, the anxiety grows. Some individuals are so affected, they become ill. They perceive public speaking as a threatening experience.

On the other hand, seasoned speakers look forward to speaking engagements as an opportunity to share their ideas, challenge the crowd, and explore things about which they are most passionate. To them, speaking in public is just part of their job or a means to advance a social cause. To them, speaking is exhilarating, not stressful.

One important influence on our perception and how we experience stress is our sense of control. A now-classic study illustrates how profoundly control may affect us. Two groups of people were exposed to an annoying, stress-inducing noise. One group was exposed to the noise with no means to reduce or control it. The other group was told that if they pushed a button on the arm of their chair, the noise would be reduced.

Subjects in the second group were unaware that the button had no affect on the noise level whatsoever. However, the stress response of the two groups was dramatically different. The group able to push the button, even though the button had no effect on the noise, suffered far fewer symptoms of stress than the other group. The apparent reason: they believed they had control over their environment and the belief translated into real bodily changes.[404]

One's susceptibility to infection may also be affected by the level of power they are given or of their perception of power in a given circumstance. Individuals who have past or present experiences being told "you won't be able to do that," or "you'll never amount to anything," or "you're no good," often feel that they have limited capability. This is often referred to as self-efficacy. When confronted with tasks that are challenging or unfamiliar, such persons come under extreme emotional stress. Fearful that they will not perform or that they will be reprimanded if they perform poorly, they withdraw. In one study, such persons with a low feeling of self-efficacy were found to produce increased levels of adrenal hormones when asked to perform a difficult task. The amount of stress hormone released was often dependent upon the person's *perceived* ability to perform the task.[405]

Perception of our own health status can have an equally dramatic effect on our well-being. Researchers posed the following question to 2,800 people over the age of 65, "At the present time, how would you rate your health: excellent, good, fair, poor or bad?" It was discovered that men who answered "excellent" were nearly seven times as likely to be alive four years later than men in apparently similar states of health who answered "poor" or "bad." Women who answered "excellent" were more than seven times as likely to be alive as similar women who answered "poor" or "bad."

According to Dr. Ellen Idler, health and aging researcher at Rutgers University, similar studies comparing self-perception with the results of complete physical exams have led to similar findings in people of all ages.[406,407] These findings suggest, in essence, that even though two people might be similar in their "actual" physical health, one who perceives her health as excellent may live longer and experience better health, while one who perceives her health as "poor" or "bad" may suffer more illness and die sooner.

Coping and the Art of Letting Go

One of the most successful tools for coping with our lives appears to be the ancient but simple act of confession. James W. Pennebaker, professor of psychology at Southern Methodist University (SMU) in Dallas, has made a career of studying the effect of disclosure on health. He has shown that those who share their deepest feelings about past or present trauma are better able to cope and are healthier than those who do not share such feelings.

The two most common means of confession are talking and writing. In a study at SMU, Dr. Pennebaker asked his freshmen students to write about their deepest anxieties and their feelings about the dramatic changes involved in beginning college. He calls this "power coping." Those students who wrote about their current anxieties had fewer illnesses and visits to the doctor over the next four months. Those who wrote about only trivial or superficial topics showed a gradual increase in visits to the doctor.

Pennebaker wondered if such a decrease in illness was due to an actual increase in immune vigilance. In another study, he and his colleagues actually measured the activity of T-cells, important in protecting us from infectious disease. His group found that those who wrote about past trauma had an increase in T-cell activity. Subjects who wrote about trauma they had not previously shared with anyone had the most dramatic rise in T-cell activity. As expected, those who wrote about traumas also had a decrease in visits to the health center.

Dr. Pennebaker has also investigated the role of using words such as I, me, my, or mine (personal pronouns) in expressive writing. He has shown that this has additional benefits to health. Dr. Pennebaker wrote that "Flexibility in the use of common words—particularly personal pronouns—when writing about traumatic memories was related to positive health outcomes. The findings point to the importance of the role of discussing the self and social relationships in writing . . ."[408]

Our General Emotional Expressiveness

While confession seems to have powerful effects on the body, our general emotional expressiveness deeply influences how we heal. Mind/body researcher Lydia Temoshok, PhD, examined the psychological factors associated with the skin cancer malignant melanoma. She discovered that emotional expressiveness was directly related to the thickness of the patients' tumors as well as the course of their disease.[409]

Temoshok's research revealed that:[410]

- Patients who were less emotionally expressive had thicker tumors and more rapidly dividing cancer cells.
- Patients who were more emotionally expressive had thinner tumors and more slowly dividing cancer cells.
- Patients who were less expressive had relatively fewer lymphocytes invading the base of the tumor (suggesting weaker defenses)
- The more emotionally expressive patients had a much higher number of lymphocytes (immune cells) invading the base of the tumor.

So what happens when we deliberately try to suppress emotions? Scientists studying this question in healthy men found that deliberate suppression of emotion led to significant decreases in a white blood cell called CD3T lymphocytes—a sign that the immune system suffers when we suppress our emotions. Those who wrote about their feelings experienced an increase in CD4 cells called T-helpers.[411]

What Do Optimists Know That Others Don't?

A pessimist has been described as "someone who, when confronted with two unpleasant alternatives, selects both."[412] Taking this definition a step further, you might say that an optimist is one who, when confronted with these alternatives chooses neither, diminishes their significance, or finds the positive possibilities in each. *The American Heritage Dictionary* defines an optimist as one who usually expects a favorable outcome.

Optimism is increasingly being viewed as an important part of a healthy immune system, while pessimism appears to be associated with lowered immunity. In an oft-cited study, researchers at the University of Michigan studied the effects of optimism and pessimism on the health of Harvard University graduates who were first interviewed in 1946 and followed for thirty-five years. Subjects were asked about difficult experiences encountered in World War II. The accounts were classified as global ("It will ruin my whole life"), stable ("It will never go away"), or internal ("It was all my fault"). Those with negative or pessimistic interpretations of their experiences were found to be consistently sicker than their more optimistic peers.

The leader of this study, Dr. Christopher Peterson, listed a number of reasons why pessimism may contribute to more frequent illness:

- Pessimism may be linked to poor problem-solving ability and therefore to serious problems—hence, vulnerability to illness.
- Pessimism may lead to social withdrawal, behavior also associated with illness.
- Pessimism-related helplessness may affect immune function.

There is also direct evidence that optimists enjoy better immune function than pessimists. In their book *Healthy Pleasures,* David Sobel, MD, and Robert Ornstein, PhD, report that when the blood of optimists is compared with that of pessimists, the optimists have higher levels of T-helper cells in relation to T-suppressors. Recall that T-helper cells stimulate immune function while T-suppressors suppress immune function. A high "helper" to "suppressor" ratio is desirable since resistance to infection and other illness would be enhanced.[413]

Martin Seligman, PhD, director of the University of Pennsylvania Positive Psychology Center, is a leading researcher in the study of the effects of optimism on immune function. His observations after decades of extensive research include the following:

- Pessimists make twice as many visits to the doctor as optimists.
- Pessimists have *twice* as many infectious diseases as optimists.
- Optimists have more active and more efficient immune systems.
- Pessimism often leads to depression, which causes a downturn in immune function.
- Major life changes can cause a decrease in immune function. In optimists the effects are less severe than in pessimists.
- Statistically, pessimists encounter more negative life events. The

> more bad life events we encounter, the more illness we will likely experience.

According to Seligman, "If your level of pessimism can deplete your immune system, it seems likely that pessimism can impair your physical health over your whole life span."[414]

Our Changing View of Optimism, Pessimism, and Immunity

Through the late '90s, it seemed as though optimism was winning out as a trait that bolstered immunity and forestalled disease. But the cautionary voices of that time have gained momentum, showing that the matter is not so simple. It seems that optimism can sometimes have a *negative* effect on the immune system.

Dr. Suzanne Segerstrom at the University of Kentucky has proposed that the complex response of the immune system in optimists may be related to the so-called *engagement* hypothesis. She summarizes the hypothesis as follows:

> Under difficult circumstances, more optimistic people remain engaged with those circumstances, whereas more pessimistic people disengage, avoid, or give up. Giving up can be a physiologically protective response because stressor exposure is minimized in the short term by giving up rather than remaining engaged (although the reverse is true in the long term).
>
> [T]he engagement hypothesis states that when circumstances are easy or straightforward, optimism will be positively related to immunity because engagement can lead to termination of the stressor (e.g., via problem-solving). However, when circumstances are difficult or complex, optimism will be negatively related to immunity because it leads to ongoing engagement with persistent stressors.[415]

To illustrate, we might contrast two individuals in a hostile work environment with a critical, punitive boss and little social support. For each individual, the work may be highly stressful. The pessimist may be more likely to see the situation as hopeless and leave the job before the effects on his or her health become too severe. The optimist might, however, expect that with time and hard work, the situation could be improved or conquered in some fashion. While this is sometimes the case, not all situations can be fixed. The optimist may remain engaged in the work situation far longer, with the whole circumstance taking a greater toll on his health than on the pessimist who may have left the job long ago.

Does Optimism Help or Hinder Immunity?

It would seem, then, that the effect of optimism on immunity is related to circumstances, our perception of those circumstances, and to our choices within those circumstances. According to the work of Drs. Seligman, Segerstrom, and others, optimism can surely bolster and support the immune system in the face of many types of psychological stressors. Segerstrom writes,

> How optimism affects the immune system critically depends on the circumstances being examined. Under many circumstances, both dispositional optimism and specific expectancies appear to buffer the immune system from the effects of psychological stressors. However, there is sometimes a physiological cost to be paid for the optimistic strategy of engaging difficult stressors rather than disengaging and withdrawing. This physical cost is reflected in higher cortisol as well as lower cellular immunity. This especially appears to be true in the short term. Whether optimism appears to hinder or impair the immune system, seems related to circumstances in which the person remains engaged—when withdrawal and disengagement might be best.

Thus, to the question of whether optimism helps or hinders the immune system, Dr. Segerstrom replies with a definitive "Yes."

Positive Emotional Style

Psychologists constantly try to refine their description of human personality traits in an effort to better understand human beings. This is one reason why there are varying schools of thought and varying definitions of human attributes. In the last chapter, we explored the effect of stress on those exposed to the common cold virus. In an ongoing series of studies, Dr. Cohen and his colleagues made a number of refinements to consider something called Positive Emotional Style (PES) and Negative Emotional Style (NES).

According to Dr. Cohen's group,

> We found that the tendency to express positive emotions was associated with greater resistance to developing a cold. We also found that PES was associated with fewer self-reported symptoms after removing the possible contributions of objective illness. Both of these associations were independent of negative emotional style (NES), the cognitive and social dispositions associated with PES, and self-reported health. These results indicate that positive emotions play a larger and more important role in disease risk and health complaints than previously believed.[416]

Following these studies, colleagues expressed concerns about the claim that emotional style had the strength of effect claimed by Dr. Cohen's group, so his study was replicated with additional controls. Dr. Cohen's follow up work added confirmation to their theory on the effects of positive emotional style. They wrote,

> For both viruses, increased positive emotional style (PES) was associated with lower risk of developing an upper respiratory illness as defined by objective criteria and with reporting fewer symptoms than expected from concurrent objective markers of illness. These associations were independent of pre-challenge virus-specific antibody, virus type, age, sex, education, race, body mass, season, and NES. They were also independent of optimism, extraversion, mastery, self-esteem, purpose, and self-reported health. We replicated the prospective association of PES and

colds and PES and biased symptom reporting, extended those results to infection with an influenza virus, and "ruled out" alternative hypotheses. These results indicate that PES may play a more important role in health than previously thought.[417]

Love and Trust

Our capacity for love and trust may also influence our defenses. One of the most prominent researchers in this area was the late Dr. David McClelland of Harvard and Boston University. McClelland set out to unravel some of the health effects of love and intimacy, and through many years of scientific study had discovered that some of the effects can be quantified.

McClelland found that people who pursued relationships without excessive anxiety or fervor, something called *relaxed desire for affiliation,* had stronger immune systems. Those who prioritized relationships also suffered from fewer and less severe bouts of illness.

McClelland then studied three different groups of people looking at immune cells called natural killer cells (NK), sentinels that eliminate cancer cells and microbes. Higher NK cell activity is a desirable trait. McClelland found that people with relaxed affiliation had much higher NK cell activity compared to those in whom personal power was more important than relationships.

McClelland and his colleague James McKay unearthed a new (at that time) force in their attempt to describe the biological effects of love, which they called affiliative trust. Affiliative trust was defined as *the desire for positive, loving relationships based on mutual respect and trust.* Individuals with high affiliative trust were found to have higher T-helper/suppressor ratios. This, again, is a sign of a robust immune system. They also found these same people had significantly less illness.[418]

In one of the most interesting studies, McClelland and his colleagues followed a group of adults for ten years. Of those with affiliative *mis-*

trust, a striking 59 percent contracted a major illness over the ten-year period. Affiliative mistrust reflected a more cynical view of relationships and was common among those who preferred personal power over loving relationships. Only 30 percent of those with high affiliative trust contracted a major illness over the same period. In essence, McClelland found that those motivated by loving relationships had half the rate of major illness.[419]

Staying Connected: Social Support and Meaningful Relationships

Human beings have always relied on a close-knit social structure for survival. Social groups were important for gathering food and for protection. But there was more to the social group than fulfillment of physical needs. Close social networks provided stability and support for every group member during good times as well as during times of pain and deprivation. Following the death of a loved one, grieving tribal members were supported by the group. During illness, the sick were cared for not only by the healer (or shaman), but by parents, grandparents, and other tribal members. During childbirth, mothers were supported by the "wise women" of the tribal group. This social support network provided the greatest insurance for survival of individuals and the group as a whole.

Having stable social ties apparently helps us resist disease even when known risk factors to disease are present. In the Surgeon General's report on smoking released in 1975, it was shown that there were 1,560 deaths per 100,000 people in those who smoked 20-plus cigarettes per day compared to only 762 deaths for nonsmokers. After careful analysis of the data, biophysicist Harold Moskowitz made a startling discovery. Divorced *nonsmokers* suffered nearly the same death rate (1,420) as did married smokers. In smokers who were divorced, the death rate climbed to 2,675.[420] What was it about marriage that seemed to be protective?

For many years, we've known that the Japanese had lower rates of heart disease than Americans. It was shown decades ago that Japanese moving to the United States developed heart disease at roughly the same rate as their American counterparts. This has been attributed primarily to differences in dietary habits between Americans and Japanese and has been supported by much research.

However, recent studies of the Japanese provide a surprising twist. Japanese men who emigrated to the United States, *but retained strong social ties and links to Japanese culture,* suffered from far lower rates of heart disease than their Japanese cohorts who did not retain such ties. This was despite a relatively high-fat diet, high serum cholesterol, high blood pressure, cigarette smoking, and alcohol consumption among many of the Japanese emigrés.[421]

It is clear that close personal relationships are important to good health and even the number of relationships may bear on our health. Scientists at Carnegie-Mellon University infected 276 healthy volunteers with rhinovirus, a virus that causes the common cold. All people became infected, but not all people became sick. Those reporting the fewest types of relationships (only one to three types of relationships) were more than four times as likely to develop a cold than those with six or more types of relationships.[422]

Relationships were broken down into the following types: relationship with a spouse, a parent, in-laws, children, schoolmates, religious groups, etc. Having multiple kinds of relationships was more important than the actual number of people with whom an individual had a relationship.

In a now-famous Harvard study, students were asked back in the mid-fifties about how they felt about their parents. Questionnaires were scored based on a scale of 1 (strained and cold) to 4 (very close). Feelings about mother and father were considered separately and together.

A startling 100 percent of those who rated both mother and father low in warmth were diagnosed with diseases in mid-life. Of those who rated both parents high in warmth, only 47 percent had diagnosed disease. The researchers offered this assessment: "The perception of love itself may turn out to be a core biopsychosocial-spiritual buffer . . ."

Students were also asked, "What kind of person is your mother (or father)?" Ninety-five percent of those who used few positive words and rated their parents low in parental caring had diseases diagnosed in mid-life. Of those who used many positive words and rated their parents high in parental caring, only 29 percent were diagnosed with a disease in mid-life.[423]

The powerful effect of close personal relationships on health may even be strong enough to overshadow some of the traditional disease risk factors such as high-fat diets and smoking. In the landmark Roseto study, residents of that town had strikingly lower rates of heart disease even though they shared the very same risk factors as adjacent communities. Roseto had been settled in the late 1800s by Italian immigrants who retained very close social, religious, and community ties. In the sixties and seventies, the face of the community and its cohesive social structure changed dramatically. With this shift came a significant increase in death due to heart disease, which became similar to that of neighboring towns.[424]

The power of connection may explain the results of a study of 350 men and 192 women in which scientists measured cortisol and looked at coping styles. The study showed that people who had *adaptive coping styles* had lower levels of cortisol over the course of a day. Adaptive coping was described as coping by problem engagement and by seeking support from others.[425]

We should also remember the work of Dr. Steve Cole and his team at UCLA, who studied gene expression in a group of people described as either "high-lonely" or "low-lonely." He found that gene expression was different in 209 sites on the genome of lonely people compared to those not classified as lonely. A large portion of these sites were associated with immune cell and immune protein regulation.[426]

While strong social ties and a close-knit support network appear to protect us from illness, there are obvious risks as well. According to Robert Ornstein, PhD, and David Sobel, MD,

> . . . social support is not a cure-all. Maintaining one's health is not as simple as four hugs a day or to smile and say 'have a nice day' to everyone. In fact, relationships can have their negative side. The more family members or close friends one has, the more vulnerable one is to experience the loss of a loved one. Relationships can be financially and emotionally draining; just ask the spouse of an alcoholic or children caring for invalid parents.[427]

The Power of Beliefs

Perhaps nothing illustrates the influence of mind over bodily function more aptly than the placebo effect. Placebo means literally "to please." A placebo is a substance that lacks intrinsic or remedial value, done or given to pacify or satisfy someone. It works because the recipient believes it has value. The placebo effect has long been considered a nuisance in medical research. It "gets in the way" of our attempts to study drugs and medical procedures. Only recently have scientists begun to investigate the implications of the placebo response as it relates to how and why we become ill. In reality, we should understand the mystery behind the placebo effect and harness its power to our advantage, much like the shamans of old.

Two cases illustrate nicely the power of the mind working through the placebo effect. Surgeons in Denmark performed an endolymphatic sac shunt on fifteen patients with Meniere's disease, a disease of the inner ear with symptoms of dizziness, deafness, and buzzing in the ear. These doctors also performed a placebo (sometimes called "sham") operation on fifteen more patients suffering from Meniere's disease.

After three years, roughly 70 percent of the subjects in each group experienced almost complete relief of their symptoms. According to the surgeons, the placebo effect was the most likely cause for improvement in these patients. The patients believed they were undergoing a beneficial surgery, thus there was a favorable outcome.[428,429]

In another instance, a patient suffering from nausea was told he would be given a new drug that would take care of his symptoms. Without his knowledge, he was given syrup of ipecac, a substance commonly used to *induce* nausea and vomiting. Within fifteen minutes his symptoms disappeared.[430] Beliefs can drive the immune system so severely that some people with asthma suffer full-blown attacks as a result of looking at artificial flowers.[431]

Beliefs are critical to the placebo effect. They are critical to the healing response. When we realize that we have control over our belief systems, we can begin to exert greater control over our lives and over our health.

Giving Mirth: Can Laughter Influence Immunity?

A short article about the health benefits of laughter appeared in *Mothering* magazine with the title "Giving Mirth."[432] It is a curious title because it associates laughter with the birth process. Giving birth is a jubilant event that brings new life into the world. When we "give mirth," do we also breathe new life into our cells, our mind, our outlook? The definition of mirth even sounds uplifting: Gladness and gaiety, especially when expressed by laughter; rejoicing or enjoyment, especially when expressed in merrymaking.[433] Giving mirth stimulates the senses. It relieves pain, reduces stress. It helps us, if only temporarily, forget our troubles.

For some, giving mirth has literally meant bringing a new life into the world. Norman Cousins, author of *Anatomy of an Illness,* attributed his recovery from a "terminal" disease in part to laughter. Hour after hour, day after day, Cousins viewed old comedy movies. Through his laughter, he claims to have given birth to a new body and mind from what was once a diseased and dying human being.[434]

Researchers from all walks of medicine are beginning to examine the healing powers of humor and laughter. Lee S. Berk, DHSc, MPH, of Loma Linda University, has discovered some of the reasons why laughter so efficiently reverses the adverse effects of stress. He has found that levels of adrenaline (epinephrine) and cortisol drop significantly following a good laugh. This results in relaxation of muscles and blood vessels and improvement in immune function. Laughter, it appears, activates natural killer cells and T-lymphocytes, cells that help destroy harmful microbes. Laughter also seems to increase the production of the immune protein gamma-interferon. The research of Lee and others shows that humor contributes to greater optimism, cooperation, and socialization—all aspects of a healthy self and a healthy society.[435]

Dr. Kathleen Dillon of Western New England College measured the levels of salivary IgA (an immunoglobulin) concentrations in students before and after viewing humorous and nonhumorous video tapes. Salivary IgA is a substance that protects against viral infections. Her work showed that those viewing humorous videos increased their IgA levels, while those viewing nonhumorous videos experienced no change. Dr. Dillon also observed that those who used humor as a means of coping with difficult life situations had higher levels of IgA initially.[436]

Laughter was also studied in relation to antimicrobial peptides (AMPs). Recall that AMPs are proteins naturally produced by the cells of our skin, lungs, digestive tract, and immune system that kill bacteria. It is part of our natural or innate immunity. Dermicidin (DCD) is an AMP produced by the sweat glands and is known to be depleted in some conditions like eczema, rendering people more susceptible to skin infection. In this study, twenty patients with eczema volunteered to have their sweat collected before and after viewing an 87-minute humorous video. Levels of dermicidin-derived peptide were found to be significantly higher after viewing the video, when compared with the starting levels. This study raises an interesting question of whether humor or laughter could be used to raise the competency of the skin barrier defenses in eczema, but also begs the question as to the merits of humor and laughter as a means of fostering stronger immunity as a preventive measure.[437]

So, can laughter be transferred to the cells of our immune system? Are there sad and happy cells? Consider the remarks of author and physician Deepak Chopra:

> Outfitted with a vocabulary to mirror the nervous system's in its complexity, the immune system apparently sends and receives messages that are just as diverse. In fact, if being happy, sad, thoughtful, excited, and so on all require the production of ehydroepiand and neurotransmitters in our brain cells, then the immune cells must also be happy, sad, thoughtful, excited—indeed, they must be able to express the full range of 'words' that neurons do.[438]

Forgiveness: Freedom to Live in the Present

In Chapter 10, I explored the effects of stress on immune function and I noted in this chapter that circumstances can be stressful or not depending upon the way in which we meet those circumstances. Quite often, this involves the way in which we internally translate, interpret, or describe a situation. Resentment and an urge for vengeance can cloud such translation.

According to Dr. Michael McCullough in his book *Beyond Revenge,* forgiveness and revenge exist as a natural part of human nature (though he acknowledges the high cost of acting out on the impulse for revenge). He argues that while revenge is a problem today, for our ancestors it was a solution, potentially serving protective functions. His work supposes that if we exclude the notion of revenge as a "disease" or a "poison," with forgiveness as the "antidote," we are free to put both in an appropriate context and better recognize where forgiveness fits in.[439]

While his view may seem counter to the prevailing view, his positions are well-documented with studies across disciplines. In recognition of the inherent value of forgiveness, McCullough takes the position that the capacity to forgive arose "because it helped our ancestors preserve relationships with genetic relatives and other valuable relationship partners." He merely argues that we recognize the evolutionary value of both revenge and forgiveness, and take those into consideration when dealing with difficult issues.

Psychologist Marshall Rosenberg has been a strong advocate of the view that the impulse for vengeance is a "plea for empathy."[440] Dr. Rosenberg has mediated and negotiated with groups in some of the most strife-torn regions of the world; Rwanda, South Africa, Bosnia, Palestine, East Timor, and many others. In recognition of "vengeance as a plea for empathy," Dr. Rosenberg has used empathic listening, finding that the urge for vengeance is softened when empathy is shown to those who are in pain. His view is that lying beneath all urges for vengeance are unexpressed and unmet needs, such as a need for safety, a need for connection, a need to be heard, and potentially many other needs.

He has also noted that forgiveness becomes a more natural process when someone has received empathy and had the opportunity to express their needs. This view is consistent with the improvement in well-being experienced by those who express themselves through writing or talking, as in Dr. Pennebaker's experiments above. This is also not inconsistent with Dr. McCullough's view that revenge has some survival value. Perhaps the urge for vengeance is reminding us of the depth of our pain and the strength of unmet needs. If we are wise enough to recognize that it is our emotional pain that drives our urge for vengeance and that empathy may be what's needed, the powerful urge of vengeance could then be taken as a sign of our profound need for empathy and to express the depth of that pain. As Nelson Mandela has stated "Resentment is like drinking poison and then hoping it will kill your enemies."

So what does this all have to do with immune defense, energy, and repair? First, resentment, the urge for vengeance, and the pain that lies beneath them have the capacity to dramatically alter our ability to cope with many different circumstances. They can cause one to perceive a situation as threatening when the same situation may be perceived as entirely nonthreatening to another. Stress is strongly related to perception. Perhaps, then, there is merit in exploring forgiveness as means to ease our way through a stressful world.

Reasons We Forgive

How we forgive may be central to truly releasing us from the past. It may also be necessary to experience the most significant health benefits. Based on her interviews with divorced men and women, psychologist Mary Trainer has outlined three principle motives that people have for forgiveness. She labeled them expedient forgiveness, role-expected forgiveness, and intrinsic forgiveness.[441]

Expedient forgiveness is forgiving in order to get something. Examples might include wanting to get healthy, wanting a better reputation, or wanting to be perceived as generous.

Role-expected forgiveness is motivated by the expectations of others or God. We are told we "should" forgive. This kind of motivation is still outside ourselves, dictated by a higher authority. It is not internalized.

Intrinsic forgiveness is a free decision that flows from the heart. It is rooted in empathy—an understanding of the other person's struggles and humanity, an understanding that we too hurt others and are capable of doing what the one who has hurt us has done.

Trainer has argued that if we attempt to forgive for the first two reasons—expedient and role-expected—we will not experience true freedom from the pain of past injury. We will not experience the health benefits or the fullness of life if our motivations are not from deep within.

Dr. E. Worthington and colleagues have described their contemporary view of forgiveness as follows:

> One key distinction emerging in the literature is between *decisional* and *emotional forgiveness.* **Decisional forgiveness** is a behavioral intention to resist an unforgiving stance and to respond differently toward a transgressor. **Emotional forgiveness** is the replacement of negative unforgiving emotions with positive other-oriented emotions. Emotional forgiveness involves psychophysiological changes, and it has more direct health and well-being consequences. While some benefits of forgiveness and forgivingness emerge merely because they reduce unforgiveness, some benefits appear to be more forgiveness specific.[442] [emphasis added]

Decisional forgiveness could be viewed as being part of a strategy. Emotional forgiveness would seem to arise out of a process of receiving empathy and genuine expression, which leads to a more natural state of change. As Dr. Rosenberg is fond of saying, empathy must always precede strategy. So it is not surprising that emotional forgiveness, receiving empathy, or emotional expression must all be a part of the process of being freed from the vengeance impulse.

The Health Effects of Forgiveness

Dr. Judith Strasser studied the health effects of forgiveness in fifty-nine adults. Each described the painful hurts they had suffered in relation to a parent, a child, spouse, friend, or others. She discovered that the more her participants had forgiven the people who had hurt them, the better their physical health in older adulthood. She also learned that *expedient forgiveness* and *role-expected forgiveness* were not associated with health benefits. Only intrinsic forgiveness was related to improved health.[443]

The Templeton Foundation for Forgiveness Research has commissioned numerous studies on forgiveness and health. In one study, those who cultivated vengeful thoughts experienced increased blood pressure, muscle tension, and heart rate. When they focused on forgiveness, these measures of stress decreased. Scientists at VA Medical Center and Medical College in Tennessee found that people who suffered from chronic anxiety, depression, and anger had thicker blood due to higher red blood cell counts.

In a study at the University of Tennessee, people were separated by their scores on the Forgiving Personality Inventory. Those considered low forgivers experienced higher blood pressure (diastolic) and higher mean arterial pressure. The lower forgivers were also more aggressive. High forgivers, on the other hand, more freely expressed positive emotions, were more likely to give social support, and showed greater empathy.

Two key factors that foster forgiveness are closeness and empathy. Researchers have recently found that relationships that are closer, more affectionate, and more committed before a betrayal or hurt are more motivated to forgive. In addition, the ability to put oneself in the offending party's shoes, to experience empathy, is crucial to forgiveness.

The Practice of Gratitude

If perception influences our response to stressful life circumstances, then surely the capacity for gratitude influences our perception. While much of what I have explored previously has been put to the test in relation to its effect on immunity and infection, studies in the practice of gratitude are relatively few. But I believe that gratitude merits serious consideration because of its ability to redefine all of our experiences.

My own belief in this emerges from a spiritual upbringing, where gratitude was practiced every day through words and action. In fact, many prayers of thanks that are central to all religious traditions are practices of gratitude. Whether one is spiritual, religious, agnostic, or otherwise, the practice of gratitude seems to have a tremendous power to contribute to the enrichment of life. More recent research into the subject hints at positive biological effects of gratitude.

Dr. JoAnn Tsang and her colleagues at Baylor University have been studying gratitude in an effort to see how daily gratitude affects the well-being of the relatives and caregivers of people with Alzheimer's. First, recall the study shared earlier about the shortened telomeres of immune cells in those who must care for chronically ill children. Giving care to the chronically ill can be a deeply stressful experience with apparent immunological consequences.

Dr. Tsang recruited a group of caregivers of Alzheimer's patients and divided them into two groups. One group was to write daily about simple gripes and hardships they experienced each day. The other group was to write about things for which they were grateful. The study lasted two weeks. Those in the "gratitude" group wrote about simple victories such as being recognized or being called by name. At the end of this brief two-week period, those in the gratefulness group had an increased sense of well-being, with a reduced level of depression.[444]

In another study of gratitude, Dr. Barbara Frederickson of the University of Michigan had fortuitously collected emotional data on students four months prior to the New York City attacks of September 11, 2001. Students were asked to "think back to the September 11th attacks and the days that have passed since then," and report on how often they experienced each of twenty different emotions. This included emotions related to the attacks and those not related. The emotions included such things as anxious, angry, sad, joy, hope, and love. It should be noted that 72 percent of the participants evidenced clinically significant symptoms of depression following 9/11.

Of the twenty different emotions, gratitude was the second most commonly experienced (compassion was first). The resilient people were more likely to have expressed emotions of compassion and gratitude. Those expressing these emotions were least likely to have experienced symptoms of depression after the events.[445]

As mentioned previously, Kenneth Kendler has been studying twins for a very long time. In one study, his group looked at the risk for lifetime psychiatric disorders in almost three thousand pairs of twins. Kendler's group found that high levels of thankfulness were associated with a reduced risk of internalizing disorders, such as depression, phobias, and bulimia. Interestingly, thankfulness was also associated with reduced risk of externalizing disorders, such as drug dependence, alcoholism, and antisocial personality.[446]

Perhaps this time-honored practice that is so commonly summoned in the face of adversity is revealing itself to science as a practice of profound influence. From this and similar work, we might argue that a formal practice of gratitude be considered as a daily journey to both celebrate life and to cope with its challenges. Dr. Robert Emmons has spent a career studying gratitude. His recent book, humbly titled *Thanks: How the New Science of Gratitude Can Make You Happier,* brings the work of the people in this field to light and gives us a glimpse into his thoughts on the power of gratitude.

Is There an Immune-Competent Personality?

There are now some three hundred studies, comprising nearly twenty thousand individuals, which have attempted to clarify the link between stress, immunity, and infection. Doctors Suzanne Segerstrom, PhD, of the University of Kentucky, and Gregory Miller, PhD, of the University of British Columbia recently undertook the daunting task of performing a meta-analysis on 293 of these studies. While the report of their analysis was filled with detail, what follows is a short summary of their findings:[447]

Acute Stressors

The types of stressors that are time-limited and that produce an active "fight or flight" response can actually boost immunity in preparation for defense against microbes that might invade via bites, cuts, punctures, or other types of wounds. This type of response is needed in almost all animal species that must fight for mates or defend themselves against predators. The natural form of immunity predominates in the immediate stages of fight or flight. If such acute stressors are extreme, however, and consume too great an amount of energy, then suppression of defenses can occur. Recall the critical role of energy in defenses.

Cumulative Stressors

There does seem to be some relationship with cumulative stressors and the immune response. However, the effect on immunity has a link to coping.

Chronic Stressors

In the face of chronic stressors, numerous measures of immune function tended to fall. This was especially true if the chronic stressors were life-changing, if they were persistent, if matters seemed beyond control, or if there was no obvious end in sight. The longer the stress period, the more likely it was that the immune system would shift into an adaptive and, often, maladaptive or detrimental mode. It is this type of chronic, seemingly inescapable stressor that appeared to have the most damaging effects on the immune system. Chronic stressors are also responsive to coping.

Age and Disease

It was also clear from the accumulated research that having a chronic disease affected how a person's immune system responded to stress. In addition, aging had a pronounced effect on the immune response to stressful circumstances.

This leads us to wonder whether there is such a thing as an immune-competent personality type. Today, there are more psychologists, physicians, and researchers that are willing to say that there may be attributes that constitute an immune-competent personality.

One such investigator is George F. Solomon, MD, one of the pioneers in the study of mind and immunity, known as psychoneuroimmunology. When pressed to describe the immune-competent personality, he was quick to acknowledge that there are no simple equations. He then went on to describe several questions outlined below:

1. Do I have a sense of meaning in my work, daily, activities, family, and relationships?
2. Am I able to express anger appropriately in defense of myself?
3. Am I able to ask friends and family for support when I am feeling lonely or troubled?
4. Am I able to ask friends or family for favors when I need them?
5. Am I able to say no to someone who asks for a favor if I can't or don't feel like doing it?
6. Do I engage in health-related behaviors based on my own self-defined needs instead of someone else's prescriptions or ideas?
7. Do I have enough play in my life?
8. Do I find myself depressed for long periods during which time I feel hopeless about ever changing the conditions that cause me to be depressed?
9. Am I dutifully filling a prescribed role in my life to the detriment of my own needs?

Closing Thoughts

We have come full circle. It once appeared that we were winning the war on germs. Our leaders declared with certainty that the microbes had been defeated—the war had been won. Today, it is clear that they cannot be defeated. This new realization that the war on germs cannot be won is really quite extraordinary. It has humbled us as a great and technologically advanced society.

Fortunately, this crisis coincides with tremendous developments in nutritional biochemistry, immunology, genetics, neuropsychology, and other fields that have permitted us to better understand the response of the host—our response. In the final section, we will explore how these findings can be woven into a strategy that can be used each day to live in this world of the microbe. We will also explore how specific testing can be used as the core of a personalized medicine strategy aimed at tailoring a program to anyone's particular needs. These ideas can then be used to develop a personal prevention strategy, to address illness when illness occurs, or to recover from the complications of antibiotic use.

PART III

The Way Forward

Chapter 12

Strategies for Living in the Microbe's World

By now it is clear that the lives of humans and microbes are woven together like a rich tapestry. Our new understanding of the mysterious blending of human cells, microbial ancestors, onboard bacteria, and viral genes into the so-called superorganism—the human-microbe hybrid—will change the way we live in our world.

The adaptation of the human is driven by the microbe and that of the microbe is driven by the human. We change together, we live together, and, as some now argue, we are one organism living a marriage of certain interdependence. This may be why we will never eradicate infectious disease and why many attempts to strike down microbes with advanced molecular weapons yield mixed results.

This chapter is a humble attempt to simplify strategies that may be helpful in our effort to coexist within the turbulent world of microbes. I say humble in recognition of two facts: First, while we have a great deal of information, we do not know all there is to know about factors that influence immune defense, energy, and repair. Second, there is a wide variation between individuals, which means that general recommendations will not necessarily suit everyone or every circumstance. Nevertheless, there do appear to be general recommendations that can be very helpful in our efforts to support our immune defense and repair capabilities.

This begins with the ability to recognize circumstances in which we may be at greater risk to the adverse impact of the microbes in, on, and around us. Once we better understand the circumstances of increased risk, we can proceed with either general or specific steps to improve our defenses. The specific responses can be developed by using the approaches of personalized medicine described in Chapter 14. Some general strategies are summarized below.

Knowing When You Might Be at Greater Risk

It is important to remember that we are living in a microbe's world. For the most part, we move through this undulating domain of unseen companions with surprising ease and safety. One component of intelligent living lies in understanding the circumstances in which our susceptibility to these microbes may arise. How do we know when we might be at increased risk to succumbing to the microbes around us? How do we know when special caution or special effort must be applied in attention to our defenses?

As noted throughout this book, seemingly healthy young people have fallen ill or died from MRSA. If we look more closely at our seemingly "healthy" population, say of young people or athletes, we find that their resistance to infection may have been compromised by poor nutrition, lack of sleep, overtraining, prescription drugs, the stress of school, or other factors. In other words, they may not have been as healthy as they were thought to be. For instance, we have come to learn that the rigors of athletic training can lower immune function to such an extent that the apparently robust and healthy athlete is actually someone at risk of infections.

This is just one example of increased vulnerability. Given the myriad influences on our defenses, it merits paying attention to the circumstances in which we ourselves might become more vulnerable.

Infants and Small Children

The immune system of young children is immature and emerging. Because infants and small children have not been exposed to many of life's germs, they have not developed the rapid defensive capabilities of adults. So, we must recognize the vulnerability of early childhood and work to support children during their vulnerable periods. However, we must also recognize the need for young children to be exposed to a wide range of microbes in order that they may develop a robust immune system. Thus, while we need to protect young children, we must not needlessly shelter them.

High School and College Students

Students are beset with stressors, such as sleep deprivation, peer pressure, homework, school exams, extracurricular activities, family difficulties, drug use, alcohol use, poor dietary habits, and many others. These can bear collectively or individually to wear down defenses. Some studies have found increased gut permeability during psychological stress, so analysis of gut integrity should be considered. This should be given specific attention if gut symptoms are present. Chronic sleep deprivation, common in students, should be considered a key contributor to lowered immune defense, energy, and repair.

The Elderly

Immune defense and repair typically declines with age. Moreover, the Th1/Th2 balance tends to shift toward one of an inflammatory profile, making the elderly more susceptible to certain types of infection. Some reasons for increased susceptibility to infections in the elderly include:

- Nutrient deficiency (commonplace in the elderly)
- Lowered physical activity
- Declining muscle mass

- Declining cellular and humoral immunity
- Poorer barrier defenses (such as in the skin, digestive tract, and lungs)
- Slower capacity to recover and repair
- Lowered stomach acidity
- Diminished or poor sleep
- Presence of chronic illness
- Use of multiple prescription drugs
- Slower or poor elimination (bowel, bladder)
- Diminished cough reflex (and diminished ability to expel mucous and microbes)

Many of the items on the above list can be modified or improved by dietary, nutritional, lifestyle, and psychosocial intervention.

Pregnant Mothers

During pregnancy there is a shift in the Th1/Th2 immune balance, favoring Th2 in an effort to protect the fetus. This renders the mother more susceptible to infection. Also, the intense energy demands of growing a fetus demand that the nutritional, sleep, and other needs of a mother be closely attended. Pregnancy is a time of increased susceptibility.

People with Chronic Diseases

Many chronic diseases involve excessive, deficient, or imbalanced activity of the immune system, which can render one susceptible to microbes. For example, white blood cell function in people with diabetes is altered, which can render them more susceptible to infection or to more severe infections, should one be contracted. In diabetes, barrier defenses can be compromised throughout the body. Women with polycystic ovary syndrome are among those with insulin and glucose abnormalities who can have altered immunity.

Thyroid disorders can lead to widespread suppression of defenses. There are many other chronic diseases in which immunity and repair is altered and for which supportive measures can be helpful.

People with Digestive Symptoms and Digestive Disorders

Anyone with digestive symptoms, irritable bowel syndrome, Crohn's disease, inflammatory bowel diseases, or abdominal discomfort related to stress or diet should be very suspicious of altered gut flora balance. It is now well known that small intestinal bacterial overgrowth is associated with leaky gut, the passage of bacteria into the bloodstream, and the passage of gut bacterial endotoxin into the bloodstream.[448] Sugar intolerance may also be a sign of bacterial overgrowth or dysbiosis.[449]

People with Recurrent Infections

It is not uncommon for children or adults to suffer from recurrent infections. In children, two common types are recurrent ear infections or recurrent throat infections. In adults, recurrent bladder infections or vaginal infections are other examples. When recurrent infections exist, it should be taken as a sign that lowered immune defense and repair mechanisms may exist.

People with Specific Genetic Conditions

All aspects of the immune defense, repair, and recovery system are under genetic control. Some of these genes exert more forceful control than others. Some genes are quite responsive to lifestyle influences and alter their expression under pressure from things like diet, nutrition, exercise, sleep, psychological stress, and environmental exposure. Anyone with a known genetic disease or a specific gene mutation may be at increased risk to alterations in immunity. A person who seems to succumb to frequent infections, may wish to explore genetic testing to see whether his or her genotype contributes to the susceptibility.

Children with Developmental Delays

It is not unusual for children with developmental delays (such as Down syndrome, autism, ADHD, Asperger's, Fragile X syndrome, etc.) to have altered host defenses. Experience has shown that children with developmental delays almost always have unique biochemical profiles that can best be sorted out through personalized laboratory testing.

People on Long-Term Medication

Prescription drugs can have widespread effects on immune function and susceptibility to infection. Drugs can also impact repair and recovery functions. This may not be significant when one is on short-term drug therapy, but long-term drug therapy is another matter. Prescription drugs may lower immunity directly. They may also deplete nutrients essential to immune defense and repair. In *The Drug-Induced Nutrient Depletion Handbook,* Dr. Jim LaValle, an associate professor at the University of Cincinnati, provides a concise overview of the direct effect of prescription drugs on specific nutrients. This book can serve as a guide to understanding how your specific medication may need to be coupled with specific nutrients in order to avoid deficiency.

Long-Term Immunosuppressive Drugs

As would be expected, people who are on long-term immunosuppressive drugs because of transplants or other conditions are especially at risk of infection. In these cases, even mundane organisms can prove threatening or lethal. Those on such drugs are wise to consider the many factors that can bolster some of the barrier components of the host defenses so that simple microbes can be defended against.

Physical Trauma

Any physical trauma increases demands on the body's repair functions that naturally shift metabolic resources away from immune defenses.

In addition, many types of trauma involve damage to the body's barriers, where microbes can gain access, triggering an infectious process directly. Anyone who has experienced physical trauma would be wise to consider the additional metabolic needs. This would be a situation in which customized laboratory profiling would be extremely helpful in taking the guesswork out of a health recovery plan.

Emotional Trauma

The effects of emotional trauma can be persistent and long-lasting. Left unattended, the impact can last years, decades, or a lifetime. It is well known that many of the coping skills that develop in response to a traumatic event are supportive in the short term but may not serve an individual over the long term. This is one reason emotional trauma can have a lasting impact. During and after a traumatic event (regardless of how far in the past), it is important to seek the help of friends and professionals. Many factors that would otherwise typically strengthen immune defenses can be less effective when there is a history of significant emotional trauma that has not been addressed.

Persistent or Prolonged Stress

We have reviewed the effects of stress on immune defense and repair. The kinds of stressors that can impact immunity are wide and varied. Levels of cortisol can be elevated during stress and contribute to immune suppression. Cortisol levels can be measured in saliva to give a picture of the daily fluctuations of this steroid hormone.

The Stress of Surgery

Surgery represents a considerable biological and psychological stressor. If surgery is accompanied by extensive time in the intensive care unit, the effects can be even more pronounced and lasting. In fact, it is not uncommon for a return to normal to take a year or more from the time one is released from the ICU. All the support systems described in this book should be considered after surgery, especially those concerned with nutritional status.

Athletes in Training

We've shown that exercise can enhance or inhibit immunity. Athletes under a heavy training schedule must pay close attention to nutrition, sleep, and other needs. This is especially true of college and high school athletes, who have the added stress of class, homework, and exams. Endurance athletes such as those training for marathons, triathlons, or iron-man competitions are among the high-risk athletes.

People are frequently shocked when healthy, young athletes succumb to infections that are expected to affect the very young and the very old—not the robust athlete. But we must understand that the rigors of training, lack of sleep, nutrient deficiency (very common in some sports), and emotional demands of competition can combine to lower immunity in fit individuals in training. In reality, athletes in training should be considered among those who are potentially at greater risk to infection due to the high demands they put on their bodies.

Signs of Overtraining

- Insomnia
- Elevated heart rate
- Weight loss
- Mild leg soreness, general aches and pains
- Muscle and joint aches (pain)
- Sudden reduction in performance
- Poor recovery
- Washed-out feeling, tired, drained, lack of energy
- Headaches
- Increased number of coughs, colds, or sore throats
- Decrease in training capacity / intensity

- Moodiness
- Anxiety
- Irritability
- Lack of motivation
- Loss of enthusiasm for the sport
- Depression
- Decreased appetite
- More frequent injuries

Overweight and Obesity

As noted throughout this book, being overweight is linked to changes in gut integrity, insulin regulation, blood glucose control, immune regulation, and inflammation. Being overweight can be measured in several different ways including 1) weight, 2) body mass index (BMI), 3) percent body fat, and 4) waist-to-hip ratio. There are standard measures of each that suggest one is past an ideal threshold.

Eating Disorders and Underweight

Being underweight also poses significant problems for immune defenses. This is especially true if there is an eating disorder. In a study of intestinal permeability in anorexia nervosa, intestinal permeability was actually shown to be impaired. In other words, there was not a leaky gut, but there was evidence of poor absorption.[450] If one is underweight without having an eating disorder, a physician should be seen to rule out a range of medical conditions. Being underweight can signify low calorie intake or intestinal malabsorption. It can also signify cytokines that have shifted toward an inflammatory state. In general, being underweight should be followed with a full medical evaluation that includes a comprehensive metabolic evaluation.

Smoking

Smoking is associated with depressed immunity that can shift toward an inflammatory state. Smoking also damages barrier defenses in the upper respiratory tract.

Where You Live: Environmental Exposure, Industrial Plants

Chemicals released into the environment can have complex effects on immune defense and repair. People living around or near industrial plants of all kinds may be exposed to a wide variety of heavy metals and volatile compounds through the air and water. If you live in a community with manufacturing plants that discharge into the air and water (as most do), extra attention on detoxification is likely needed.

Where You Live: Feedlots and Animal Farms

Antibiotics and antibiotic-resistant bacteria have been found to be more concentrated on and near feedlots and farms that raise animals for food. If you live near one of these facilities, there could be an increased chance that you harbor more antibiotic-resistant intestinal bacteria or that you might be exposed to harmful organisms that are antibiotic-resistant. Hog farms have been particularly noteworthy for their contribution to this, though other animal farms contribute as well. The risk to any given individual is hard to assess at this time, so if you live in such an environment, it may be wise to use some of the strategies for strong immune defense, energy, and repair.

Wise Use of Antibiotics

Minimizing exposure to unnecessary antibiotics requires that we recognize the potential sources of exposure and make wise choices about use of these products. Below is a brief discussion of how we might limit exposure under specific circumstances.

Personal Care Products

Limit the use of antibacterial (antibiotic, antimicrobial, anti-infective, etc.) personal care products. Triclosan is a common compound added to antibacterial personal care products. Many doctors working with antibiotic-resistance research are convinced triclosan is problematic and must be reduced. According to the Centers for Disease Control and Prevention (CDC), vigorous hand washing in warm water with plain soap for at least ten seconds is sufficient to fight germs in most cases, even for healthcare workers.

Smart Meat Selection

While an individual cannot control the use of antibiotics in farming, it is possible to reduce exposure to these drugs by choosing beef, poultry, pork, and fish carefully. Refer to product labels that carry claims related to antibiotics, such as those from the USDA noted below:

Natural Products

A product containing no artificial ingredient or added color and is only minimally processed (a process which does not fundamentally alter the raw product) may be labeled natural. The label must explain the use of the term natural (such as "no added colorings or artificial ingredients; minimally processed.")

No Hormones (Pork or Poultry)

Hormones are not allowed in raising hogs or poultry. Therefore, the claim "no hormones added" **cannot be used** on the labels of pork or poultry unless it is followed by a statement that says "Federal regulations prohibit the use of hormones." This does not mean that antibiotics were not used.

No Hormones (Beef)

The term "no hormones administered" may be approved for use on the label of beef products if sufficient documentation is provided to the agency by the producer showing no hormones have been used in raising the animals. This does not mean that antibiotics were not used.

No Antibiotics (Red Meat and Poultry)

The terms "no antibiotics added" may be used on labels for meat or poultry products if sufficient documentation is provided by the producer to the agency demonstrating that the animals were raised without antibiotics.

No Antibiotics Added, Raised without Antibiotics

Animals are not fed antibiotics at any point in their life cycle, including for veterinary treatment. If an animal is sick and must be fed antibiotics, it cannot be sold under this label.

No Subtherapeutic Antibiotics Administered

Antibiotics are not used for growth promotion, but may be used to treat sick animals. This label can be confusing and it is often misused. If one is truly concerned about absolutely restricting antibiotics in the diet, the previous definition is more reliable.

Free Range and Free Roaming

This applies to poultry. It only requires that animals be "allowed access to the outside." It is subject to many abuses and is the source of confusion among consumers. It does not imply that animals have been raised free of antibiotics. This label also does not apply to beef, pork, or eggs.

Organic

Organic meat, poultry, eggs, and dairy products come from animals that are given no antibiotics or growth hormones. Organic food is produced without using most conventional pesticides; fertilizers made with synthetic ingredients or sewage sludge; bioengineering; or ionizing radiation. Before a product can be labeled organic, a government-approved certifier inspects the farm where the food is grown to make sure the farmer is following all the rules necessary to meet USDA organic standards. Companies that handle or process organic food before it gets to the local supermarket or restaurant must also be certified.

Smart Fruit Selection

The U.S. Food and Drug Administration has not restricted the use of antibiotics on fruit trees. Selecting organic fruit or fruit that is declared to be free of antibiotics is a preferred way to reduce exposure to antibiotics through this means.

Choosing Probiotics

There are many ways to frame the issue of probiotics. For our purposes, the three general areas of use are 1) general consumption in foods, 2) consumption of supplements for health maintenance, and 3) consumption of probiotic supplements for the purpose of treating or managing a health condition. This section is meant to address selection of probiotics for treating or managing a health condition.

Rather than describing specific probiotics, it is more broadly useful to outline a series of key points that should be considered when purchasing or using a probiotic:

- Specific bacterial strain (genus-species-strain), e.g. *Lactobacillus plantarum* 299v, *Lactobacillus rhamnosus* GR-1.
- Strains must be live or viable, not attenuated or killed

- Number of viable organisms per dose volume
- Use-by date
- Batch or lot code
- Evidence of clinical studies from *the specific strain* being sold
- Company information and contact numbers
- Supplement facts

If you have a specific condition, it is important to use a strain of probiotic that has been specifically tested in that disorder. Key points about specific strains of probiotics and research should be considered, as below:

- The product being purchased for a specific use should have studies in which the specific probiotic strain has been tested in that condition.
- The product being purchased for a specific use should be at the dose used in studies for that condition.
- Articles or scientific papers that discuss studies of a specific tested strain of probiotic should not be used as evidence to support health claims of an untested probiotic.
- Probiotic strains that are tested in one disease or disorder should not be considered to have been proven to work in a disorder in which they have not been tested.
- Strains that have been tested to modify as specific feature, such as improving intestinal barrier defenses (which is not a disease), may not be successful in all cases of weakened barrier defenses.
- Strains that have been tested alone in clinical studies cannot be expected to behave the same when combined with other strains. Combination products should have studies specific to those combination products. If they do not, there would be uncertainty about whether the product would perform the same as in the individual studies. On the other hand, such combinations could likely work quite well.

Talking to Your Doctor about Antibiotics

Doctors and patients are now in an uneasy relationship when it comes to antibiotics. Patient pressure to prescribe antibiotics can often lead to unnecessary antibiotic prescriptions. On the other hand, some doctors may pressure a patient into unnecessary antibiotic use. In order to lessen the likelihood of inappropriate antibiotic use, you should be prepared to have a very concise office visit so you can quickly inform the doctor of what is wrong so you can optimize your time during the office visit, and so you are prepared to answer certain types of responses (especially related to antibiotic prescribing).

In preparation for any office visit, it is best to have things written down as a guide.

1. **Study your condition**. With Internet resources, you can be well prepared for the office visit.
2. **Make a list**. Bring a list of your main symptoms and your main concerns. Include the circumstances in which symptoms began, when they began, and how they have progressed over time. Keep the list very brief and succinct.
3. **Medications and supplements.** Make a list of prescription medications, over-the-counter drugs, herbs, probiotics, and nutritional supplements. Include dose and frequency of use.
4. **Questions**. Make a list of questions that you wish to ask the doctor. Identify which questions are of greatest importance to you, understanding the limited time of most office visits.
5. **Take notes**. Write down key points of the conversation immediately after the visit.

Antibiotic Questions

First, do not pressure your doctor to prescribe antibiotics. Should your doctor recommend antibiotics, you may consider responding along the lines of the statement below followed by a series of questions:

"Doctor, I understand that you have my best interests in mind and that both of us have an interest in using antibiotics only if necessary. I respect your opinion and I am wondering if you would be willing to answer a few short questions about antibiotics in my case."

- Are you certain it is a bacterial infection and not a viral infection?
- Will you perform a culture to be certain it is a bacterial infection?
- Will you perform a susceptibility test to identify the antibiotic that will be most effective against this bacterium?
- Will you perform a test to determine if the bacterium is resistant to this antibiotic?
- Can we use the antibiotic with the narrowest spectrum of action? (Avoid broad-spectrum antibiotics whenever possible.)
- What is the shortest possible duration I must take this antibiotic?
- Are there supportive measures I can use *in conjunction with* the antibiotic?
- What are the risks if I do not take the antibiotic?
- Are there measures I can use *instead* of the antibiotic?
- What probiotic do you recommend I take and for how long?
- Should I be concerned about yeast infections? If so, how will we follow up on this?
- What can we do in the future to improve my defenses against infections?
- Are there other tests you recommend to better understand my health status?

Remember, in many busy medical practices, it is not always easy to get all of these questions answered, and in smaller clinics, the laboratory facilities may not exist for comprehensive testing. Your goal is not to enter into a struggle with your doctor, but to try to establish a partnership of mutual respect. Some doctors will find the above communication uncomfortable; others may welcome such participation. You will have to gauge the circumstances of your medical provider. If you find that your doctor is not interested in such partnership, you may wish to seek another provider.

It is important to respect the doctor's dilemma. Infectious disease is a complex area of medical practice. Doctors have been given new practice guidelines that urge more judicious use of antibiotics, so the situation is improving somewhat. At the same time, office visits are short, patient demands are high, and the liability that goes along with not treating an acute infection that leads to complications can influence prescribing. Doctors often prefer to err on the side of caution, believing that patient injury and a malpractice suit is more likely if they do not give an antibiotic when it was indicated. However, the doctor's decision to give an antibiotic might be the *right* decision in a given situation.

Can Avoiding Antibiotics Be Harmful?

Thus far, I have given ample attention to the difficulties with antibiotic use and overuse. I have also stressed the importance of fundamentally changing how we think about living in the microbe's world. Having made these points clearly, it is important to remember that antibiotics are life-saving drugs. There are times and circumstances in which the right drug, for the right condition, given at the right time is crucial. An example is tuberculosis, for which the right antibiotic must be taken for months to years in order to achieve the intended result in the individual and to protect others. In cases of hospitalization for critical illness, deaths have been shown to drop sharply when the appropriate antibiotics are given early enough in the crisis.

Many disorders of bacterial overgrowth in the gut that are not emergency in nature might actually have to be treated with antibiotics. This can be the case even when the disorder may have been caused by or made worse by antibiotics. In these cases, genetic analysis of gut bacteria can pinpoint the harmful bugs, so that a selective antibiotic can be chosen for treatment. Ironically, then, those who suffer from irritable bowel syndrome, Crohn's disease, inflammatory bowel disease, or other disorders of the gut, may actually *need* antibiotics in order to eliminate harmful bugs and give their body a chance to recover. If we confirm that obesity is linked to overgrowth of certain families of microbes (as discussed in Chapter 3), we may also one day use selective antibiotics in the early stages of managing this disorder.

We must also not forget what doctors now refer to as *stealth infections.* These are hidden infections that might contribute to chronic diseases not typically linked to microbes. The discovery of a stealth infection linked to gastric ulcers resulted in a Nobel Prize for Barry Marshall and Robin Warren in 2005. This appears to be only the beginning, as evidence of stealth infection continues to grow for diseases such as atherosclerosis, schizophrenia, some forms of arthritis, chronic bronchitis, chronic fatigue, menstrual cramping, prostatitis, skin conditions, developmental delays in children, and many others. We may likely find that some of these conditions benefit from some form of targeted antibiotic use (though a healthy host must remain foremost).

Without question, there is a long list of circumstances in which antibiotics might be needed. So, the concepts put forth in *Beyond Antibiotics* should not been seen as a rejection of antibiotic drugs. This should be very clearly understood. *Beyond Antibiotics* is about the wise use of antibiotics, the appropriate use of antibiotics, and the avoidance of their use whenever possible.

Simple Strategies to Support Defense and Repair

As noted above, general strategies can often prove helpful, though their very nature means that they will not apply to everyone in all situations. Below is a set of general considerations that may contribute to improved health and immunity. Many of them may also make life more enjoyable.

Diet and Nutrition

Consider:

- Reducing your intake of refined sugar. Excess sugar can make the immune system sluggish. Elevated blood sugar (as in diabetes) has been linked with poor white blood cell function.
- Reducing your intake of high glycemic (high GL) carbohydrates.
- Reducing your intake of fat (unless it is already at or below 20 percent of your total calories). Avoid margarine and hydrogenated fats. If your triglycerides are high, work to lower them. Elevated blood fats can slow immune function.
- Increasing your intake of omega-3 essential fatty acids such as those found in flax oil, fish oil (salmon, mackerel, herring, sardines, trout), and krill oil. You may also wish to take a perle of evening primrose oil or borage oil daily, which contain the omega-6 oil gamma-linolenic acid (GLA). Those in the industrialized world often consume too little of these oils.
- Ensuring adequate amounts of dietary protein. The protein content of muscle may be one important determinant of the strength of the immune response during infection.
- Avoiding white bread and refined flour products. They are devoid of essential nutrients including the essential fatty acids mentioned above.
- Including fiber in your diet in the form of fruits, vegetables, nuts, seeds, legumes, and whole grains. These foods are also high in vitamins and minerals.
- Reducing your intake of pastries, doughnuts, French fries, chicken nuggets, candies, and other foods containing transfatty acids.
- Eating several smaller meals a day as opposed to three large meals a day. It is easier on all aspects of your body.
- Restricting coffee intake to early in the day. Coffee consumption

too late in the day (after lunchtime) may interfere with sleep, which can alter immunity.

- Reducing your intake of soft drinks, especially those containing fructose and aspartame.
- Following the rhythms of your body. Eat when you're hungry, stop when you're full. Don't let the clock rule mealtime. Try mealtime without the paper, TV, or radio.
- Rotating your foods to avoid boredom and monotony.
- If you have a health problem, consider the possibility that the foods you consume might be part of the problem. These may be due to poor food quality, intolerance to certain foods, or excess of certain macronutrients (such as protein, fat, or carbohydrate).
- Not obsessing about nutrition. While a healthy, balanced diet is important to wellbeing, fretting about it may negate much of the good you've accomplished.
- Splurging on your favorite treats now and then. If you've followed the guidelines above, reward yourself. Rigidity and abstinence are not the order of the day—just moderation.

Lifestyle

Consider:

- Getting regular exercise, even if it's only walking for thirty minutes each day. Those who exercise moderately are more resistant to infection. Make sure the exercise is fun. Do it with a friend if at all possible. Heavy exercisers can be *more* susceptible to infection. If you are a heavy exerciser who gets ill frequently, modify your workouts. **Exercise may be one of the most important of all influences on immune function.**
- Building muscle mass by using resistance exercises. Muscle is increasingly being viewed as an important component of the immune response. Greater muscle mass may aid in defense

against microbes, and in recovery from infection, trauma, or surgery.

- A weekly or biweekly sauna (especially during the high-risk winter months). It appears to help cleanse the body of waste products and impurities, and may cut the incidence of infection. If you have heart disease, are pregnant, or have circulatory problems, see your doctor before proceeding.
- Getting more touch in your life. Treat yourself to a weekly therapeutic massage. Touch your spouse more often. Touch and hug your kids throughout the day. Babies especially love touch.
- Getting adequate sunlight, especially if you live in a northern climate, during winter, or if you work indoors under artificial lights. Get outside on sunny winter days. Sun exposure on your hands and face is often enough, but full body is better. Avoid excessive sun exposure during summertime.
- Giving up smoking, if you smoke. If there is a smoker in your home, encourage them to quit. Smokers and those who live with smokers get more respiratory infections.
- Being more attentive to your rhythms of work and life. If you find work intruding more strongly into your life than you would like, consider restructuring your working life.
- Limiting Internet and TV hours. It may contribute to a more sedentary life, obesity, and poor nutrition. It takes time away from interacting with family and friends, and from introspection. Late-night viewing can interfere with sleep.
- Designating a "quiet room" in the house—especially if you have children. This is a room that allows you to escape from stressful noise and chatter. The room should contain no TV or radio and should be off-limits to others while you are inside. Try arranging quiet time for your kids as well.
- Finding daily time for meditation, prayer, reflection, or whatever quietude meets your personal needs.

- Looking at the health of your parents and siblings. If they are prone to certain types of illness, you may be likewise. Take preventive steps regarding lifestyle and nutrition.
- Drinking alcohol in moderation.
- Avoiding overuse of prescription drugs.
- Avoiding use of illicit drugs.
- Getting deep, sound, and abundant sleep. It cannot be stressed enough. **Sleep may be one of the most important of all influences on immune function.** A short nap in the afternoon is often helpful, provided it does not disrupt your evening sleep. Evening sleep that begins by 9 or 10 p.m. is considered by many to be most productive in supporting immune defense and repair.

Environment

Consider:

- Limiting your use of synthetic materials.
- If you suffer from chronic or recurrent infections, it may be due to an excessive body burden of toxic metals or compounds. Have an evaluation done by a doctor familiar with environmental medicine. Certain blood and urine tests can detect exposure to toxins you may not be aware of.
- Regular checkups and having blood and urine analysis to detect toxic exposure, if you work in an occupation in which chemicals are used.
- Your exposures might be affecting your health if you live in an area near industrial plants.
- That antibiotic-resistant microbes or antibiotics may be present in your environment in increased amounts, if you live near a feedlot or farm that raises animals for food.
- Minimizing or avoiding synthetic personal hygiene products.
- A filtration system or use of bottled water (provided the bottled

water is known to be pure and documented by testing) if you live in an area with heavily chlorinated, fluoridated, or contaminated water.

- Wearing protective gloves and clothing whenever working with toxic chemicals at home or at work. This includes common lawn and garden products.
- Consuming organic fruits and vegetables as a means to lower pesticide, herbicide, and fungicide exposure.

Mood, Mind, and Emotions

Consider:

- Working at becoming more of an optimist. Optimists appear to have healthier immune systems, suffer from fewer infections, and are not as adversely affected by stressful life events. They in fact experience fewer negative events.
- That optimism can have downside, if one remains in a difficult situation too long, hoping that a better outcome will eventually emerge. Recognize your tendencies.
- Guarding against cynicism and hostility. Rates of premature death in people who are hostile, cynical or suspicious are four to seven times higher than in people who are not. If you or others might describe you as cynical or hostile, consider working toward retranslating your view of the world. It may help your resistance to disease and also cause life to become more of a celebration.
- Seeking empathy. Express your feelings and emotions with someone you trust. Suppressed anger, sadness, grief, or other emotions can lead to suppressed immunity.
- Keeping a daily journal of your feelings, especially during important life events. It gives the immune system a boost that can be verified as long as six weeks after the journal-keeping has been discontinued.

- Giving to others. One of the most profound features of being human is the need to contribute to the well-being of others.
- Expressions of gratitude. Studies have now begun to show that finding things for which to be grateful, even in difficult situations, improves markers of well-being.
- Forgiveness. Many describe improved well-being after forgiving another. Studies have begun to show that forgiveness can alter physiology in positive ways.
- Taking more control. If you are in a situation that seems outside your control, find little things over which you can exert control. A sense of control seems to help our immune systems function more efficiently.
- Asking for and accepting support from friends and loved ones.
- Seeking a deeper sense of meaning and purpose in your relationships, work, and daily activities.
- Learning to say "no" (when you need to) when others ask for your help or services. While service and giving are important parts of a healthy life, being unable to assert yourself and claim your needs can compromise well-being.
- Taking classes in relaxation. Self-relaxation techniques have been shown to boost immunity, relieve pain, and improve life in general.
- If you are depressed, seek help from a professional. Seek out people you trust. Get moderate exercise. People suffering from depression have weakened immune systems and are more susceptible to infection.
- If you are a caregiver for a chronically ill spouse, child, or friend, seek other means of support. Take breaks. Find other outlets. Caregiving can be immensely draining and can take a toll on immune function.
- Laughing as much as you can. Attend funny movies, read funny stories, socialize with funny people, and try to see the humorous things in life.

- Limiting or avoiding entertainment that is graphic, violent, or harsh. Studies with soldiers have found altered immune cell function when exposed to such imagery.
- When stressful life events strike, take extra time, do relaxation exercises, write in a journal, discuss your feelings with someone you trust, stay away from junk food, take extra vitamins. During high-stress periods, we are vulnerable. The extra effort spent caring for yourself will pay off.
- Rating your health high and beginning to view yourself as healthy. Those who do actually live longer and feel better.
- Avoiding rigidity. Rigidity or inflexibility in one's beliefs may translate into a rigid and inflexible immune system. In studies, rigid routines have been associated with increased infection duration and severity.
- The sanctity of seasonal rituals, whatever your religious or spiritual conviction.
- Taking greater control of your health. Do not rely on doctors. When you use doctors, try to form a health partnership. Find a doctor whose philosophy of care is similar to your own. You will be more likely to trust his/her advice and follow through with recommendations. In such a relationship, doctors are less likely to respond negatively to your questions.

Social

Consider:

- Finding a community with whom you share interests. Close social ties are important to our resistance to disease. Loneliness has been linked to declining immunity and changes in genes associated with immunity.
- Cultivating interpersonal relationships. Those with more close personal ties have healthier immune systems. Those who isolate

themselves are more susceptible to illness that is more severe and long-lasting.

- Play, play, play. The less we play, the more somber and serious our world becomes. Play is an absolute necessity for health and well-being.
- Planning an outing with your spouse or mate at least once a week. Plan regular outings with your children where they get your undivided attention.
- Taking vacations. It doesn't have to be far, just a change of scenery.

Chapter 13

Common Conditions: Are Antibiotics Warranted?

As noted previously, the Centers for Disease Control and Prevention (CDC) have an aggressive plan in place to reduce the use of antibiotics. Their main objective is to reduce unnecessary use of these drugs so that antibiotics remain a viable tool in the future. Another reason for their aggressive campaign is to minimize adverse effects in patients who might receive these drugs unnecessarily.

Below is a brief overview of some common conditions for which antibiotics are routinely prescribed. Some of these may contain more technical detail than you think necessary. However, the guidelines and commentary are meant to help you understand the data that doctors must they consider, as they wrestle with the decision of whether to use antibiotics. It is my belief that this knowledge is also helpful as consumers of health care evaluate their doctor's recommendations. To fully grasp the ramifications of antibiotic use, we must consider the following:

- The most common conditions for which antibiotics are now used
- The likelihood of a condition being due to bacterial infection (vs. viral infection)
- The potential for success or failure in using antibiotics in these conditions
- The current recommendations of organizations like the Centers for Disease Control regarding appropriate antibiotic use in these conditions

The following examples should allow all of us to participate in reducing the use of antibiotics in an effort to curb antibiotic resistance and to limit the adverse effects that can be associated with unnecessary antibiotic use. Of course, decisions about any individual case can only be made after consultation with a doctor or appropriate licensed healthcare provider. The management of infections can be complex and individual circumstances (such as children with autism or adults with cancer) can require special approaches. Therefore, the following should be considered general comments, which include summaries promulgated by the Centers for Disease Control.*

Sore Throats in Children

There are more than seven million pediatric visits each year to treat sore throats alone, and inappropriate use of antibiotics for this condition continues to be a serious problem. Despite concerns about excessive antibiotic use, doctors still prescribe antibiotics for one-half to two-thirds of children with sore throats.[451] Only about 12 percent of cases are bacterial infections related to group A beta-hemolytic streptococcus (GABHS).[452] Most others are likely viral. According to CDC guidelines, clinical findings alone do not adequately distinguish strep from non-strep sore throats.[453] Sore throats with other symptoms including significant runny nose, cough, hoarseness, conjunctivitis, or diarrhea are likely viral.[454] It is recommended that the Rapid Strep test be positive before beginning antibiotic therapy. Experts recommend confirming negative Rapid Strep test results with a strep culture.[455]

According to CDC guidelines, the following procedure should be followed in diagnosis and treatment of a bacterial sore throat. It is use-

*Note: Treatment guidelines for any illness undergo continual review and revision as new studies improve diagnosis and treatment. The guidelines above should be considered current as of the time of this writing. Further information can always be found on the websites of the Centers for Disease Control and Prevention, the Infectious Diseases Society of America, or other trusted medical sources.

ful to note such guidelines, since it helpful to understand what your doctor is being asked to follow.

- Diagnose as group A streptococcal pharyngitis using a laboratory test in conjunction with clinical and epidemiological findings.
- Antibiotics should not be given to a child with pharyngitis in the absence of diagnosed group A streptococcal infection.
- Penicillin remains the drug of choice for treating group A streptococcal pharyngitis.

Sore Throats in Adults

Most cases of pharyngitis or tonsillitis in adults are viral infections. According to the CDC, only about 5 to 15 percent of adult cases of sore throat are due to bacteria (group A beta-hemolytic strep.[456] There is no need for antibiotics except when GABHS is the causative pathogen. Lab testing is not necessary in all patients with pharyngitis (sore throat). Instead, all adults should be screened for the following:

- History of fever
- Lack of cough
- Secretions of the tonsils
- Tender lymph nodes in the front of the neck

People with none or only one of these findings should *not* be tested or treated with antibiotics for GABHS.

Acute and Chronic Earaches in Children

Earache is the number one reason for doctor visits in childhood, and the number one reason for antibiotic prescriptions in children. Key factors in understanding the effectiveness and wise use of antibiotics in ear infections include:

- Whether the earache is acute or chronic
- The age of the child

- Illness severity
- Certainty of the diagnosis

The terms acute otitis media is used to describe an earache of rapid onset, sometimes with severity, without an ongoing history of the condition. In the year 2000, there were 16 million office visits for acute middle-ear problems in the U.S. Antibiotic prescriptions numbered 802 for every 1,000 office visits, continuing the trend in which roughly 80 percent of children with acute earaches receive antibiotics. This accounts for some 13 million antibiotic prescriptions each year.[457]

Chronic earache (or chronic otitis media with effusion—fluid) describes an earache that is lingering, lasting, or constant (commonly without painful symptoms). Chronic earaches have usually been thought to be sterile, or free of bacteria, which would explain why antibiotics are typically not helpful in chronic middle earaches. However, recent studies suggest that some cases of chronic earache have bacterial biofilms (see Chapter 1), which are generally impervious to antibiotics.[458] The presence of bacterial biofilms was recently shown in a study of twenty-six children undergoing surgery for the placement of tubes.[459] However, there are still many doctors who believe that most cases of chronic earaches are not bacterial at all and do not warrant antibiotic use.[460]

Guidelines of the CDC and American Academy of Pediatrics

As a point of reference, it is helpful to understand the current treatment guidelines for treatment of earaches in the United States. While these guidelines are suggested, it is important to note that some experts in the field recommend more aggressive antibiotic therapy, whereas others recommend a more conservative approach and greater avoidance of antibiotic therapy.

Principles of Appropriate Use of Antibiotics According to the CDC and AAP[461,462]

1. Classify episodes of otitis media (OM) as **acute** otitis media (AOM) or otitis media with effusion (OME). **Only treat *certain children* with proven AOM.**
2. A certain diagnosis of AOM meets three criteria:
   - History of acute onset of signs and symptoms
   - Presence of middle ear effusion
   - Signs or symptoms of middle-ear inflammation

   Severe illness is moderate to severe earache or fever greater than 39°C.

   Non-severe illness is mild earache and fever less than 39°C in the past 24 hours.
3. Children with AOM who should be treated as follows:

■ Table 13.1. **Treatment Guidelines for Children with Acute Otitis Media (CDC)**

Age	Certain Diagnosis	Uncertain Diagnosis
< 6 months	Antibacterial therapy	Antibacterial therapy
6 months to 2 years	Antibacterial therapy if severe illness	Observation of non-severe illness
> 2 years	Antibacterial therapy if severe illness; observation if non-severe illness	

Don't prescribe antibiotics for initial treatment of OME:

- Treatment may be indicated if fluid in both ears persists for 3 months or more.

Changing Opinions

While the CDC guidelines advocate a more conservative approach (less antibiotics) than in the past, some doctors urge even greater caution with these drugs. In the *American Family Physician,* Dr. John McConaghy wrote a brief entitled "Controversy in Otitis Media Management: Should We Follow the CDC Recommendations?" In this paper he notes that:

- More than 80 percent of cases of acute otitis media resolve spontaneously.
- This is compared with a 93 percent resolution rate with antibiotic therapy.
- Antibiotics only shorten the course of acute otitis media by one day in one out of eight children treated.
- The only short-term advantage of using antibiotics to treat otitis media is a modest decrease in the number of children with continued pain at two to seven days from diagnosis. Use of antibiotics has not affected the long-term outcomes.
- Narrow-spectrum antibiotics are still the recommended and effective treatment for acute otitis media and, in most children, a shortened course (five days) is adequate treatment with no negative impact on clinical outcomes.

Dr. McConaghy states that "These recommendations by the CDC and the DRSP* Therapeutic Working Group may be useful in some patient subpopulations, but we believe that they should not be generalized to primary care and family practice populations without solid, clinical, patient-oriented outcomes data to support them. Rather than throwing more antibiotics at ear infections, we should be focusing efforts on reducing their indiscriminate use and identifying subsets of children who truly need antibiotics."[463]

These thoughts echo the sentiments of a great many physicians. More cautious guidelines on treating earaches have evolved because, over the years, strong opinions have emerged based on critical reviews of the evidence. For instance, in an article in the *Journal of the Ameri-*

---

*DRSP: drug-resistant *Strep. pneumoniae*

can Medical Association, researchers reported that children with chronic otitis media with effusion who received amoxicillin fared no better than those on placebo and, in fact, suffered two to six times greater recurrence than those on placebo. Similar findings were reported for Pediazole and cefaclor.[464]

Dr. John Bailar, the Scholar-in-Residence at the National Academy of Sciences' Institute of Medicine and editorial board member of the *New England Journal of Medicine,* reported on his analysis of the data regarding antibiotic treatment of otitis earache. Commenting on the pattern of ineffectiveness he wrote, "This remarkable trend . . . seems to demolish the conclusion that antibiotics improve the outcome [of otitis media]."[465]

In Sweden, antibiotic treatment of earache is viewed with great caution. According to Karin Prellner, MD, of the Swedish Medical Research Council, it would be difficult to conduct a placebo-controlled trial using antibiotics in otitis media in Sweden because antibiotics are viewed as an ineffective and potentially harmful form of therapy. She suggested that doctors there would be faced with a serious ethical conflict if they were forced to give antibiotics for what they consider a benign disorder, i.e. otitis media without complications.[466]

Robert Ruben, MD, while president of the American Society for Pediatric Otolaryngology, gave an address in which he seriously questioned the value of antibiotics for treating earache on three grounds: lack of effectiveness, antibiotic-resistant bacteria, and safety. He stated, "It would appear that the widespread use of antibiotics for otitis media with effusion has added to the creation of antibiotic-resistant organisms throughout the world. . . . The creation of antibiotic-resistant organisms is now a medical and social problem that needs to be addressed and regulated."[467]

Regarding effectiveness he states, "Overall, the effectiveness of antibiotics for all of the types of morbidities [illnesses] associated with otitis media with effusion is marginal or equal to that of placebo."

He expressed great concern over side-effects of antibiotics when he remarked, "The sequelae [consequences] resultant from the use of antibiotics is substantial to both patient and society. Analysis of the data indicates that antibiotics are an ineffective and dangerous form of care for otitis media with effusion."

According to the Agency for Health Care Policy and Research, it is estimated that avoiding unnecessary treatment of OME (chronic middle earache with effusion) would save up to 6 to 8 million courses of antibiotics each year.[468]

According to CDC practice guidelines, without specific signs of infection or with non-specific signs and symptoms (runny nose, cough, diarrhea), antibiotic treatment "has not been demonstrated to be effective in long-term resolution of OME."

When Parents Are Informed

Doctors writing in the journal *Family Practice* wanted to see whether educating parents about the wise use of antibiotics for treating acute middle earache would have any bearing on antibiotic use. At the time of the first visit, each parent received an antibiotic prescription, with the instruction that it could be given if their child did not improve over the next 24 to 48 hours. The decision on whether to use the drugs was left to the parent (who could contact the physician at any time if needed).

Doctors then gave a short explanation about earache and antibiotics to the parents of 44 children, while the parents of 37 children received no explanation. The explanation included the following points:

- Acute otitis media (AOM, or acute middle earache) is part of an upper respiratory tract infection.
- It has been well established that in most cases children will recover regardless of antibiotic prescription.
- Dangerous late complications from AOM unfortunately may occur

regardless of whether antibiotics were or were not delivered in the course of the acute illness.

- Parents were recommended in cases of high fever or severe pain to administer paracetamol (acetaminophen, Tylenol) prescribed according to the child's weight.

Of the parents who received this explanation about earaches and antibiotic treatment, only 37 percent gave their children the antibiotic. Of those who did not receive the explanation, 63 percent administered the antibiotic. Of those who did not receive the explanation, 77 percent who used the antibiotic did so on the first day. According to the doctors, "In children with AOM [acute otitis media], a brief explanation by the family physician to the child's parents about the disease and its expected spontaneous recovery could significantly decrease antibiotic use by about 50 percent."[469]

Sinusitis in Adults

Approximately 40 million Americans are affected by sinusitis every year, with 33 million cases of chronic sinusitis reported annually to the U.S. Centers for Disease Control and Prevention. According to CDC practice guidelines:

- Most cases of acute sinusitis are due to uncomplicated **viral,** upper respiratory tract infections.
- Bacterial and viral rhinosinusitis are difficult to differentiate on clinical grounds.
- The clinical diagnosis of acute bacterial rhinosinusitis should be reserved for patients with rhinosinusitis symptoms lasting seven days or more and who have facial or tooth pain or tenderness (especially when one-sided) and nasal secretions.
- People who have rhinosinusitis symptoms for less than seven days are unlikely to have a bacterial infection.

- Acute bacterial rhinosinusitis resolves without antibiotic treatment in the majority of cases.
- Antibiotic therapy should be reserved for patients meeting the criteria for the clinical diagnosis of acute bacterial rhinosinusitis who have moderately severe symptoms, and for those with severe rhinosinusitis symptoms—especially those with unilateral face pain—regardless of duration of illness.
- Initial treatment should be with the most narrow-spectrum agent that is active against the most likely microbes.

A study of 252 adults was recently undertaken to compare antibiotic use and a placebo in sinusitis. All patients had a history of nasal discharge and maxillary or frontal sinus pain for at least 48 hours. All patients also had evidence of pus. Each patient received a topical decongestant along with acetaminophen (Tylenol). The group of 252 was divided in half, where one half received a placebo and the other half received a broad spectrum antibiotic (amoxicillin/clavulanic acid) twice a day for six days.

These doctors found no difference in the cure rates at one week and two weeks. Diarrhea was almost four times more likely in the antibiotic group. According to the authors, "A broad spectrum antibiotic was ineffective in relieving symptoms faster than placebo in patients diagnosed with acute sinusitis in general practice."[470]

Acute Cough in Children (Acute Bronchitis)

The Centers for Disease Control stress that in the well-appearing child with cough illness, "antibiotics are NOT the answer." The following key points about coughs in children should be noted:

- Cough illness/bronchitis is principally caused by viruses.[471]
- Airway inflammation and sputum production are non-specific responses and do not imply a bacterial cause.

- An examination of six studies (in adults) concluded that antibiotics were ineffective in treating cough illness/bronchitis.[472]
- Antibiotic treatment of upper respiratory infections does not prevent bacterial complications such as pneumonia.[473]

According to the CDC, antibiotics should not be used for a cough of less than 10 to 14 days' duration in a well-appearing child who does not have physical signs of pneumonia. Consider antibiotics only for:

- Suspected pneumonia, based on fever with focal exam, infiltrate on chest x-ray, rapid breathing, or toxic appearance.
- Prolonged cough (greater than 10 to 14 days without improvement), which may suggest specific illness that warrants antibiotic treatment.[474]
- Mycoplasm (pneumonia) or pertussis (whooping cough). Treatment with antibiotics such as erythromycin, may be warranted in a child older than 5 years when mycoplasm or pertussis is suspected.[475]

Acute Cough in Adults (Acute Bronchitis)

According to CDC summaries, more than 90 percent of cases of acute cough illness in adults are nonbacterial. Viral causes of acute cough include influenza, parainfluenza, respiratory syncitial virus, and adenovirus. According to the CDC, pneumonia in adults is unlikely if all of the following are absent:[476]

- Fever greater than 38°C (99°F)
- Rapid breathing, greater than 24 breaths per minute
- Rapid heart rate, greater than 100 beats per minute
- Evidence of consolidation (fluid) on chest exam

According to a review published in the *New England Journal of Medicine*,[477] "Antimicrobial agents are not recommended in most cases of acute bronchitis. Systematic analyses of clinical trials have suggested that antibiotics may reduce the duration of symptoms, but at best modestly."[478]

Common Cold or Mild Upper Respiratory Tract Infection in Children

The CDC brochure for physicians on guidelines for treatment of the common cold begins with the following: "When parents request antibiotics for rhinitis or the 'common cold' . . . Give them an explanation, not a prescription." The CDC notes that children have two to nine viral respiratory illnesses per year.[479]

A recent study of parental beliefs noted that "Some parents believe that antibiotics are useful for conditions *where no benefit has been proven,* including acute bronchitis and upper respiratory infections.[480] [emphasis added] According to Dr. Sherif Mossad of the Cleveland Clinic, "Antibiotics have no role in the management of the common cold or any mild upper respiratory tract infection." He further remarks that "Sixty-eight percent of those receiving antibiotics are given non-recommended or more expensive broad-spectrum drugs."

According to the CDC, in a small percentage of cases the common cold can be complicated by bacterial sinusitis. This diagnosis should be undertaken carefully. When bacterial sinusitis is identified, the following should be considered:

- Target likely organisms with first-line drugs such as amoxicillin, amoxicillin/clavulanate.
- Use the shortest effective course. Should see improvement in 2 to 3 days. Continue treatment for 7 days after symptoms improve or resolve (usually a 10 to 14 day course).
- Consider imaging studies in recurrent or unclear cases.

Common Cold or Mild Upper Respiratory Tract Infection in Adults

Despite clear evidence that antibiotics are not appropriate for most cases of upper respiratory tract infections, almost 75 percent of adults with upper respiratory tract infections are prescribed antibiotics by their doctors. This accounts for some 41 million antibiotic prescriptions—roughly 20 percent of all antibiotics given to adults.[481] Unnecessary antibiotic prescriptions given for treatment of upper respiratory tract infections cost approximately $700 million per year.[482]

Addressing the matter, Michael Pichichero, MD, at the University of Rochester Medical Center, framed it in this way: "Are physicians who use antibiotics for most upper respiratory tract infections (URIs) providing any significant benefit for their patients? The short answer is no, but let us examine the data."[483] Dr. Pichichero went on to cite studies in which antibiotics were compared to placebo and where bacterial and viral cultures were performed. The doctors reported that "the groups did not differ in their response to the treatment regimens in terms of mean duration of fever, failure to improve, the development of complications, or the persistence of bacterial pathogens in the nasopharynx."[484]

According to recent CDC summaries:

- Studies have found the common cold resolves without antibiotic treatment.
- Treatment with an antibiotic does *not* shorten the duration of illness or prevent bacterial rhinosinusitis.
- Patients with purulent green or yellow secretions do not benefit from antibiotic treatment.

Urinary Tract Infection

Urinary tract infections account for about 8.3 million doctor visits in the United States each year.[485] They are distinctly different from the illnesses above in that there is a high prevalence of bacterial infections, when compared to the high prevalence of viral infections in other disorders.

Urinary tract infections are more common in women than in men. One reason is because a woman's urethral opening is close to sources of bacteria from the vagina and the anus. For some women, sexual intercourse seems to trigger an infection. This is also commonly due to vaginal and colonic bacteria. In adult women, the rate of urinary tract infections gradually increases with age.

People with diabetes have a higher risk of urinary tract infections because of changes in their immune system. The effect of diabetes on immune function will be explored in later chapters. Other disorders that suppress the immune system also raise the risk of a urinary tract infection.

Use of antibiotics can be appropriate in urinary tract infections. This is especially true when urine cultures have been performed and sensitivity tests to antibiotics have been performed. Since *Mycoplasma* or *Chlamydia* are difficult to culture by standard methods, special methods must be used to test for these.

Urinary tract infections may occur because bacteria are more able to adhere to the urethra or the bladder in some people. Some studies (discussed previously) have shown that certain foods can reduce the rate of attachment of bacteria to the bladder wall.[486]

Teenage and Adult Acne

It is estimated that up to 90 percent of teenagers will show some evidence of acne.[487] For this, physicians will prescribe substantial amounts of antibiotics, often keeping a child on them for years. The evidence that such antibiotics are effective for acne is inconclusive, and many doctors believe that antibiotics used in this way contribute to ill health in teenagers. While antibiotics can be of short-term benefit to some with acne, one must also be aware of the risks of these drugs. Any time long-term use of antibiotics is being considered, it should be done with full awareness of the potential consequences.

One concern that has been raised in regards to antibiotics and acne surrounds the adverse effects of the drug minocycline. This drug is used to treat moderate to severe acne in adolescents. A case has been reported of a fifteen-year-old boy who had taken minocycline for fourteen days.

He was initially treated by his primary physician on the fifteenth day of minocycline therapy "for symptoms of fever, joint swelling, and a rash." A pediatric rheumatologist subsequently diagnosed the boy as having drug-induced lupus. According to the treating physician, "The patient's myalgia [muscle pain] and arthralgia [joint pain] subsided within six weeks, but his strength, coordination, and endurance did not reach their prior levels for three to four months."[488]

Minocycline used for acne has also been linked with liver damage. A large database analysis was undertaken to look for reports of minocycline-associated liver damage. People taking minocycline for reasons other than acne were not included in the study. The researchers found 65 reported cases of liver damage, which were classified as 1) having insufficient information to classify, 2) autoimmune hepatitis with lupus-like symptoms, and 3) hypersensitivity reaction associated with dermatitis. The authors wrote, "Severe cases of minocycline-associated hepatotoxicity appear to be a hypersensitivity reaction and occur within a few weeks of commencing therapy. An autoimmune hepatitis usually presents after exposure to minocycline of a year or more, is more common in women, and is sometimes associated with lupus-like symptoms."[489]

At the Dentist

For many years, it has been routine dental practice to treat people with a history of rheumatic fever, heart valve abnormalities, or other heart conditions with antibiotics. It was believed that bacteria in the mouth could enter the bloodstream during routine dental procedures such as teeth cleaning and lodge themselves in the heart, leading to a condition known as endocarditis (called infective endocarditis).

This practice exposes many thousands of patients to antibiotics each year who are not ill. In their ongoing effort to reduce unnecessary antibiotic use and at the same time appropriately protect patients who may be at risk of infective endocarditis, the American Heart Association has developed new guidelines that have been endorsed by other groups such as the American Dental Association, the Infectious Diseases Society of America, and the Pediatric Infectious Disease Society.[490]

The guidelines say that **patients who have taken preventive antibiotics routinely in the past but no longer need them** include people with:[491]

- mitral valve prolapse
- rheumatic heart disease
- bicuspid valve disease
- calcified aortic stenosis
- congenital heart conditions such as ventricular septal defect, atrial septal defect, and hypertrophic cardiomyopathy

The new guidelines are aimed at patients who would have the greatest danger of a bad outcome if they developed a heart infection.

Preventive antibiotics prior to a dental procedure are advised for patients with:[492]

- artificial heart valves
- a history of infective endocarditis
- a cardiac transplant that develops a problem in a heart valve
- certain specific, serious congenital (present from birth) heart conditions, including
  - unrepaired or incompletely repaired cyanotic congenital heart disease, including those with palliative shunts and conduits
  - a completely repaired congenital heart defect with prosthetic material or device, whether placed by surgery or by catheter intervention, during the first six months after the procedure
  - any repaired congenital heart defect with residual defect at the site or adjacent to the site of a prosthetic patch or a prosthetic device

The conditions above represent just a fraction of illnesses related to microbes. They are the conditions for which the vast majority of antibiotics are given. Attention to the appropriate care and caution in these kinds of conditions will reduce the exposure of common bacteria to antibiotics, which will contribute mightily toward a reduction in antibiotic-resistant bacteria.

Chapter 14

Personalized Medicine and Strong Defenses

Personalized medicine involves understanding a person's disease or disease susceptibility by first using molecular or biochemical analysis, which is followed by the development of therapies that are based on these molecular analyses. It is typically meant to involve genomic, proteomic, and metabolomic analysis. Stated more simply, it involves the measurement of genes, proteins, and small molecule metabolites, with the intent to better describe the genetic and biochemical events taking place within a person. This knowledge can then be used to develop a treatment that is tailored to the person's unique biochemistry at that point in time.

In some circles, personalized medicine includes using biochemical assessment in order to arrive at the preferred drug therapy. *Beyond Antibiotics* is oriented in a distinctly different direction, focusing on ways in which drug therapy might be avoided and identifying underlying metabolic deficiencies that might weaken our defenses against microbes. In other words, we are trying to fortify the immune defenses as a means to improve health and avoid antibiotic drugs wherever possible.

This chapter places a heavy emphasis on nutritional biochemistry as the foundation of personalized medicine. We must understand that all fundamental biochemistry in the human body is fueled by and interacts with the small molecules that we encounter in the diet. All energy, all synthesis of DNA, synthesis of proteins, synthesis of small molecules, synthesis of cells, construction of barrier defenses, and any activity one might describe, are wholly and completely dependent upon the essential materials derived from the diet.

These deficiencies necessarily give rise to alterations in biochemistry over time and to a breakdown of our defense and repair capabilities. It can be no other way. In the future, we will think it unconscionable that a physician would revert to drug therapy without determining whether the patient's health condition is due to an underlying deficit of a fundamental precursor (typically a nutrient molecule).

Why Immune Defense, Energy, and Repair?

To make the best use of this chapter on personalized medicine, it is important to understand another distinction that I have made throughout this book. Many popular books written for the purpose of "immune building" or "immune boosting" are centered on the immune system proper—the network of white blood cells and immune proteins. While I include this very same attention to the immune system proper, the approach in this book is to broadly expand our discussion to that of immune defense, energy, and repair. This, necessarily, also includes a vast network of genetic and biochemical events that are involved in energy, muscle metabolism, the anti-inflammatory system, the barrier defenses (such as those in the skin, lungs, and digestive tract), the neurochemistry of mood (so as to improve our coping abilities), gut bacterial balance, and so on.

In my twenty years of experience with laboratory assessment and personalized medicine, it has become evident that a wide variety of deficiency patterns exist within the general population. Personalized medicine is a way to focus supplementation where it is needed by performing a detailed assessment of nutritional status using a combination of blood and urine tests.

Chapter 5 explored some of the basic ways in which vitamins, minerals, and other small molecules influence the immune system, as well as all of the supportive energy and repair systems. Personalized medicine based on laboratory analysis allows us to take a broad picture of nutrients that influence these systems, removing the guesswork associated with supplementation. With this approach, we can personalize the use of diet and nutrition to, hopefully, arrive at a nutrient balance that is optimum for a robust defense system. (See Appendix C for a discussion of why nutrients are critical for defense, energy, and repair.)

Nutrients can be measured in blood plasma, blood serum, whole blood, blood cells, and urine by direct and indirect methods. Direct methods are just as they sound, wherein we measure the concentration of the nutrient in blood or in blood cells. Indirect methods take advantage of our knowledge of vitamins and minerals in metabolism. For example, vitamin B12 is required to convert methylmalonic acid to succinic acid. If elevated levels of methylmalonic acid appear in urine, we know that vitamin B12 levels are low because the factor needed to facilitate the conversion (B12) is not present in adequate amounts.

In our approach to personalized medicine, we can measure a large number of vitamins, minerals, amino acids, fatty acids, and accessory food factors known to be important to immune defense, energy, and repair. This may include measuring some fifty to two hundred compounds, which can be used to develop a kind of metabolic map.

This chapter is designed to be a practical tool for use in developing a personalized health maintenance or health recovery plan.* There are also tests described that may indicate the need for specific drug therapy.

*Personalized medicine and functional medicine include a wide range of assessments beyond the molecular laboratory assessment presented here. These would include, for instance, assessments of mood, temperament, personality, coping styles, and many others within the field of psychology. However, due to the profound influence of molecular changes and the need for a certain brevity in this book, I have chosen to focus on assessment of biochemical changes. It should also be noted that lifestyle and psychological factors impact heavily on biochemical measures, so the measures described herein often reflect other aspects of life.

The emphasis is on tests that will allow an accurate assessment of your nutrient status so that you can proceed, with the help of a professional, to tailor a preventive or therapeutic plan to your needs. This section also contains a set of profiles that can help assess immune status, gastrointestinal function, and the presence of specific types of infections.

This section, then, is designed to give you information about available tests and permit you to speak intelligently with a health care professional about how to best tailor a program to suit your needs.

All attempts to understand a health challenge begin with a thorough history and an understanding of current concerns. This provides important context into which the laboratory tests can be placed and gives some direction to the laboratory testing that should be pursued.

Many physicians working in the field of personalized medicine will approach an assessment in the following manner.

Step 1. General Metabolic Profile (GMP). This is a profile that includes a set of targeted essential and nonessential molecules that are fundamental to metabolism, without which the natural defenses cannot function. This profile can be universally applied to any person, with any health condition, at any stage of illness or recovery. Such a profile typically involves measuring some one hundred or more biomarker compounds, which immediately yield information about basic metabolism. This alone can often be used to develop an appropriate personalized plan.

Common tests ordered as part of the General Metabolic Profile include:

Amino acids (blood or urine)
Fatty acids (plasma or red cell)
Organic acids (urine)
Trace elements (red blood cell, white blood cell)
Vitamins (whole blood, plasma, or serum)
Accessory nutrients (like coenzyme Q10, carnitine, etc.)

Step 2. Early Targeted Metabolic Profile. If the history clearly suggests that specific tests are needed beyond the general metabolic profile, these can be performed immediately and in parallel to the GMP (without waiting for the results of the GMP). For example, a history of extensive antibiotic use or significant intestinal symptoms would likely cause a physician to want to investigate intestinal function early in the process—perhaps at the same time as the GMP. A history or suspicion of a hormonal disorder would argue in favor of doing a specific hormone profile early in the testing process.

Step 3. Conditional Targeted Metabolic Profile. The first phases of testing will often show abnormal results that will point the direction toward specific follow-up testing. In this way, the general metabolic profile is used to guide future testing in the personalized medicine assessment. This profile might include tests mentioned in this section and may also include tests not described here.

This chapter is designed as a guide in the fundamental tests of personalized medicine. In the field of clinical chemistry and personalized medicine, the number of biochemical and genetic markers is tremendous and would take an entire book to describe. Thus this chapter, while detailed, must necessarily omit the tests that are more specialized or less frequently used.

Personalized Medicine and Assessment of the Nutrient Families

Personalized medicine, with nutritional biochemistry at it core, permits us to measure key nutrients and nutrient families that influence our immune defense, energy, and repair systems. Common nutrient families that can be measured include:

Vitamins	Minerals
Trace elements	Fatty acids
Amino acids	Accessory nutrients

Assessing Vitamin Status

Vitamins are well known for their essentiality. There are two main considerations in assessing vitamins. First, the specimen type, whether it be whole blood, plasma, serum, red cells, white cells, urine, or sweat, stool, hair, or some other specimen. The second is the means to determine the vitamin levels. For instance, direct assessment of the vitamin may be useful, as in serum vitamin B12, but better tests may be more functional in nature, such as holotranscobalamin or methylmalonic acid. Since these are primarily decisions the health care provider must make, I will not complicate our discussion by describing the advantages and disadvantages of each.*

The vitamins include:

Vitamin A	Vitamin D
Vitamin E	Vitamin K
Vitamin C	Thiamin (B1)
Riboflavin (B2)	Niacin (B3)
Pantothenic Acid	Pyridoxine (B6)
Biotin	Folic acid
Cobalamin (B12)	

Semi- or quasi-vitamins include carnitine, choline, inositol, and coenzyme Q10.

*A discussion of laboratory methods can be found in Sauberlich, HE. Laboratory Tests for the Assessment of Nutritional Status, CRC Press; Lord, RS, Bralley, JA. Laboratory Evaluations for Integrative and Functional Medicine, Institutes for Advancement in Molecular Medicine.

Testing for Vitamin D Status

It may seem like vitamin D is being given undue attention by being singled out while other vitamins are discussed as panels. This is for two reasons. First, it is increasingly clear that vitamin D is more hormone than vitamin. Scientists have known for decades that vitamin D has a steroid structure similar to testosterone, estrogen, and cortisol (at least in its backbone). In recent years, it has become clear that the biological effects of this powerful steroid go well beyond vitamin status. The second reason for this attention to vitamin D is that vitamin D excess can trigger negative metabolic changes, especially in people with certain autoimmune disorders. Vitamin D status is often assessed using only one marker. Many doctors now suggest that both markers below be assessed.

Vitamin D Markers

- 1,25-Vitamin D3
- 25-Vitamin D3

Testing for Trace Elements

Testing for trace elements is one of the more nuanced assessments in personalized medicine. This is because trace element compartments in the body vary in their usefulness as a reflection of mineral status. For instance, serum magnesium is widely used in the clinic to assess magnesium status. However, only a small portion of body magnesium lies in blood, so serum is not a good indicator of whole body magnesium status (though it is useful to detect when falling magnesium levels begin to threaten the heart). Red blood cell magnesium or a magnesium loading test would be considered better indicators of magnesium status.

Minerals and Trace Elements to Be Analyzed:

Calcium	Chromium
Cobalt	Copper
Iodine	Iron
Magnesium	Molybdenum
Phosphorous	Potassium
Selenium	Sulfur
Zinc	

Testing for Iron Deficiency and Overload

Iron deserves special attention since both iron deficiency and iron excess can alter defenses against bacteria. Moreover, the presence of the genetic mutation for hemochromatosis is common and strongly influences immunity. Detecting iron deficiency or your tendency (or risk) to accumulate iron in excess involves four standard biochemical tests and two genetic tests:

Biochemical Tests for Iron Status

Serum iron	Serum ferritin
Transferrin saturation	Total iron binding capacity (TIBC)

Genetic Tests for Inherited Disease of Iron Accumulation

Hfe mutation C282Y	Hfe mutation H63D

Techniques for evaluating brain iron content have been developed through advancements in magnetic resonance imaging (MRI) via the effect of iron on transverse relaxation rates (R_2). Essentially, the field-dependent R_2 increase (FDRI) method is a specific measure of the total iron contained in ferric oxyhydroxide particles that form the mineral core of ferritin molecules within the brain.[493] An adult with a chronic neurodegenerative disease, particularly Parkinson's or Alzheimer's, may wish to request this test to determine whether iron accumulation is present. This should be coupled with the iron status and genotype tests mentioned above.

Determining Blood Fatty Acid Levels

Fatty acids are the fundamental building blocks of almost all cell membranes in the body (except bone, for example). Fatty acids also form the foundation for a cascade of signaling molecules bewildering in their complexity. It has become clear that fatty acids can up-regulate and down-regulate different aspects of immunity. Through their influence on lipoxins, defensins, and resolvins, compounds associated with recovery and repair, fatty acids are central to the recovery process.

Therefore, becoming specific in our assessment of fatty acid status allows us to tailor any program to our needs. Also, inborn errors of fatty acid metabolism occur with some frequency. These can often be detected with a blood profile. Moreover, fatty acid metabolism is highly dependent upon cofactor vitamins and minerals. Selected fatty acid patterns encountered in a blood test can often point us toward these deficiencies. Finally, fatty acid profiles will often reveal that fatty acid values are low even though the individual is ingesting fatty acid supplements. This is how we frequently discover that the person is not absorbing nutrients and likely has an intestinal absorption deficit. This is an all too common finding in people with an extensive history of antibiotic use.

Below is a list of specific fatty acids that should be considered a component of any blood profile of fatty acids. Fatty acids are commonly measured in red blood cells or in plasma. There is some debate about which tissue is best used to assess fatty acids. It is commonly believed that plasma yields a better picture of current dietary intake, while red blood cells yield a better picture of the fatty acid status over time.

Polyunsaturated Omega-3

alpha-Linolenic
Eicosapentaenoic
Docosapentaenoic
Docosahexaenoic

Polyunsaturated Omega-6

Linoleic
gamma-Linolenic
Dihomogammalinolenic
Eicosadienoic
Arachidonic
Docosapentaenoic
Docosadienoic
Docosatetraenoic

Polyunsaturated Omega-9

Mead

Monounsaturated (Omega-7, Omega-9)

Myristoleic
Palmitoleic
Vaccenic
Oleic
11-Eicosanoic
Erucic
Nervonic

Saturated Fatty Acids (even numbered)

Capric
Lauric
Myristic
Palmitic
Stearic
Arachidic
Behenic
Lignoceric
Hexacosaenoic

Saturated Fatty Acids (odd numbered)

Pentadecanoic
Heptadecanoic
Nonadecanoic
Heneicosanoic
Tricosanoic

Trans Fatty Acids

Palmitelaidic
Elaidic
Total C:18 trans

Fatty Acid Ratios

Linoleic Acid/Dihomogammalinolenic acid

Eicosapentaenoic Acid/ Dihomogammalinolenic acid
Arachidonic Acid/Eicosapentaenoic acid
Triene/Tetraene

Comprehensive Cholesterol Profile

Standard tests for blood fats include cholesterol, HDL, LDL, VLDL, and triglycerides. More specific tests are available that measure subgroups of lipids important in health and disease. This is sometimes called the VAP.

HDL cholesterol
LDL cholesterol
VLDL cholesterol
Total cholesterol
Triglycerides
HDL_2
HDL_3
Total HDL cholesterol
Total non-HDL
Non-HDL/HDL ratio
LDL-R-Cholesterol
Total LDL cholesterol
LDL-R subclass pattern: A, A/B, B
$VLDL_{1,2}$ (Buoyant)
$VLDL_3$ (Dense)

Amino Acids Assessment

Chapters 4 and 5 addressed the role of protein and muscle in immune defenses. Muscle mass and strength are associated with enhanced immunity, resistance to infection, better response when an infection occurs, better recovery from infection, and better recovery from trauma. The reservoir of protein that exists in our muscle is based on the building blocks, the amino acids. One way to promote strong defense, recovery, and repair is to maintain an ample amino acid pool within muscle. Also, amino acids are required for all proteins involved in immunity, in metabolism, in building receptors, and more. In short, without adequate amino acids, systemwide errors can occur that affect all aspects of human function.

Assessment of amino acid status can be helpful to determine if reserves might be low during states of health. During illness, amino acid levels in blood can be assessed to understand the severity of deficiency. Tests can also be performed once the acute stage of illness has passed to determine how amino acid supplementation might best be used to speed recovery.

Amino acid analysis is performed on blood plasma or on a 24-hour urine specimen. Plasma is considered to yield a picture of amino acids with inferences about amino acid status. It allows one to compare measured values with established reference ranges. Urine is expected to yield information about relative amino acid levels over a 24-hour period, and provides valuable insight into metabolic pathways involving amino acids. Urine amino acids can also help determine if cofactors needed for amino acid metabolism might be low. Amino acid interpretation is a complex matter and requires an assessment of patterns that may emerge on testing.

Under ideal circumstances, combining the data from plasma and urine amino acid measurement can be expected to yield the most complete information about a person's state of health. However, if one were to perform a single test to look at amino acid status, blood plasma would be the preferred source.

Amino acids and amino acid metabolites commonly measured in urine and plasma include the following. Those in bold are considered essential amino acids. They cannot be made by the body and must be obtained from the diet. These are commonly found to be deficient in profiles we've run on patients:

Arginine	Asparagine
Aspartic acid	Histidine
Isoleucine	**Leucine**
Valine	**Lysine**

Methionine	**Phenylalanine**
Threonine	**Tryptophan**
Serine	Glycine
Taurine	Tyrosine
Cysteine	Cystine
Citrulline	Glutamic acid
Glutamine	Ornithine

Additional compounds derived from amino acids include:

Alanine	beta-Alanine
Anserine	Carnosine
Sarcosine	alpha-Aminoadipic acid
Cystathionine	gamma-Aminobutyric acid
homocysteine	beta-Aminoisobutyric acid
Hydroxylysine	Hydroxyproline
Methionine sulfoxide	1-Methylhistidine
2-Methylhistidine	Phosphoethanolamine
Phosphoserine	Proline
Urea	

Organic Acid Analysis

Organic acids are small molecules that are central to a vast network of metabolic events within the body. The measure of organic acids in urine has been used for decades to detect errors in metabolism and also to detect nutrient deficiencies that might disrupt metabolism. Since there are literally hundreds of compounds present in urine, each laboratory selects the specific analyte panel on which they focus.

The following table includes molecules commonly measured in organic acid profile include:

■ Table 14.1. Molecules Commonly Measured in Organic Acid Profile

Organic Acid	Metabolic Role/Clinical Significance
Energy Production	
Citrate	Citric acid cycle/energy metabolism
Cis-aconitate	Citric acid cycle/energy metabolism
Isocitrate	Citric acid cycle/energy metabolism
alpha-ketoglutarate	Citric acid cycle/energy metabolism
Succinate	Citric acid cycle/energy metabolism
Fumarate	Citric acid cycle/energy metabolism
Malate	Citric acid cycle/energy metabolism
Lactate	Aerobic/anaerobic energy Oxidative phosphorylation
Pyruvate	Aerobic/anaerobic energy Oxidative phosphorylation
Cofactor Markers	
Xanthurenate	Tryptophan metabolism
alpha-ketoisovalerate	Amino acid metabolism using B-vitamins
alpha-ketoisocaproate	Amino acid metabolism using B-vitamins
alpha-keto-methylvalerate	Amino acid metabolism using B-vitamins
Glycolate	Oxalate-ascorbate
Methylmalonate	B12, BCAA input into Kreb's cycle
beta-hydroxyisovalerate	Enzymes requiring biotin
Hydroxymethylglutarate	Coenzyme Q10 synthesis
Carbohydrate Metabolism	
beta-hydroxybutyrate	Balance of fat and CHO metabolism, indication for chromium
alpha-hydroxybutyrate	Balance of tat and CHO metabolism, indication for chromium
General Detoxification Markers	
Glucarate	Liver enzyme activation, glycine, glutathione, NAC
Pyroglutamate	Kidney amino acid recovery required for glutathione synthesis

Fatty Acid Oxidation	
Adipate	Fatty acid metabolism, which may reflect the following nutrient needs: carnitine, riboflavin, pantothenate ascorbate,
Suberate	Fatty acid metabolism, may reflect riboflavin need
Ethylmalonate	Fatty acid metabolism, may reflect coQ10 need
Neurotransmitter Metabolism	
Vanilmandelate	Epinephrine and norepinephrine metabolism
Homovanillate	Dopamine metabolism
5-hydroxyindoleacetate	Serotonin metabolism; may reflect tryptophan need
Kynurenate	Tryptophan metabolism; may reflect pyridoxine need
Quinolinate	Tryptophan metabolism; may reflect magnesium need
Dysbiosis Markers	
Benzoate	These markers can be products of gut microbial metabolism that have the potential to interfere with energy metabolism.
Hippurate	
p-cresol	
p-hydroxybenzoate	
p-hydroxyphenylacetate	
p-hydroxyphenyllactate	
Dihydroxyphenylpropionate	
Tricarballylate	
beta-ketoglutarate	
Hydrocaffeeate	
Tartarate	
Arabinitol (D/L-Arabinitol ratio)	
Arabinose	
Citramalate	

Oxidative Stress Profile

Measures of oxidative stress can provide information about how a disease process or health condition may be affecting oxidative balance in the body. They can also be considered an indirect reflection of antioxidant defenses.

Table 14.2. Tests for Assessment of Oxidative Stress

Plasma Variable	Specific Biomarkers
Lipid peroxidation	Malondialdehyde, F2-isoprostane, 4-hydroxynonenal
NO synthesis	Nitrite, nitrate, nitrotyrosine
Circulating antioxidants (unconjugated)	Uric acid, protein SH groups, bilirubin
	Ascorbic acid, alpha-tocopherol, beta-carotene, lycopene Antioxidant enzymes (GSHPx, catalase) Selenium, Zinc Glutathione (GSH), glutathione disulfide (GSSG) GSH to GSSG ratio (GSH:GSSG)
Xanthine oxidase activation	Plasma xanthine oxidase

Assessment of Gut Microbes

It is now clear that the forest of bacteria that inhabits our intestinal tract is strongly influenced by dietary intake, stress, injury, antibiotic drugs, and a host of other factors. Antibiotics are one of the most powerful classes of substances that shape our interior microbial landscape, thus anyone with a history of antibiotic use would be wise to pay attention to the integrity of her gut bacterial population. In addition, any strategy to build overall immune defenses, foster healing, and prevent infections must attend to the complex dynamics at work within the intestinal tract. More specifically, any attempts to restore health when there is a history of antibiotic use would be wise to include the gut.

While there are general strategies that can be helpful, such as consumption of prebiotics and probiotics, the vast complexity of the gut flora and intestinal metabolism require that we proceed with at least some measure of specific information.

Looking Inside

There are two major tools we can use to approach personalized medicine applied to the gut: genomics and targeted metabolomics. Within the latter, there are two major ways in which scientists can "image" the metabolism taking place within the intestinal tract. In general, this is done by testing the metabolic footprints (small molecules) associated with microbial metabolism in the gut and selected measures of gut function. There are two primary specimens from which to gather these "footprints" of gut metabolism. One is by examination of stool and the other by examination of urine.

Examination of the stool for bacterial types and the byproducts of their metabolism can tell us much about what has gone wrong and how to proceed with a personalized recovery plan. Biochemical analysis of urine can give us additional information about the gut bacteria, since the biochemical footprints of the gut bacteria make their way into the bloodstream and are excreted into the urine.

The modern tools we now use to reveal these details include genetic and biochemical fingerprinting. The process going on in the gut is enormously complex. The tests now in use will likely one day seem limited and overly simplistic, but we currently possess enough knowledge and the basic tools to make some very precise measurements that can lead to nicely tailored, personalized wellness plans. The tests for devising a personalized medicine effort aimed at intestinal wellness are explored below.

Genetic Testing and Gut Bacteria in Stool

One of the first steps to improving immune health via the intestinal tract is through the identification of the predominant "normal" and "abnormal" flora residing in the gut. Another way of viewing this is that we wish to understand whether beneficial gut microbes have diminished or overgrown while likewise determining whether harmful microbes are present in excess. This has always proven a complex task since most of the gut microbes grow without oxygen (called anaerobes). Culturing for microbes in an oxygen-free environment is costly and complex, making it difficult to get an accurate reflection of the resident populations in the gut.

New genetic tests have emerged on the scene that look for the genes of specific bacteria in stool specimens. These tests do not require complex culturing techniques, but rely upon standard amplification techniques refined during the human genome project. Laboratories can now locate, classify, and quantify the bacterial types within a stool specimen based on an assessment of what's called 16S ribosomal RNA (16S rRNA) or 16S rDNA. Typical microbes include, but are not limited to:

Normal or Predominant Bacteria

Obligate Anaerobes (cannot grow in the presence of oxygen)

Bacteroids sp — Clostridia sp
Fusobacteria — Mycoplasma
Prorotelia — Streptomyces
Firmicutes

Facultative Anaerobes (can grow in the presence of some oxygen)

Bifidobacterium sp — Lactobacillus sp

Obligate Aerobes (must grown in the presence of oxygen)

Escherechia coli

Opportunitstic Bacteria

Enterobacteria

Pathogens

C. dificile — *Campylobacter j.*
EHE coli — *Helicobacter pylori*

Parasites

E. histolytica	*G. lamblia*
Cryptosporidium	

Drug-Resistance Genes

aacA, aphD	mecA
vanA, B, C	gyrB, pare
PBP1a, ZB	

Gut Bacterial Footprints in Urine

With any good mystery in search of a culprit, we look for fingerprints, footprints, and other tell-tale signs of the perpetrator. Urine contains an array of such footprints, but in order to understand why, a brief detour into the world of diet and the gut is warranted.

As noted earlier, we share our food with the resident microbes of our colon. We take most of the good stuff, extracting vitamins, minerals, amino acids, fatty acids, and the like, before the bolus of food gets to the colon. Once in the colon, the remnants of our meal are greeted by the all-too-eager forest of resident microbes—the colonic flora. They gleefully gobble, churn, and digest the parts of the meal that are undigestible to us and those that may have passed too quickly for our internal systems to respond. As the gut bacteria metabolize these foodstuffs, they produce waste products—some good and some not so good.

Whether harmful or helpful, some of the waste products released from gut bacteria (waste products generated from their digestion of our meal) slowly make their way across the gut barrier and into the bloodstream (even when there is no leaky gut). These compounds can circulate in the bloodstream (sometimes causing harm, but that's another story) and eventually appear in the urine. With sophisticated but standard analytical techniques we can measure these compounds in the urine. Some of the footprints are very general and tell us only that there is dysbiosis (imbalance of gut bacteria). Others are quite specific and alert us to the presence of harmful organisms such as *Clostridium dificile,* a bug whose numbers explode in the presence of excessive antibiotics and which is associated with bloody diarrhea.

■ Table 14.3. Selected Gut-Bacteria-Derived Molecules Found in Urine

Ammonia	Benzoate
Butyrate	Enterolactone
Enterodiol	Valerate
Propionate	Hippurate
p-cresol	p-hydroxybenzoate
p-hydroxyphenylacetate	p-hydroxyphenyllactate
Dihydroxyphenylpropionate	Tricarballylate
beta-ketoglutarate	Hydrocaffeate
Tartarate	Arabinitol
Arabinose	Citramalate

Intestinal Parasites

If you are a microbe (bacteria, yeast, fungi, parasite) you are in a life and death competition for space and resources (food, nutrients). A healthy gut flora, well populated with Firmicutes and Bacteroidetes goes a long way to preventing parasitic organisms from gaining a foothold, which they do by the simple act of occupying space on the colon wall. If the colon wall is carpeted with vast amounts of beneficial bacteria, there is little or no space available onto which harmful organisms can attach and siphon off nutrients. You might liken it to a bad patch of grass on the lawn. When the grass is fertilized, watered, and gets adequate sunlight, a lush carpet emerges that is resistant to weeds. But allow your grass to thin and develop barren patches, and weeds will aggressively move in and begin to take over the lawn. Such is life in the colon. The harmful bacteria are like weeds. In the colon, a healthy population of "good" bacteria results in production of antimicrobial peptides and other molecules that create a hostile environment in which harmful organisms cannot easily grow.

The beneficial, semiharmful, and harmful organisms are always engaged in this battle. When beneficial organisms are reduced by antibiotics, the harmful organisms, such as parasites, are free to rise up. A colonic version of gang warfare ensues. In recognition of this time-honored fact, we often test for parasites in cases of heavy or frequent antibiotic use, lowered immunity, or gut symptoms.

The list below contains just some of the parasites commonly found in the colon. The more exotic forms have been left out for brevity. If discovered through stool testing, these parasites require specific treatment, often drug treatment, in order to restore gut microbial balance, gut barrier defenses, gut immune defenses, and general host immune defenses.

Giardi lamblia
Blastocystis hominis
Dientamoeba fragilis
Entamoeba histolytica
Cryptosporidium

Digestive Function

Stool samples can be used to assess certain aspects of digestive function, such as fat digestion, fat absorption, protein digestion, and others. Components of these profiles include:

Short-Chain Fatty Acids

Total SCFA
Propionate
Butyrate
Valerate

Long-Chain Fatty Acids

Total LCFA
Cholesterol
Total Fat
Triglycerides

Testing for Leaky Gut

As discussed previously, the intestinal membranes are selective about what they allow to pass through. Damage or injury to the lining of the small or large intestine can occur from infection, trauma, food intolerance, antibiotic use, and other factors. When the lining is damaged, molecular fragments that should be prevented from crossing the gut barrier are allowed to pass through, resulting in biochemical and immune reactions that have a persistent negative affect on health.

A simple test called the lactulose / mannitol test can be administered to determine if a leaky gut is present. Lactulose is a disaccharide (two sugars hooked together) that is not easily absorbed. When we consume lactulose, it should pass through the bowel and end up in the stool. It should *not* appear in the urine in appreciable amounts. Mannitol is a simple, monosaccharide (one sugar) that is easily absorbed across the gut lining. When we consume it, it should be absorbed into the bloodstream and end up in the urine.

When lactulose and mannitol are given together, mannitol should show up in the urine and lactulose should not. When lactulose appears in the urine, we conclude that the gut is leaky, permitting molecules to "leak" across the gut barrier that should not be permitted. The ratio of lactulose to mannitol gives an idea of the extent of the leaky gut phenomenon.

Leaky Gut Test[494]

- Swallow a solution of 5 grams of mannitol and 5 grams of lactulose
- Collect urine for 6 hours
- Laboratory analysis of lactulose and mannitol; calculate lactulose / mannitol ratio
- Interpretation:
  - Less than 14 percent mannitol recovered = malabsorption of carbohydrate

- Greater than 1 percent lactulose recovered = Leaky gut (increased intestinal permeability)
- Lactulose and mannitol values are plotted on a graph

Other agents are also sometimes used, including polyethylene glycol PEG400, PEG1000, 51CrEDTA, 99mTcDTPA, 51CrEDTA/14C-mannitol, rhamnose, and cellobiose.

Small Intestine Bacterial Overgrowth

In many different illnesses, bacteria from the colon can migrate upstream and colonize the small intestine—a location where these microbes do not belong. This is referred to as small intestine bacterial overgrowth. When this occurs, bacteria in the small intestine have access to food much earlier and produce gases such as hydrogen and methane.[495] This frequently occurs with long-term antibiotic therapy or with use of very powerful antibiotics. A simple test to detect small intestinal bacterial overgrowth can be administered to quickly identify how significant the migration of colon microbes into the small intestine might be.

- No antibiotics permitted for 7 days before the test.
- Ingestion of a sugar (disaccharide) lactulose.
- Collect exhaled breath every 30 minutes over a period of 2 to 4 hours. Sometimes collection is done from 6 to 24 hours.
- Analyze for hydrogen gas and methane gas.

Testing for Food Allergy

Gut integrity and general health can be negatively impacted by intolerance to food. An important example is that of celiac disease, in which intolerance to wheat gluten results in severe compromise of the intestinal tract. Gluten intolerance may also result in endocrine disruption, affecting the thyroid gland. Gluten intolerance is even known to contribute to degeneration of a portion of the brain known as the cerebellum in some people. Below is a brief list of blood tests that can be used to measure immune reactivity to foods:

Gluten Intolerance and Celiac Disease

Some doctors believe that a person must be consuming gluten while collecting specimens for testing. Other doctors contend that this is not necessary:

- IgA antihuman tissue transglutaminase (TTG)
- IgA endomysial antibody immunofluorescence (IgA-EMA)
- HLA-DQ2 (gene test from mouth swab)
- Antigliadin antibody (IgG and IgA) stool
- Antigliadin antibody (IgG and IgA) blood

Note: there is disagreement about whether antigliadin antibodies in blood are useful. A recent NIH consensus panel suggested that they not be routinely used because of low sensitivity and specificity. But pilot studies in which blood antigliadin antibodies were correlated with measures of leaky gut have demonstrated significance. Also, antigliadin antibodies in stool appear to be highly sensitive.

IgE Food Antibodies

Immunoglobulin E (IgE) is produced as part of the acute or rapid response to foods. Reactivity to foods through the IgE mechanism is usually abrupt and occurs within about 20 minutes from the time of consuming the food. These types of reactions are often noticeable because of the close proximity in time to the time of ingestion.

IgG Food Antibodies

Immunoglobulin G (IgG) is produced as part of a delayed response to foods. Reactivity to foods through the IgG mechanism commonly takes many hours to several days. Because of this delayed response, these types of reactions are more difficult to detect without testing, and may not be easily associated with consumption of a given food. IgE and IgG food antibody panels are often both used in order to detect reactivity to food by either means.

Testing for Heavy Metals

Testing for heavy metals is usually done by assessing blood, urine, or hair. The best specimen for assessment is determined by the element, time of exposure, and duration of exposure. In general, blood is used when metal exposure is thought to be recent or ongoing. For example, children exposed to lead in the home on an ongoing basis can be tested by measuring lead levels in blood. A child who may have eaten paint chips three days ago is best tested using blood. However, one whose exposure was two years ago is best assessed using urine, hair, fingernails, or toenails. Blood is preferred for acute exposure since the body removes toxic elements from the blood in a very short period.

When exposure to a toxic element has occurred at some time in the past, tissue element analysis or urine analysis are typically used. Hair element analysis is widely used in forensic medicine to isolate toxic elements. Clinically, hair is an inexpensive and easily obtained substance that gives a good picture of metal exposure.

Urine is also often used to assess metal toxicity. This is usually done by first challenging with a drug or nutrient known to bind heavy metals. These are called chelating substances and the test is called a *provocation*. The chelating substance enters the body and binds to the heavy metal that has been stored in the body tissue. Once bound together, the chelating substance-metal complex is flushed out through the kidney and can be collected in the urine.

The best nutrient chelating substances for heavy metals are those that contain a sulfur group (-SH). These groups cling tightly to metals such as mercury, arsenic, and lead. Glutathione is a small sulfur-containing peptide that is often used to reduce the body's load of heavy metals.

Drugs are often used as chelating substances since they bind tightly to certain metals and are readily excreted. Those commonly used include:

- D-penicillamine
- DMSA (dimercaptosuccinic acid)
- DMPS (dimercaptopropane sulfonate)
- EDTA (ethylenediaminetetraacetic acid)

Whenever a challenge (chelating) substance is considered for assessment of heavy metals, kidney clearance must first be assessed. A minimal assessment should include urinary creatinine clearance and a measurement of 24-hour urine volume. Provocation with a chelating substance is contraindicated during pregnancy, lactation, or kidney disease.

Elements such as aluminum are not easily bound by chelating substances, but can be displaced from the body by nutrients such as magnesium, malic acid, and vitamin C.

Toxic Elements Assessed in Blood, Urine, or Hair

Lead	Mercury
Cadmium	Arsenic
Antimony	Aluminum
Barium	Beryllium
Bismuth	Boron
Lithium	Nickel
Strontium	Thallium

Chemical Pollutants

The measurement of chemical pollutants is not part of standard practice in most clinics. This would likely be an assessment that would be most available in a research setting, an environmental medicine clinic, or occupational health clinic. Specific toxic molecules can be measured in blood or urine. Examples include, but are not limited to, the following:

Chlorinated (organochlorine) pesticides
Chlordane and related compounds
Aromatic volatile solvents
Chlorinated volatile solvents
Aliphatic volatile solvents
Chlorophenoxy herbicides
PCBs (polychlorinated biphenyls)

Assessment of Immune Status

Assessment of immune system status consists of many different tests. This section will focus on the primary measures of immunity (excluding the more exotic and complex).

White Blood Cell Profile

Total white blood cells
Lymphocytes
Eosinophils
Neutrophils
Monocytes
Basophils

Basic Immune Antibody Panel

Ig refers to immunoglobulin.

IgG (total)
IgG-1
IgG-2
IgG-3
IgG-4
IgA
IgM
IgE

T-Helper/T-Suppressor Ratio

Total and % T-Cell	Total and % T-Helper
Total and % T-Suppressor	T-Helper/T-Suppressor Ratio

C-Reactive Protein

Serum high sensitivity C-reactive protein (hs-CRP) is used as a general measure of inflammation and immune activation. C-reactive protein can be elevated during infection, which is a normal response. However, when CRP is elevated during non-infection periods, it indicates that the immune system is hyperactive. This occurs in diabetes, obesity, some forms of arthritis, and a variety of other situations.

Th1/Th2 Balance

Many studies discussed in this book have focused on the importance of the Th1/Th2 balance. The Th1/Th2 balance is really a measure of the immune proteins called cytokines. Some of the cytokines included in a Th1/Th2 profile are listed below.

Table 14.4. Testing for Th1/Th2 Balance

	Th1	Th2
Type of Immunity	Cell-mediated	Humoral
Cytokines Measured	IL-12 ↑ INF-γ ↑ TNFα ↑	IL-3 ↑ IL-4 ↑ IL-5 ↑ IL-6 ↑ IL-10 ↑ IL-13 ↑

Secretory IgA

As mentioned throughout this book, secretory IgA is an immunoglobulin (immune protein) that protects the mucosal surfaces of the respiratory tract and intestinal tract. Low sIgA is associated with increased susceptibility to pathogenic microbes. Because low sIgA is often linked with stress and cortisol, sIgA profiles are often included along with a cortisol profile. In addition, both are measured in saliva, so it is possible to do only one saliva collection and measure both molecules.

Immune System Energy: ATP and ADP

In Chapter 4, we discussed a test called the ATP/ADP ratio, which has been shown to be altered in some people with recurrent infections or susceptibility to infections. Though not widely used in clinics as yet, the ATP/ADP ratio could be a helpful indicator of energy deficits. In my opinion, if the ATP/ADP ratio is reduced, the next step is to ask why energy is reduced. Energy production may be impaired because of a deficiency of:

- Precursors needed to use as fuel (amino acids, sugars, fatty acids)
- Cofactors needed to drive the conversion of energy (magnesium, iron, copper, etc.)
- Coenzymes needed to drive the conversion of energy (based on vitamins such as thiamin, riboflavin, pyridoxine, etc.)

Energy production may also be impaired because of excess or toxicity, including but not limited to:

- Heavy metal exposure (mercury, lead, cadmium, etc.)
- Environmental exposure to toxic molecules (PCBs, etc.)
- Exposure to toxic molecules from gut bacteria (arabinitol, beta-ketoglutarate, cresol, etc.)
- Infections by bacteria, viruses, yeast, fungi, molds, or parasites

If the ATP/ADP ratio is altered, it is important to understand what has impaired energy production. Laboratory assessment of those items listed above can help uncover changes in biochemistry that might be responsible for the reduced energy.

Adrenal Stress Profile

Given the impact of stress and coping on immunity, it is often helpful to use laboratory tests to measure the extent to which stress related biochemical events have been altered.

Measurement of cortisol in saliva over the course of an entire day can give a picture of the stress response, as reflected in the cortisol curve. A collection of urine over 24 hours can be used to measure catecholamines like epinephrine and norepinephrine (adrenalin). A comprehensive stress profile such as the one below can reveal much about the stress response.

Cortisol (saliva or blood) collected at 8 a.m., 12 noon, 8 p.m., and 12 midnight
DHEA/DHEAS (dehydroepiandrosterone)
Testosterone
Estrogen
Progesterone
Estrogen/Progesterone ratio
Pregnenalone
24-hour urinary catecholamines (epinephrine and norepinephrine)

Hormone Testing

The endocrine, or hormonal, system plays a powerful role in regulating the immune system, as well as all energy, barrier defense, and repair systems. While a full discussion of endocrine tests is not warranted here, a basic review of certain tests that should be considered is helpful.

Thyroid Hormone Panel

TSH
Free T4
Free T3
Reverse T3
Thyroperoxidase
Antithyroid antibodies

Male Hormone Panel

Testosterone, Total
Dihydrotestosterone
Sex Hormone Binding Globulin
Free Androgen Index
Estradiol
Follicle-stimulating hormone (FSH)
Luteinizing hormone (LH)

Female Hormone Panel

2-hydroxy-estradiol
4-hydroxy-estradiol
16-hydroxy-estradiol
2/16-hydroxy-estradiol ratio
Follicle-stimulating hormone (FSH)
Luteinizing hormone (LH)
Progesterone
Estrogen/Progesterone ratio
Pregnenalone
Testosterone, Total
Sex Hormone Binding Globulin

Obesity and Insulin Resistance Profile

Conditions that linked to abnormal blood sugar metabolism can significantly affect defense and repair. The following should be measured.

Glucose
HbA1c
Insulin
Lipid profile (VAP above)

Closing Thoughts

The tests described here represent only a portion of those that might be included in a personalized medicine profile. Whether the most basic of these is chosen or whether more comprehensive testing is preferred, these measures will give extraordinary insight into the metabolic state as it relates to immune defense, energy, and repair.

Epilogue

Darragh had scored the winning basket at the buzzer against archrival Mullen, keeping Fairview in contention for a possible state tournament run. The game seemed to ebb and flow along with the fierce Colorado snowstorm rushing in from the mountains to our west. This was Darragh's night.

Just six days later, Darragh was on life support after falling sick with a sore throat. Darragh was a beloved teammate of my son Julian and of all those at Fairview High School in Boulder, Colorado. Robust, intense, strong, and gifted, there seemed to be no limit to the fire that Darragh brought with him to the court. Now he would need that fire to wage the most intense battle of his life—a battle for life itself.

As we sat in the bleachers, Darragh's teammates trotted onto the floor, each wearing a green t-shirt in solidarity with their fallen brother. Basketball was surely the last thing on the minds of these teenage boys who displayed Darragh's number 3 sketched in marker and a four-leaf clover, representing his beloved Irish heritage. Life should not hang in the balance like this.

But here we were. What began as an "ordinary" sore throat gave way to a cascade of bacteria crashing through the tonsil wall, seeding the bloodstream, and rushing through Darragh's body. The signs led the doctors to the diagnosis: Lamierr's disease.

Lamierr's disease is caused by a bacterium called *Fusobacterium necrophorum* (and occasionally *F. nucleatum, F. mortiferum,* and *F. varium*). A normal inhabitant of the throat area, Fusobacteria (which are nonoxygen-loving) nestle into the airless crypts of a tonsillar abscess caused by strep bacteria. Here, the Fusobacteria multiply and penetrate from the tonsils into the nearby jugular vein in the neck. Clots begin to form, which can clog the jugular vein, then break lose and cause blood clots to form in the lungs. These clots also carry massive arsenals of bacteria, which get seeded throughout the bloodstream, spreading the infection. As bacteria disseminate and clots fill the branches of the lung's vessels, shortness of breath, severe chest pain, and pneumonia follow with terrifying speed.

With Darragh in a coma and on full life support, his parents were told it was "in God's hands." One doctor suggested taking out a portion of Darragh's lung. Another argued that they use more potent drugs. Still another opinion came forward: "Do nothing." As the first hours of this life-and-death crisis played out, we sat and watched a game played by young men with heavy hearts, hoping that prayers would be answered and that a beloved brother would find the strength to rise against untenable odds.

Darragh finally arose from the coma and his crisis. Antibiotics, anticoagulants, critical care, and the love of many saved his life. Through his ordeal, he had lost twenty-five pounds. His body seemed to yield those twenty pounds of muscle and fat in order to feed the immune defenses that would eventually draw him back to life—a true testament to the intelligence of a human body.

We will never know why Darragh fell to this aggressive bacterial illness. But his ordeal surely reminds us that we are living in a world where invisible bacteria, even seemingly harmless ones, may breach our defenses at any time. We are also reminded that our antibiotic drugs are extraordinary gifts—gifts to be used with great care.

Doctors are alarmed by the fact that our antibiotics are failing and the development of new antibiotics has slowed to a trickle. This has spawned a search for new antibiotics in all corners of the earth. Scientists are looking to creatures with uncanny abilities to fight off infections. Alligators living in bacteria-infested waters possess a remarkable defense against all manner of dangerous bugs. In the laboratory, these novel proteins in alligator blood appear to kill certain forms of antibiotic-resistant bacteria, fungi, and viruses. Compounds from plants scattered across the planet have been found to harbor vast libraries of molecules that kill dangerous microbes in test-tube experiments. Frogs from remote forests of the Amazon harbor fragile but potent molecules on their skin that seem to thwart microbes that cause hospital-acquired infections such as *Staph aureus* and *Acinetobacter.* Scientists across the globe have begun to engineer *phages,* natural virus-like entities that are common enemies of bacteria.

Out of this new frontier will arise many promising agents. But we must be certain that we learn from our past encounters with the microbial world. Bacteria have shown they can win at almost any game. They are masters of adaptation that will likely find ways to defeat our new drugs and perhaps even learn to feed off them, as before. This has already been shown to be true with antimicrobial peptides like those found in alligators and frogs. One breakthrough compound has, sadly, now proven to elicit resistance in twenty-two of twenty-four bacterial strains tested, suggesting that the low levels of these antimicrobial peptides in nature may be effective, but the concentrated amounts needed in medicine foster resistance.[496]

This is not a surprising finding. Most early drugs of promise are guaranteed to fail because of ineffectiveness, resistance, toxicity, or cost. As a result, our ancitipated new arsenal may dwindle as the complexity of nature reminds us of her dominion.

These stark realities of drugs and bugs return us to ourselves—the host. Our dance with the microbe is not simple. But knowing that this is a dance and not a war gives us the vision to move forward in more thoughtful ways. Our blueprint for living in the microbe's world will still require antibiotics, old and new. But the foundation of this effort must now turn to the host.

Individuals who take it upon themselves to live in a way that fosters strong defenses will likely be able to reduce their vulnerability to microbes and thus their need for antibiotic drugs. Should doctors choose to practice medicine that is centered on host defenses, we will likely see reduced infections and improved recovery when infections do occur. Doctors practicing in this way would also help us to reduce reliance on antibiotics, which will reduce resistance and cause old antibiotics to return to the arsenal.

We will never defeat the microbes. We cannot completely insulate ourselves from infection, nor can we be certain that our efforts will protect us against unknown exposures. Infections will occur. Outbreaks will occur. Epidemics will occur. But if we are to gamble our future on antibiotics or strong defenses, nature would seem to favor strong defenses.

Appendix A

Antibiotics That Interfere with Nutrients

Below is a brief list of nutrients that may be depleted by the use of antibiotic drugs. When antibiotic courses are short (ten days or less), direct nutrient interactions may not be severe unless diarrhea has occurred. Anytime diarrhea occurs with antibiotic use, significant depletion in nutrients should be suspected.

Anytime an antibiotic acts to significantly alter normal intestinal bacteria, overgrowth of harmful organisms in the gut can lead to widespread changes in nutrient utilization. This can occur even with short courses of very strong or broad-spectrum antibiotics. Long-term courses with antibiotics can have pronounced effects on nutrient levels.

■ Table A.1. Effect of Antibiotics on Selected Nutrients

The following information has been reprinted with permission from *Natural Medicines Comprehensive Database.* For more information, please go to www.naturaldatabase.com

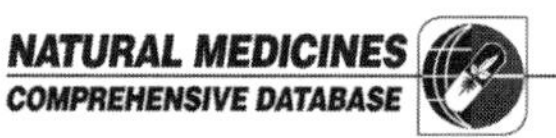

Drug Influences on Nutrient Levels and Depletion

Some medications can affect the levels of certain nutrients in the body. There is considerable interest in using nutritional supplements to counteract these possible drug-induced "nutrient depletions." The chart below shows the current scientific understanding of these relationships, and suggested actions.

Antibiotics	Nutrient Depleted	Possible Mechanism	Comments & References
Antibiotics, General: Cephalosporins, Fluoroquinolones, Isoniazid, Macrolides, Penicillins, Sulfonamides, Tetracyclines, Trimethoprim/ Sulfamethox azole	Biotin Dibencozide Pantothenic Acid (B5) Pyridoxine (B6) Riboflavin (B2) Thiamine (B1) Vitamin B12 Vitamin K	Destruction of normal intestinal microflora may lead to decreased production of various B vitamins and vitamin K. Some cephalosporins interfere directly with vitamin K-dependent clotting factor production.	The intestinal microflora is reduced by antibiotics. However, the B vitamins are mainly obtained from the diet, and any changes in their production by intestinal bacteria is unlikely to be clinically significant.[4434-43,6243,9502,9530] Reduction in vitamin K-dependent clotting factor production may be significant in people with other risk factors for low vitamin K levels. Monitor these patients closely.[4437,4439,7135,9502,11513-6]
Antibiotics, General	Folic Acid	Disruption of normal intestinal microflora decreases enterohepatic circulation and reabsorption of folic acid, and may reduce synthesis. Trimethoprim inhibits conversion of folic acid to its active form.	Folic acid synthesized by intestinal microflora probably doesn't contribute significantly to overall folate status, and supplements aren't necessary with normal courses of antibiotics.[2677,4436-7,6243]

Antibiotics	Nutrient Depleted	Possible Mechanism	Comments & References
Antibiotics, General, (cont.)	Folic Acid		Prolonged courses of high-dose trimethoprim rarely cause megaloblastic anemia, and folic acid supplements have been used to prevent this. However, some evidence suggests folic acid supplements can reduce the efficacy of trimethoprim. Avoid supplements unless recommended by a physician.[2677,4468,4531,9382-7,9398-9]
Aminoglycosides: Amikacin (*Amikin*) Gentamicin (*Garamycin*) Kanamycin (*Kantrex*) Netilmicin (*Netromycin*) Streptomycin Tobramycin (*Nebcin*)	Magnesium Potassium	Increased urinary excretion, associated with drug-induced renal damage.	Monitor patients for electrolyte disturbances and declining renal funciton. Give intravenous electrolyte replacement if necessary, and consider dose reduction/discontinuation of the aminoglycoside.[9519]
Cefditoren Pivoxil (*Spectracef*)	Acetyl-L-Carnitine L-Carnitine Propionyl-L-Carnitine	Chronic use of cefditoren can induce carnitine deficiency.	Long-term use of cefditoren might require supplementation, but short-term use does not seem to have a clinically significant effect on carnitine levels.[12759]
Chloramphenicol (*Chloromycetin*)	Niacin and Niacinamide	Chloramphenicol may interfere with the actions of nicotinamide adenine dinucleotide (NAD).	Deficiency is unlikely unless therapy is prolonged.[14514,14530-3]

Antibiotics	Nutrient Depleted	Possible Mechanism	Comments & References
Fluoroquinolones: Ciprofloxacin (*Cipro*), Enoxacin (*Penetrex*), Gatifloxacin (*Tequin*), Levofloxacin (*Levaquin*), Lomefloxacin (*Maxaquin*), Moxifloxacin (*Avelox*), Norfloxacin (*Noroxin*), Ofloxacin (*Floxin*), Sparfloxacin (*Zagam*), Trovafloxacin (*Trovan*)	Calcium Iron Magnesium Zinc	Formation of insoluble complexes (prevents absorption of both nutrient and fluoroquinolone).	A significant effect on levels of these nutrients is unlikely when fluoroquinolones are taken at least 2 hours before, or 4–6 hours after calcium, iron, magnesium, or zinc.[828,2682,3046,4412,4531]
Neomycin *(Mycifradin)*	Beta-Carotene Dibencozide Vitamin A Vitamin B12	Reduced absorption.	Not clinically significant with short-term use of neomycin.[3046,5916,8434,10565-6]
Pivampicillin (*Pondocillin*)	Acetyl-L-Carnitine L-Carnitine Propionyl-L-Carnitine	Chronic use of pivampicillin can induce carnitine deficiency.	Long-term use of pivampicillin might require supplementation, but short-term use does not seem to have a clinically significant effect on carnitine levels.[12759]
Penicillins (sodium-containing): Carbenicillin (*Geocillin*), Mezlocillin (*Mezlin*), Penicillin G sodium (*Pfizerpen*), Piperacillin (*Pipracil*), Ticarcillin (*Ticar*)	Potassium	A large sodium load is presented to the kidneys, resulting in sodium reabsorption and potassium excretion.	Monitor potassium levels, and give supplements or switch to a different antibiotic if necessary.[9519]
Sulfadiazine	Acetyl-L-carnitine L-carnitine Proprionyl-L-carnitine	Not known.	A single case report describes symptomatic L-carnitine deficiency in a patient treated with pyrimethamine plus sulfadiazine which reversed when both drugs were stopped.[14600]

Antibiotics	Nutrient Depleted	Possible Mechanism	Comments & References
Tetracyclines: Tetracycline *(Achromycin V, Panmycin, Robitet, Robicaps, Sumycin, Teline, Tetracap, Tetracyn, Tetralan),* Demeclocycline (*Declomycin*), Doxycycline (*Bio-Tab, Doryx, Doxy Caps, Doxychel, Doxychel Hyclate, Monodox, Periostat, Vibra-Tabs, Vibramycin),* Minocycline (*Dynacin, Vectrin*), Oxytetracycline (*Terramycin, Uri-Tet*)	Calcium Iron Magnesium Zinc	Formation of insoluble complexes prevents absorption of both nutrient and tetracycline. Doxycycline does not reduce zinc absorption.	A significant effect on levels of these nutrients is unlikely when tetracyclines are taken at least 2 hours before, or 4–6 hours after food or supplements containing calcium, iron, magnesium, or zinc.[4412,4531,4549-50,4945]
	Potassium	Increased renal excretion associated with nephropathy.	Due to a toxic degradation product in outdated tetracyclines. Avoid outdated drugs.[4425]

Antifungals

Amphotericin B (*Abelcet, AmBisome, Amphocin, Amphotec, Fungizone*)	Magnesium Potassium	Increased urinary excretion, associated with drug-induced renal damage.	Monitor patients for electrolyte disturbances and declining renal function. Give intravenous electrolyte replacement if necessary, and consider changing to a different antifungal.[9519]
Fluconazole (*Diflucan*)	Potassium	Increased urinary excretion, associated with drug-induced renal damage.	Monitor potassium levels and renal function in people on prolonged fluconazole therapy, and in those with other risk factors for hypokalemia. Consider a supplement and discontinuation of fluconazole if necessary.[9519]

Antifungals	Nutrient Depleted	Possible Mechanism	Comments & References
Pyrimethamine (*Daraprim*)	Folic Acid	Folate antagonism. Pyrimethamine binds to dihydrofolate reductase, preventing conversion of folic acid to its active form.	At lower pyrimethamine doses, the need for supplementation has not been adequately studied. Advise patients to maintain good dietary folate intake. People receiving larger pyrimethamine doses (those required to treat toxoplasmosis), should receive folinic acid (leucovorin) to prevent megaloblastic anemia. Avoid folic acid, which antagonizes the therapeutic effects of pyrimethamine.[4425,4532,9380]
	Acetyl-L-carnitine L-carnitine Proprionyl-L-carnitine	Not known.	A single case report describes symptomatic L-carnitine deficiency in a patient treated with pyrimethamine plus sulfadiazine which reversed when both drugs were stopped.[14600]
Quinacrine	Riboflavin (B2)	Can interfere with conversion to the active form flavin adenine dinubleotide (FAD).	May cause riboflavin deficiency. Clinical significance is not known.[505,10521-2]
Antituberculosis Agents			
Aminosalicylic Acid (Para-aminosalicylic Acid, *Paser*)	Folic Acid	Inhibits absorption in the gastrointestinal tract.	May worsen the folic acid deficiency associated with tuberculosis. Recommend supplements if diet is folate-deficient.[4459,8441,9363,9388,9395-7]

Antituberculosis Agents	Nutrient Depleted	Possible Mechanism	Comments & References
Aminosalicylic Acid (cont.)	Iron	Reduced gastrointestinal absorption.	Monitor for signs and symptoms of iron deficiency and give supplements if needed.[9574]
	Dibencozide Vitamin B12	Reduced gastrointestinal absorption.	Monitor vitamin B12 levels if treatment lasts more than one month.[4558,9395,9397,9574]
Cycloserine (*Seromycin*)	Folic Acid	Possibly reduces absorption or increases metabolism.	Rare cases of megaloblastic anemia reported, but usually with other factors contributing to folate deficiency. Recommend supplements only if dietary intake is deficient.[4531,4536,9363]
	Niacin and Niacinamide	Interference with conversion of tryptophan to niacin.	Encephalopathy responsive to niacinamide reported rarely, usually when cycloserine is used with other drugs which interfere with niacin.[4531;14517-8]
	Pyridoxine (B6)	Inactivates pyridoxal-5'-phosphate, increasing pyridoxine requirements.	Deficiency can contribute to the neurotoxicity and seizures associated with cycloserine. It is recommended that pyridoxine 150-300 mg/day be taken with cycloserine. [2677,3022,4459, 8894,9501]

Antituberculosis Agents	Nutrient Depleted	Possible Mechanism	Comments & References
Ethambutol (*Myambutol*)	Copper Zinc	Ethambutol and its metabolite chelate copper and zinc in the gastrointestinal tract and decrease their absorption.	It is not known if copper supplementation is beneficial.[4535,8971] Zinc deficiency may contribute to visual dysfunction associated with higher doses of ethambutol. Monitor visual function. It is not clear if zinc supplements are helpful, and there is concern they may interfere with the therapeutic effects of etha mbutol.[4453,11613,11639-41]
Ethionamide (*Trecator-SC*)	Niacin and Niacinamide	Ethionamide has structural similarities to niacinamide and may interfere with its activity.	Encephalopathy responsive to niacinamide reported rarely, usually when ethionamide is used with other drugs which may interfere with niacin.[14517-8]
Isoniazid (INH, *Laniazid*)	Pyridoxine (B6)	Interferes with pyridoxine metabolism.	Patients receiving >10 mg/kg/day of INH should be supplemented with 50-100 mg of pyridoxine per day.[4481-2]
	Niacin and Niacinamide	Isoniazid inhibits the conversion of tryptophan to niacin. It also has structural similarities to niacinamide and may interfere with its activity.	Might induce pellagra if taken for long periods, particularly in poorly nourished patients and those taking other drugs which interfere with niacin.[2677,4865-6,6243,14514,14520]
Pyrazinamide	Niacin and Niacinamide	Pyrazinamide has structural similarities to niacinamide and may interfere with its activity.	Deficiency occurs rarely, but responds to niacinamide supplements.[14529]

Drugs	Nutrient Depleted	Possible Mechanism	Comments & References
Rifampin (*Rifadin, Rimactane, Rofact)*	Vitamin D	Increased hepatic metabolism of vitamin D due to enzyme induction.	This may cause osteomalacia if therapy lasts more than 1 year and vitamin D intake is low. Monitor calcium and vitamin D levels and consider supplements if necessary. Isoniazid taken concurrently may cause liver enzyme inhibition and prevent this effect.[11561-5]
	Vitamin K	Possibly decreased gastrointestinal absorption, destruction of vitamin K-producing bacteria, and interference with regeneration of vitamin K from inactive metabolite.	Consider supplements in people with other risk factors for vitamin K deficiency.[11517-8]

Reprinted with permission from: http://www.naturaldatabase.com/(S(ajbjfavtwysl0i553wcig42m))/ce/ceCourse.aspx?s=ND&cs=&st=0&li=0&pc=08-40&cec=0&pm=5

Appendix B

Why Antibiotics May Contribute to Obesity

One of the first studies that gained our attention was one in which germ-free mice were implanted with gut bacteria from normal mice. It should be noted that germ-free mice (mice with no gut bacteria) do not grow as well as other mice that have ample gut bacteria. When the gut bacteria from normal mice were implanted into the intestines of germ-free mice, the germ-free mice gained weight better than their other germ-free counterparts who were still "germ free."[497] This raised the possibility that certain gut bacteria made the mice better at extracting energy from the food they ate. This concept of "extracting energy" would go on to generate great excitement among researchers.

The next study set out to see whether the gut bacteria of genetically obese mice were better at extracting calories from food than their genetically lean cousins. But first, what does being better at extracting calories really mean? Our diets are filled with substances that we can easily digest, but contain others that are too insoluble (many fibers) for us to break down. Thus, we cannot get the energy (via the simple sugars of which they are made) out of some fibers, so they cannot contribute to our body mass.

Think of those cellulose-digesting bacteria in the stomach of a cow or a goat. Cows and goats can eat all manner of seemingly indigestible material (like corn stalks, corn cobs, alfalfa, and such) because some of their gut microbes produce the enzyme cellulase, which breaks down cellulose. Cellulose is a polymer of sugars. It is just a complex polymer that we cannot ordinarily break down. If you've ever wondered why an elk or a bison can turn into such a hulking beast by munching prairie grass, you can thank gut bacteria.

Back to our story of energy extraction—if the gut bacterial population of a mouse becomes better at breaking down difficult to digest fibers, it becomes better at freeing up those simple sugars that make up the complex fiber. Once the simple sugars are released, they act like any other sugar—they are absorbed into the bloodstream and either burned as energy or stored as fat (to oversimplify a bit).

So, what does the gut bacteria of an obese mouse look like, when compared to a lean mouse. First off, the gut bacteria of obese mice *are* better at extracting more calories from the food they eat than are their lean counterparts. That's a good beginning to our understanding, but how do they accomplish this? It appears that genetically obese mice have 50 percent fewer Bacteroidetes and more Firmicutes than their lean cousins.[498]

Bacteroidetes and Firmicutes are among the predominant phyla of bacteria in the gut, accounting for between 60 and 80 percent of the fecal bacterial community.[499] They are generally considered "friendly." The Bacteroidetes include Bacteroides. The Firmicutes include Lactobacillus, Mycoplasma, Bacillus, and Clostridium. Members of both phyla are known to help us to break down otherwise indigestible foods.

Scientists have shown that this trait of improved energy extraction from calories can actually be transmitted from obese mice to lean, germ-free mice by transplanting the gut bacteria of the obese mice to the lean mice. When the researchers transferred gut microbes from the conventional mice to the germ-free mice, the previously lean germ-free mice increased body *fat by roughly 60% in just 14 days.*[500] In other words, lean mice got fatter when given the gut bacteria of obese mice. This holds a very compelling potential message for humans.

Follow-up studies with obese mice have also revealed one additional confirmative finding. Washington University scientists measured undigested material in the stool of obese mice that could still be "burned" as energy. It is kind of like digging through the camp fire in the morning and finding a few unburned log fragments. As the researchers expected, the obese mice had less energy remaining in their stools (fewer unburned logs in the fire pit), when compared to their lean littermates. This confirmed that the obese mice were extracting more energy from their food (which occurred by virtue of their gut bacteria that were more efficient at extracting energy).[501]

Appendix C

Why Nutrients Are Important in Defense, Energy, and Repair

Our bodies rely on two basic forms of nutrients: essential and nonessential. Essential nutrients are those the body cannot make, so they must be obtained from the diet. Nonessential means your body can make what it needs from precursor nutrients derived from the diet. Vitamins and minerals are *essential.* Eight amino acids and two fatty acids are *essential.* You cannot make these.

Just like an assembly line or baking a cake, if the key starting materials or smaller components are not available, the end product is altered. In the human body, if specific nutrients are unavailable in adequate amounts, the end product is altered. It is really that simple. Whenever we are deficient in a single nutrient, many processes can be altered. When we are deficient in several or many nutrients, large networks of our metabolism begin to falter. We can look at it this way:

A is the essential nutrient we get from the diet. **B** is what we need to make to support our defense, energy, and repair.

■ **Figure C.1.**

In order for us to make B from A, we need vitamin cofactors and usually a trace mineral of some kind.

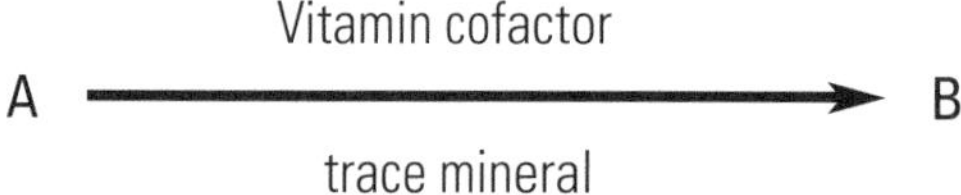

■ **Figure C.2.**

It is easy to see that if we have too little "A," too little of the vitamin, or too little of the trace mineral we cannot make B in the right amounts for metabolism to work properly. Let's look at a real example.

Serotonin is the neurotransmitter we need for proper brain function. Serotonin deficiency is a central culprit in mood and in our ability to manage stress. (Serotonin is also widespread in the gut.) We must have it to function properly and *we must make it from raw materials.*

Magnesium, Zinc

Tryptophan ⟶ Serotonin

Vitamin C

■ **Figure C.3.**

The parent nutrient tryptophan is, of course, an essential amino acid that we "must" get from the diet. If we do not get enough tryptophan, serotonin cannot be made in adequate amounts. Also, if we lack sufficient vitamin C, magnesium, or zinc we cannot make enough serotonin. The effect—mood, appetite, sleep, and a rash of other features of daily life are altered.

One Mineral Can Alter All Sugar and Energy Metabolism

Since energy is the foundation of our defenses, let's look at how we convert sugar into energy. It is a well-understood process with many steps, which is called glycolysis. Without adequate magnesium, the process of handling sugars from our diet is severely impaired. For instance, numerous studies have shown that magnesium deficiency is well-known to increase the risk to diabetes, chronic fatigue, heart disease, and other ills. It is easy to see why, when one looks at only one simple pathway of how we metabolize sugars.

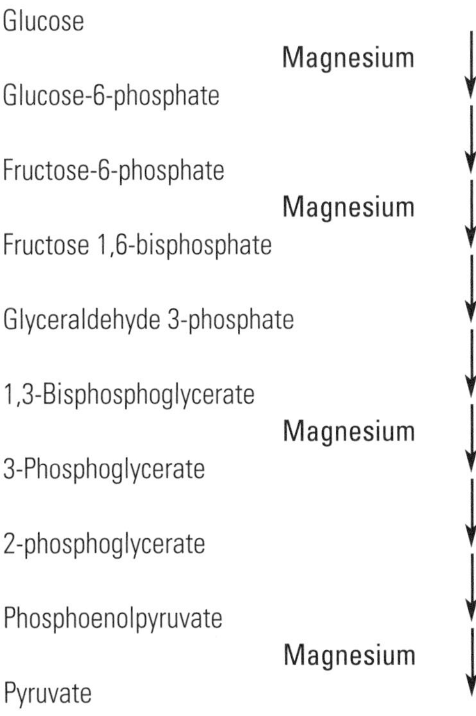

■ **Figure C.4.**

Strikingly, magnesium is involved in some three hundred enzyme systems within the body, making it one of our most vital cofactors. *All* reactions involving ATP, the body's energy currency, must have magnesium in order to proceed. This is fundamental biochemistry, but it is not widely known among doctors or among the public. In short, without adequate magnesium, our metabolism *will* suffer. The energy available to our immune defenses will suffer. Imagine, now, if deficiencies of two, three, or more nutrients occurs.

How Diet and Disease Processes Contribute to Nutrient Deficiencies

Vitamins, minerals, amino acids, and fatty acids are fundamental to our core metabolism. Deficiency of one or more nutrients can *lead* to disease. This is fundamental biochemistry as taught in all university and medical school curricula.

What we cannot forget is that once a disease process has begun, *the disease process itself* may produce higher needs for certain nutrients, or cause competition for or destruction of certain nutrients.

Let's see why a person with fatigue and impaired energy might need one important nutrient in supplement form—carnitine.

Carnitine helps us shuttle our fatty acids (fats) into a little structure called mitochondria, where the fats can be burned as fuel. Mitochondria are a little like furnaces. You might think of carnitine as the person who carries wood from out behind the house and puts it into the fireplace to be burned. The carnitine fatty-acid shuttle is how a person is able to burn fat from the diet. Too little carnitine, however, and the fats pile up as so many logs on the wood pile, waiting to be burned. Fat-burning slows, blood fats build up, and belly fat grows. Impaired energy ensues. Fortunately, we can make our own carnitine—to a point.

Humans use an amino acid from dietary protein sources called lysine to make the carnitine we need. Though it takes many steps and requires several nutrients to make, the carnitine assembly line looks like this:

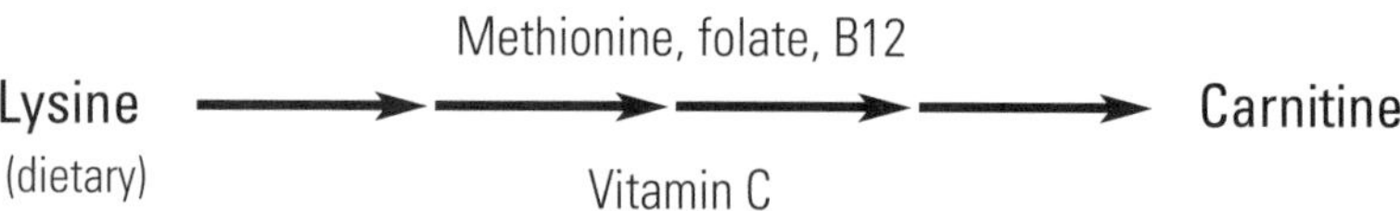

Figure C.5.

Now let's get back to someone who consumes a lot of dietary sugar or who has elevated blood sugar from diabetes. Sugars have a love affair with lysine—they stick to it and hold on tight. If dietary sugars are too high or if blood sugar gets too high, all that sugar starts tying up the lysine we need to make our carnitine. The result; the carnitine assembly line peters out.

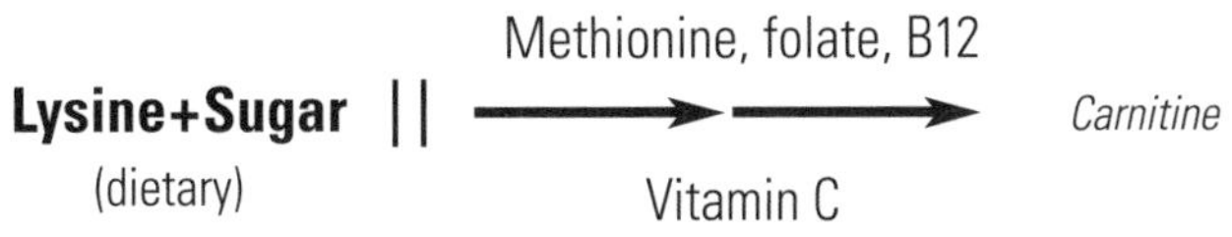

Methionine, folate, B12

Lysine+Sugar || ——→——→ *Carnitine*

(dietary) Vitamin C

■ **Figure C.6.**

Once the carnitine levels start falling, we get worse and worse at shuttling our fats into the furnace to be burned. In short, we get worse at generating energy from one of our key dietary fuels. The carnitine fatty-acid relationship is only one reason why we say people *must* manage their blood sugar and must be careful about their dietary sugars (though there are many other reasons).

Essential and Conditionally Essential Nutrients

As noted in Chapter 5, *essential nutrients* are those our bodies cannot make. Fundamental human metabolism cannot proceed without these essential nutrients. Included are:

- 21 minerals
- 13 vitamins
- 8 amino acids (10 for children)
- 2 essential fatty acids

Conditionally essential refers to compounds our bodies can make, but under various circumstances we cannot make enough of them to meet our requirements. These include are but not limited to:

- Carnitine
- Taurine
- Cysteine
- Lipoic acid
- Coenzyme Q10
- Choline
- Tyrosine
- Serine
- SAMe
- Arginine
- Betaine
- Glutamine
- Glutathione
- Glycine
- EPA (Eicosapentaenoic acid)
- DHA (docosahexaenoic acid)
- Arachidonic acid

Why Supplemental Nutrients Are Needed

These examples are helpful to understand why any program aimed at improving our defenses must rely upon certain core nutrients. Nutritional biochemistry has now matured to the point where we can use laboratory tests to see broad defects in metabolism. This enables us to design intelligent support strategies that help restore the fundamentals of our immune defense, energy, and repair system—through a state of metabolic fitness.

In the end, achieving a state of "metabolic fitness" is one critical element needed in order for any individual to best cope with the immense challenges presented by the microbial world in which we live.

Appendix D

Protective Agents Found in Human Breast Milk

A summary from the symposium on "Innate Immunity and Human Milk" outlined the large number of probiotics, prebiotics, antimicrobial peptides, fatty acids, glycans, and other molecules present in milk. A full discussion is beyond the scope of this book, but a brief summary of compounds in human milk that aid vital defenses is shown below.[502,503]

■ Table D.1. Protective Agents Found in Human Milk

Innate Immune System (Natural)	Adaptive Immune System (Acquired)
Prebiotics	
Probiotics	
Bifidobacterium longum	
Bifidobacterium animalis	
Bifidobacterium bifidum	
Bifidobacterium catenulatum	
Lactobacillus gasseri	
Lactobacillus fermentu	
Multifunctional Milk Components:	Humoral Immunity
Fatty acids	sIgA (secretory IgA)
Lactoferrin	Immunoglobulin, maternal
alpha-lactalbumin	sIgA, IgG, IgM, IgD
Cell surface receptor homologues	
Immunomodulatory Agents:	Cell-Mediated Immunity
Nucleic acids	Monocytes
Cytokines	Macrophages
Soluble cytokine receptors	PMNs
Antioxidants	Lymphocytes
Antimicrobial Compounds	
Human ß-defensin 1	
Lactoferrin	
Lactoperoxidase	
Lysozyme	
Soluble carbohydrates	
Glycolipids	

Adapted from: Newburg, D. Innate immunity and human milk. J Nutr 2005;135:1308–1312 and Phadke, SM, Deslouches, B, Hileman, et al. Antimicrobial peptides in mucosal secretions: The importance of local secretions in mitigating infection. J Nutr 2005;135: 1289–1293; Gueimonde, M, Laitinen, K, Salminen, S, Isolauri, E. Breast Milk: A Source of Bifidobacteria for Infant Gut Development and Maturation? Neonatology 2007;92:6466.

Appendix E

■ **Table E.1. Infectious Microbes Where Virulence Is Made Worse by Iron**[504,505]

Gram-negative bacteria		
Acinetobacter	Aeromonas	Campylobacter
Capnocytophaga	Chlamydia	Ehrlichia
Enterobacter	Escherichia	Klebsiella
Legionella	Moraxella	Neisseria
Pasteurella	Proteus	Pseudomonas
Salmonella	Shigella	Vibrio
Yersinia		
Gram-positive bacteria		
Bacillus	Clostridium	Corynebacterium
Erysipelothrix	Listeria	Staphylococcus
Streptococcus		
Acid-fast bacterium		
Mycobacterium		
Protozoa		
Entamoeba	Leishmania	Naegleria
Plasmodium	Toxoplasma	Trypanosoma
Fungi		
Candida	Cryptococcus	Histoplasma
Paracoccidioides	Pneumocystis	Pythium
Rhizopus	Trichosporon	

Notes

1. Bloom, BR, Murray, CJ. Tuberculosis: Commentary on a re-emergent killer. Science 1992;257:1055–64.
2. Neu, HC. The crisis in antibiotic resistance. Science 1992;257:1064–1073.
3. Cohen, ML. Epidemiology of drug resistance: Implications for a post-antimicrobial era. Science 1992;257:1050–1055.
4. Berkelman, RL, Hughes, JM. The conquest of infectious disease: Who are we kidding? Ann Intern Med 1993;119(5):426–27.
5. Kellam, P. Attacking pathogens through their hosts. Genome Biol 2006;7(1): 201.
6. Stolberg, SG. Superbugs. New York Times, August 2, 1998.
7. Lederberg, J, Shope, RE, Oaks, SC Jr.; eds. Emerging Infections: Microbial Threats to Health in the United States. Institute of Medicine. Washington, DC: National Academy Press; 1992.
8. Those overworked miracle drugs. Newsweek 1981;8(17):63.
9. Mead, PS, Slutsker, L, Dietz, V, et al. Food-Related Illness and Death in the United States. Emerg Infect Dis 1999;5(5):607–25.
10. Sahyoun, NR, et al. Trends in causes of death among the elderly. Centers for Disease Control, National Center for Health Statistics, Aging Trends, 2001;1.
11. Stalam, M, Kaye, D. Antibiotic agents in the elderly. Inf Dis Clin N Am 2000;14:357–69.
12. Birnbaum, HG. Morley, M, Greenberg, PE, Colice, GL. Economic burden of respiratory infections in an employed population. Chest 2002;122:603–611.
13. Centers for Disease Control and Prevention, National Center for Health Statistics, 1999 National Nursing Home Survey. Nursing Home Residents, number, percent distribution, and rate per 10,000, by age at interview, according to sex, race, and region.
14. http://www.who.int/gpsc/background/en/index.html
15. Mah, TF, O'Toole, GA. Mechanisms of biofilm resistance to antimicrobial agents. Trends Microbiol 2001;9:34–39.
16. Bad Bugs, No Drugs: As Antibiotic Discovery Stagnates . . . A Public Health Crisis Brews. A White Paper prepared by the Infectious Diseases Society of America, 2004.

17. Imperi, F, Caneva, G, Cancellieri, L, Ricci, MA, Sodo, A, Visca, P. The bacterial aetiology of rosy discoloration of ancient wall paintings. Environ Microbiol 2007;9(11):2894–902.
18. Dantas, G, Sommer, MOA, Oluwasegun, RD, Church, GM. Bacteria subsisting on antibiotics. Science 2008;320(5872):100–3.
19. Hood, AM, Pearson, AD, Shahamat, M. The extent of surface contamination of retailed chickens with *Campylobacter jejuni* serogroups. Epidem Inf 1988; 100:17–25.
20. Arnon, SS, et al. Botulinum toxin as a biological weapon. JAMA 2001;285: 1059–1070.
21. Socransky, SS, Haffajee, AD. Dental biofilms: Difficult therapeutic targets. Periodontology 2000;28:12–55.
22. Socransky, SS, et al. Microbial complexes in subgingival plaque. J Clin Periodontol 1998;25:134–44.
23. Wilson, M. Microbial Inhabitants of Humans: Their Ecology and Role in Health and Disease. Cambridge, UK: Cambridge University Press, 2005. 287.
24. Isolauri, E, Kirjanaiene, PV, Salminen, S. Probiotics: A role in the treatment of intestinal infection and inflammation. Gut 2002;50:54–59.
25. Vitali, B, Pugliese, C, Biagi, E. Dynamics of vaginal bacterial communities in women developing bacterial vaginosis, candidiasis, or no infection, analyzed by PCR-denaturing gradient gel electrophoresis and real-time PCR. Appl Env Microbiol 2007;73(8):5731–41.
26. Zhous, X, Bent, SJ, Schneider, MG, et al. Characterization of vaginal microbial communities in adult healthy women using cultivation-independent methods. Microbiology 2004;150:2565–73.
27. Blaser, M, Gao, Z, et al. Proc Natl Acad Sci 2007;104(8):2927–32.
28. Wilson, M. Microbial Inhabitants of Humans: Their Ecology and Role in Health and Disease. Cambridge, UK: Cambridge University Press, 2005. 117.
29. Gill, SR, et al. Metagenomic analysis of the human distal gut microbiome. Science 2006;312:1355–9.
30. Sekirov, I, Finlay, B. Human and microbe: United we stand. Nature Medicine 2006;12:736–37.
31. Cummings, JH, Rombeau, JL, Sakata, T, eds. Physiological and clinical aspects of short chain fatty acids. Cambridge, UK: Cambridge University Press, 1994.
32. Roediger, WE. Role of anaerobic bacteria in the metabolic welfare of the colonic mucosa in man. Gut 1980;21(9):793–798.
33. McDevitt, J, Goldman, P. Effect of the intestinal flora on the urinary organic

acid profile of rats ingesting a chemically simplified diet. Food Chem Toxicol 1991;29(2):107–13.
34. Tamm, AO. Biochemical activity of intestinal microflora in adult celiac disease. Nahrung 1984;28(6–7):711–15.
35. Margulis, L. Symbiosis in Cell Evolution. San Francisco: W. H. Freeman and Company, 1981. 206–227.
36. Goodacre, R. Metabolomics of a superorganism. J Nutr 2007; 137: 259S–266S.
37. Hume, ED. Pasteur Exposed: The False Foundations of Modern Medicine. Australia: Bookreal, 1989.
38. Lappé, M. When Antibiotics Fail: Restoring the Ecology of the Body. Berkeley, CA: North Atlantic Books, 1986. 17–18.
39. McKeown, T. The Role of Medicine: Dream, Mirage or Nemesis? Oxford University Press, 1976. 391.
40. McKeown, T, 391.
41. McKeown, T, 62.
42. Kass, EH. Infectious diseases and social change. J Infect Dis 1971;123(1): 110–114.
43. McKinlay, JB, McKinlay, SM. The questionable contribution of medical measures to the decline of mortality in the United States in the twentieth century. Millbank Memorial Fund Quarterly Summer 1977;405–428.
44. Lappé, M, Antibiotics, 18.
45. Weinstein, L. Infectious disease: retrospect and reminiscence. J Infect Dis 1974; 129(4):480–92.
46. Weinstein, L., Infectious disease, 480–92.
47. Stradomska, TJ, Bobula-Milewska, B, Bauer, A, et al. Urinary D-arabinitol/L-arabinitol levels in infants undergoing long-term antibiotic therapy. J Clin Microbiol 2005;43(10):5351–54.
48. Christensson, B, Wiebe, T, Pehrson, C, Larsson, L. Diagnosis of invasive Candidiasis in neutropenic children with cancer by cetermination of D-arabinitol/L-arabinitol ratios in urine. J Clin Microbiol 1997;35(3):636–40.
49. Sigmundsdottir, G, Christensson, B, Bjorklund, LJ, et al. Urine D-arabinitol/L-arabinitol ratio in diagnosis of invasive candidiasis in newborn infants. J Clin Microbiol 2000;38(8):3039–42.
50. Pirottal, MV, Garland, SM. Genital Candida species detected in samples from women in Melbourne, Australia, before and after treatment with antibiotics. J Clin Microbiol 2006;44(9):3213–3217.
51. http://www.idsociety.org/content.aspx?id=9200#cand.

52. Bolte, ER. Autism and *Clostridium tetani*. Med Hypoth 1998;51:133–44.
53. Parracho, HMRT, Bingham, MO, Gibson, GR, McCartney, AL. Differences between the gut microflora of children with autistic spectrum disorders and that of healthy children. J Med Microbiol 2005;54:987–91.
54. Shultz, SR, Macfabe, DF, Ossenkopp, KP, Scratch, S, Whelan, J, Taylor, R, Cain, DP. Intracerebroventricular injection of propionic acid, an enteric bacterial metabolic end-product, impairs social behavior in the rat: Implications for an animal model of autism. Neuropharmacol 2008 (in press).
55. Pimentel, M, Mayer, AG, Park, S, Chow, EJ, Hasan, A, Kong, Y. Methane production during lactulose breath test is associated with gastrointestinal disease presentation. Dig Dis Sci 2003;48:86–92.
56. Mannino, DM, Homa, DM, Pertowski, CA, et al. Surveillance for asthma—United States, 1960–1995. Morb Mort Weekly Rpt CDC Surveill Summ 1998;47:1–27.
57. Noverr, MC, Noggle, RM, Toews, GB, et al. Role of antibiotics and fungal microbiota in driving pulmonary allergic responses. Infect Immun 2004;72(9): 4996–5003.
58. Noverr, Role of antibiotics, 4996–500359.
59. http://www.nlm.nih.gov/medlineplus/news/fullstory_66715.html
60. Duffy, M. Side effects: When dumbbells and antibiotics clash. New York Times, March 16, 1999.
61. Sode, J, Obel, N, Hallas, J, Lassen, A. Use of fluoroquinolones and risk of Achilles tendon rupture: A population-based cohort study. Eur J Clin Pharmacol 2007;63(5):499–503.
62. Arora, R, Kulshreshtha, S, Mohan, G, et al. Estimation of serum zinc and copper in children with acute diarrhea. Biol Trace Elem Res 2006;114(1–3): 121–6.
63. Dibner, JJ, Richards, JD. Antibiotic growth promoters in agriculture: History and mode of action. Poultry Sci 2005;84:634–43.
64. Dibner and Richards, Antibiotic growth promoters, 634–43.
65. Visek, WJ. The mode of growth promotion by antibiotics. J Anim Sci 1978;46:1447–1469.
66. Ley, RE, Turnbaugh, PJ, Klein, S, Gordon, JI. Nature 2006;444:1022–23.
67. Carmen, M, Isolauri, E, Laitinen, K, Salminen, S. Distinct composition of gut microbiota during pregnancy in overweight and normal-weight women. Am J Clin Nutr 2008;88(4):894–99.
68. Harder, T, Bergmann, R, Kallischnigg, G, Plagemann, A. Duration of breast-

feeding and risk of overweight: A meta-analysis Am J Epidemiol 2005;162: 397–403.

69. Kalliomaki, M, Collado, MC, Salminen, S, Isolauri, E. Early differences in fecal microbiota composition in children may predict overweight. Am J Clin Nutr 2008;87:534–8.
70. Chandler, D, Dugdale, AE. What do patients know about antibiotics? Br Med J 1976;8:422.
71. Lee, GM, Friedman, JF, Ross-Degnan, D, et al. Misconceptions about colds and predictors of health service utilization. Pediatrics 2003;111(2):231–236.
72. McNulty, CA, Boyle, P, Nichols, T, Clappison, P, Davey, P. Don't wear me out—the public's knowledge of and attitudes to antibiotic use. J Antimicrob Chemother 2007;59: 727–738.
73. Friedman, J, Lee, G, Kleinman, K, Finkelstein, J. Child care center policies and practices for management of ill children. Ambulatory Pediatr 2004;4(5): 455–460. (AHRQ grants T32 HS00063, HS10247).
74. Kuzujanakis, M, Kleinman, K, Rifas-Shiman, J, Finkelstein, J. Correlates of parental antibiotic knowledge, demand, and reported use. Ambulatory Pediatr 2003;3(4):203–210. (AHRQ grant HS10247).
75. Friedman, JF, Lee, GM, Kleinman, KP, et al. Acute care and antibiotic seeking for upper respiratory tract infections for children in day care: Parental knowledge and day care center policies. Arch Pediatr Adolesc Med 2003;157:369–374.
76. Mangione-Smith, R, Elliott, MN, Stivers, T, et al. Ruling out the need for antibiotics: Are we sending the right message? Arch Pediatr Adolesc Med 2006;160(9):945–52.
77. van Driel, ML, De Sutter, A, Deveugele, M, et al. Are sore throat patients who hope for antibiotics actually asking for pain relief? Ann Fam Med 2006;4(6):484–5.
78. Blalock, JE, Smith, EM. Conceptual development of the immune system as a sixth sense. Brain Behav Immun 2007;21:23–33.
79. Davis, MM. Panning for T-cell gold. The Scientist 2004;18:28–29.
80. Andreas Krack, A, Sharma, R, Figulla, HR, Anker, SD. The importance of the gastrointestinal system in the pathogenesis of heart failure. Europ Heart J 2005;26:2368–2374.
81. Reikeras, O, Shegarfi, H, Wang, JE, Utvag, SE. Lipopolysaccharide impairs fracture healing: an experimental study in rats. Acta Orthop 2005;76(6):749–53.
82. Kilkkinen, A, Pietinen, P, Klaukka, T, et al. Use of oral antimicrobials decreases serum enterolactone concentration. Am J Epidemiol 2002;155:472–477.

83. Boccardo, F, Lunardi, G, Guglielmini, P, et al. Serum enterolactone levels and the risk of breast cancer in women with palpable cysts. Eur J Cancer 2004;40:84–89.
84. Vanharanta, M, Voutilainen, S, Rissanen, TH, et al. Risk of cardiovascular disease-related and all-cause death according to serum concentrations of enterolactone: Kuopio Ischaemic Heart Disease Risk Factor Study. Arch Intern Med 2003;163:1099–1104.
85. Maier, SF, Watkins, LR, Fleshner, M. Psychoneuroimmunology: The interface between behavior, brain, and immunity. Am Psychol 1994;49:1004–17.
86. Greiner, EF, Guppy, M, Brand, K. Glucose is essential for proliferation and the glycolytic enzyme induction that provokes a transition to glycolytic energy production. J Biol Chem 1994;269:31484–90.
87. Sukoyan, GV, Mamuchishvili, IG, Pagava, KI. Relationship between immune status and activity of the lymphocyte energy supply system in adolescents suffering from frequent diseases. Bul Exper Biol Med 2005;139(6):695–7.
88. Marriage, BJ, Clandinin, MT, MacDonald, IM, Glerum, DM. Cofactor treatment improves ATP synthetic capacity in patients with oxidative phosphhorylation disorders. Mol Genet Metab 2004;81(4):263–72.
89. Nelson, RJ, Demas, GE, Klein, SL, Kriegsfeld, LJ. Seasonal Patterns of Stress, Immune Function, and Disease. Cambridge, UK: Cambridge University Press, 2002. 185.
90. Khuroo, MS, Teli, MR, Skidmore, S, et al. Incidence and severity of viral hepatitis in pregnancy. Am J Med 1981;70:252–5.
91. Siegel, M, Greenberg, M. Incidence of poliomyelitis in pregnancy: Its relation to maternal age, parity, and gestational period. N Engl J Med 1955;253:841.
92. Bronson, FH. Mammalian Reproductive Biology. Chicago: University of Chicago Press, 1989.
93. Martinez-Lopez, LE, Friedl, KE, Moore, RJ, Kramer, TR. A longitudinal study of infection and injuries of Ranger students. Mil Med 1993;158:433–7.
94. Linenger, JM, Flinn, S, Thomas, B. Musculoskeletal and medical morbidity associated with rigorous physical training. Clin J Sport Med 1993;3:229–34.
95. Kramer, TR, Moore, RJ, Shippee, RL, Friedl, KE, Martinez-Lopez, L, et al. Effects of food restriction in military training on T-lymphocyte responses. Int J Sports Med 1997;18 Suppl 1:S84–90.
96. Zhang, X-J, Chinkes, DL, Wolfe, RR. The flow phase of wound metabolism is characterized by stimulated protein synthesis rather than cell proliferation. J Surg Res 2006;135:61–67.

97. Wolfe, RR. The underappreciated role of muscle in health and disease. Am J Clin Nutr 2006;84:475–82.
98. Pereira, CT, Barrow, RE, Sterns, AM, et al. Age dependent differences in survival after severe burns: A unicentric review of 1674 patients and 179 autopsies over 15 years. J Am Coll Surg 2005;202(3):536–48.
99. Tipton, KD, Borheim, E, Wolf, SE, Stanford, AP, Wolfe, RR. Acute response of net muscle protein balance reflects 24h balance after exercise and amino acid ingestion. Am J Physiol Endocrinol Metab 2002;284:E76–9.
100. Rosenberg, IH, Roubenhoff, R. Stalking sarcopenia. Ann Int Med 1995;23: 727–28.
101. Kotler, DP. Cachexia. Ann Int Med 2000;133:622–634.
102. Metter, EJ, Talbot, KA, Schrager, M, Conwite, R. Skeletal muscle strength as a predictor of all-cause mortality in healthy men. J Gerontol 2002;57A: B359–65.
103. Frost, RA, Lang, CH. Regulation of muscle growth by pathogen associated molecules. J Anim Sci 2008 Jan 11.
104. Wiendl, H, Hohlfeld, R, Kieseier BC. Immunobiology of muscle: Advances in understanding an immunological microenvironment. Trends Immunol. 2005;26(7):373–80.
105. Alba-Loureiro, TC, Munhoz, CD, Martins, JO, et al. Neutrophil function and metabolism in individuals with diabetes mellitus. Braz J Med Biol Res 2007;40:1037–44.
106. Falguera, M, Pifarre, R, Martin, A, et al. Etiology and outcome of community-acquired pneumonia in patients with diabetes mellitus. Chest 2005;128(5):3233–39.
107. Hu, Y, Block, G, Norkus, EP, et al. Relations of glycemic index and glycemic load with plasma oxidative stress markers. Am J Clin Nutr 2006;84(1):70–76.
108. Ardigo, D, Valtuena, S, Zavaroni, I, et al. Pulmonary complications in diabetes mellitus: The role of glycemic control. Curr Drug Targets Inflamm Allergy 2004;3:455–458.
109. Kurz, AD, Sessler, DI, Lenhardt, R. Perioperative normothermia to reduce the incidence of surgical wound infection and shortened hospitalization. N Engl J Med 1996;334:1209–15.
110. Torres, AR. Is fever suppression involved in the etiology of autism and neurodevelopmental disorders? BMC Pediatr 2003;3:9.
111. Jenssen, H, Hamill, P, Hancock, REW. Peptide antimicrobial agents. Clin Microbiol Rev 2006;19(3):491–511.

112. Gallo, RL. Antimicrobial Peptides in Human Health and Disease. Norwich, UK: Horizon Press, 2005.
113. Armogida, SA, Yannaras, NM, Melton, AL, Srivastava, MD. Identification and quantification of innate immune system mediators in human breast milk. Allergy Asthma Proc 2004;25(5):297–304.
114. Schauber, J, Dorschner, RA, Yamasaki, K, Brouha, B, Gallo, RL. Control of the innate epithelial antimicrobial response is cell-type specific and dependent on relevant microenvironmental stimuli. Immunology 2006;118(4):509–19.
115. Schauber, J, Dorschner, RA, Yamasaki, K, Brouha, B, Gallo, RL. Control of the innate epithelial antimicrobial response is cell-type specific and dependent upon relevant microenvironmental stimuli. Immunology 2006;118:509–19.
116. Mariani, E, Ravaglia, G, Forti, P, et al. Vitamin D, thyroid hormones, and muscle mas influence natural killer (NK) innate immunity in healthy nonagenarians and centenarians. Clin Exp Immunol 1999;116:19–27.
117. Tang, ZF, Ling, YB, Lin, N, Hao, Z, Xu, RY. Glutamine and recombinant human growth hormone protect intestinal barrier function following portal hypertension surgery. World J Gastroenterol 2007;21(15):2223–8.
118. Chavance, M, et al. Nutritional support improves antibody response to influenza virus in the elderly. Br Med J 1985;11(9):1348–49.
119. Nockels, CF. Protective effects of supplemental vitamin E against infection. Fed Proc 1979;38:2134–8.
120. Newberne, PM, Williams, G. Nutritional influences on the course of infections. In Dunlop, RH, Moon, HW. Resistance to Infectious Disease. Saskatoon, Canada: Saskatoon Modern Press, 1970. 93.
121. McKeown, T. The Role of Medicine: Dream, Mirage, or Nemesis? Princeton, NJ: Princeton University Press, 1979. 75.
122. McKeown, T, The Role of Medicine, 60.
123. Houang, ET, Ahmet, Z, Lawrence, AG. Successful treatment of four patients with recalcitrant vaginal trichomoniasis with a combination of zinc sulfate douche and metronidazole therapy. Sex Trans Dis 1997;24(2):116–119.
124. Schachner, L, et al. A clinical trial comparing the safety and efficacy of topical erythromycin-zinc formulation with a topical Clindamycin formulation. J Am Acad Dermatol 1990;22(3)489–95.
125. Chandra, RK. Effect of vitamin and trace element supplementation on immune responses and infection in elderly subjects. Lancet 1992;340:1124–27.
126. Bendich, A. Vitamin E status of U.S. children. J Am Col Nutr 1992;11(4): 441–44.

127. Blumberg, J. Assessing immunological function across the lifespan. International Symposium on Functional Medicine. Maui, Hawaii,1993.
128. Neggers, YH, Nansel, TR, Andrews, WW, et al. Dietary intake of selected nutrients affects bacterial vaginosis in women. J Nutr 2007;137:2128–33.
129. Peck, MD, Weber, JM, McManus, A, et al. Surveillance of burn wound infections: A proposal for definitions. J Burn Care Rhabil 1998;19:386–9.
130. Berger, MM, Baines, M, Faffoul, W, et al. Trace element supplementation after major burns modulates antioxidant status and clinical course by way of increased tissue trace element concentrations. Am J Clin Nutr 2007; 85:1293–300.
131. McCowen, K, Bistrian, BR. Immunonutrition: Problematic or problem solving? Am J Clin Nutr 2003;77:764–70.
132. Gæde, P, Vedel, P, Larsen, N, et al. Multifactorial intervention and cardiovascular disease in patients with type 2 diabetes. N Engl J Med 2003;348(5): 383–93.
133. Block, G, Jensen, CD, Norkus, EP, et al. Usage patterns, health, and nutritional status of long-term multiple dietary supplement users: a cross-sectional study. Nutr J 2007;6(30):1–11.
134. Field, CJ, Johnson, IR, Schley, PD. Nutrients and their role in host resistance to infection. J Leuk Biol 2002;71:16–32.
135. Thurnahm, DI, Northrop-Clewes, CA, McCullough, FSW, et al. Innate immunity, gut integrity, and vitamin A in Gambian and Indian infants. J Infect Dis 2000;182:S23–S28.
136. McDowell, EM, Keenan, KP, Huang, M. Effects of vitamin A deprivation on hamster tracheal epithelium: A quantitative morphologic study. Virchow's Archiv B Cell Pathol Incl Mol Pathol. 1984;45:197–219.
137. Hussey, GD, Kelin, M. A randomized, controlled trial of vitamin A in children with severe measles. N Engl J Med 1990;323:160–4.
138. Bauernfeind, JC. The safe use of vitamin A: A report of the International Vitamin A Consultative Group. Washington, DC: The Nutrition Foundation, 1980.
139. Zuk, M. Riddled with Life. Orlando, Florida: Harcourt, 2007. 186–90.
140. Report: Cod-liver oil treatment of tuberculosis. Brompton Hospital Records, 1849. 38.
141. Davies, PDO. Vitamin D and tuberculosis. Am Rev Respir Dis 1989;139:1571.
142. Daves, PDO. A possible link between vitamin D deficiency and impaired host defense to Mycobacterium tuberculosis. Rubercle 1985;66:301–6.

143. Rook, GAW. The role of vitamin D in tuberculosis. Am Rev Respir Dis 1988;138:768–70.
144. Davies, P, Grange, J. The genetics of host resistance and susceptibility to tuberculosis. Ann NY Acad Sci 2004:151–6.
145. Cannell, J, Hollis, B, Zasloff, M, Heaney, R. Diagnosis and treatment of vitamin D deficiency. Expert Opin Pharmacother 2008;9(1):107–18.
146. Richards, JB, Valdes, AM, Gardner, JP, et al. Higher serum vitamin D concentrations are associated with longer leukocyte telomere length in women. Am J Clin Nutr 2007;86(5):1420–25.
147. Ahuja, JKC, Goldman, JD, Moshfegh, AJ. Current status of vitamin E nutriture. Ann NY Acad Sci 2004;1031:387–390.
148. Prasad, JS. Effect of vitamin E supplementation on leukocyte function. Am J Clin Nutr 1980;33:606–8.
149. Anderson, R. Ascorbate-mediated stimulation of neutrophil motility and lymphocyte transformation by inhibition of the peroxidase-H2O2–halide system in vitro and in vivo. Am. J Clin Nutr. 1981; 34:1906–11.
150. Naidu, KA. Vitamin C in human health and disease is still a mystery? An overview. Nutr J 2003;2(7):1–10.
151. Carr, AC, Frei, B. Toward a new recommended dietary allowance for vitamin C based on antioxidant and health effects in humans. Am J Clin Nutr. 1999;69(6):1086–1107.
152. Strand, TA, Taneja, S, Bhandari, N, et al. Folate, but not vitamin B-12 status, predicts respiratory morbidity in north Indian children. Am J Clin Nutr 2007;86:139–44.
153. Dhu, A, Galan, P, Hercberg, S. Folate status and the immune system. Prog Food Nur Sci 1991;15:43–60.
154. Cantwell, RJ. Iron deficiency anemia of infancy: Some clinical principles illustrated by the response of Maori infants to neonatal parental iron administration. Clin Pediatr 1972;11(8):443–49.
155. Arnon, SS, Damus, K, Thompson, B, et al. Protective role of human milk against sudden death from infant botulism. J Pediatr 1982;100(4):568–73.
156. Murray, MJ, Murray, AB, Murray, MB, Murray, CJ. The adverse effect of iron repletion on the course of certain infections. Br Med J 1978;2(6145): 1113–15.
157. Richard, SA, Zavaleta, N, Caulfield, LE. Zinc and iron supplementation and malaria, diarrhea, and respiratory infections in children in the Peruvian Amazon. Am J Trop Med Hyg 2006;75(1):126–32.

158. Cronje, L, Bornman, L. Iron overload and tuberculosis: A case for iron chelation therapy. Int J Tuberc Lung Dis 2005;9(1):2–9.
159. Tannotti, LL, Tielsch, JM, Black, MM, Black, RE. Iron supplementation in early childhood: Health benefits and risks. Am J Clin Nutr 2006;84(6):1261–76.
160. Flemming, DJ, Jacques, PF, Tucker, KL, et al. Iron status of the free-living, elderly Framingham Heart Study cohort: An iron-replete population with a high prevalence of elevated iron stores. Am J Clin Nutr 2001;73:638–46.
161. Walker, EM, Walker, SM. Effects of iron overload on the immune sytem. Ann Clin Lab Sci 2000;30:354–65.
162. Roy, M, Kiremidjian-Schumacher, L, Wishe, HI, et al. Selenuim supplementation enhances the expression of interleukine-2 receptor subunits and internalization of interleuikin-2. Proc CosExp Biol Med 1993;202:295–301.
163. Anneren, G, Magnusson, CGM, Nordvall, SL. Increase in serum concentrations of IgG2 and IgG4 by selenium supplementation in children with Down's Syndrome. Arch Dis Child. 1990;65:1353–55.
164. Broom, CS, McArdle, F, Kyle, JAM, et al. An increase in selenium intake improves immune function and poliovirus handling in adults with marginal selenium status. Am J Clin Nutr 2004;80:154–62.
165. MAFF Joint Food Safety and Standards Group. Food Surveillance Information Sheet. London: HMSO, 1997 (No. 127).
166. Dietary reference intakes for vitamin C, vitamin E, selenium, and carotenoids. A report of the Panel on Dietary Antioxidants and Related Compounds, Subcomittees on Upper Reference Levels of Nutrients and Interpetation and Uses of DRIs, Standing Committee on the Scienticfic Evaluation of Dietary Reference Intakes, Food and Nutrition Board, Washington, DC: National Academy Press, 2000:284–324.
167. Prasad, AS. Effects of zinc deficiency on Th1 and Th2 cytokine shifts. J Infect Dis 2000;182:S62–S68.
168. Prasad, AS, Effects of zinc deficiency, 200.
169. Walsh, CT, Sandstead, HH, Prasad, AS, Newberne, PM, Fraker, PJ. Zinc health effects and research priorities for the 1990s. Environ Health Perspect 1994;102:5–46.
170. Sturniolo, GC, Di Leo, V, Ferronato, A, D'Odorico, A, D'Incà, R. Zinc supplementation tightens "leaky gut" in Crohn's disease. Inflamm Bowel Dis 2001;7(2):94–8.
171. Licastro, F, Chiricolo, M, Mocchegiani, E, et al. Oral zinc supplementation in Downs syndrome subjects decreased infection and normalized some

humoral and cellular immune parameters. J Intellect Disabil Res 1994; 38–149–62.

172. Sandstead, HH. Understanding zinc: Recent observations and interpretations. J Lab Clin Med 1994;124:322–7.
173. Ruel, MT, Ribera, JA, Santizo, MC, et al. Impact of zinc supplementation on morbidity from diarrhea and respiratory infections among rural Guatemalan children. Pediatr 1997;99:808–13.
174. Sazawal, S, Black, R, Jalla, S, et al. Zinc supplementation reduces the incidence of acute lower respiratory infections in infants and preschool children: A double-blind controlled trial. Pediatr 1998;102:1–5.
175. Prasad, AS, Beck, FWJ, Kaplan, J, et al. Effect of zinc supplementation on incidence of infections and hospital admissions in sickle cell disease. Am J Hematol 1999;61:194–202.
176. Meydani, SN, Barnett, JB, Dallal, GE, et al. Serum zinc and pneumonia in nursing home elderly. Am J Clin Nutr 2007;86:1167–73.
177. Bogden, JD, Oleske, JM, Munves, EM, et al. Zinc and immunocompetence in the elderly: Baseline data on zinc nutriture and immunity in unsupplemented subjects. Am J Clin Nutr 1987;46:101–9.
178. Prasad, AS, Beck, FW, Bao, B, et al. Zinc supplementation decreases incidence of infections in the elderly: Effect of zinc on generations ocytokines and oxidative stress. Am J Clin Nutr 2007;85(3):837–44.
179. Schroeder, JJ, Cousins, RJ. Interleukin-6 regulates metallothionein gene expression and zinc metabolism in hepatocyte monolayer cultures. Proc Natl Acad Sci USA 1990;87:3137–41.
180. Brooks, WA Santosham, M, Naheed, A, et al. Effect of weekly zinc supplements on incidence of pneumonia and diarrhea in children younger than 2 years in an urban, low-income population in Bangladesh: Randomised controlled trial. Lancet 2005;366:999–1004.
181. Bhandari, N, Bahl, R, Taneja, S, et al. Effect of routine zinc supplementation on pneumonia in children aged 6 months to three years: Randomised controlled trial in an urban slum. BMJ 2002;324:1358.
182. Coles, CL, Bose, A, Moses, PD, et al. Infectious etiology modifies the treatment effect of zinc in severe pneumonia. Am J Clin Nutr 2007;86:397–403.
183. Krones, C, Klosterhalfen, B, Fackeldey, V, et al. Deleterious effects of zinc in a pig model of acute endotoxemia. J Invest Surg 2004;17:249–56.
184. Chandra, RK. Excessive zinc impairs immune responses. JAMA 1984;252(11): 1443–46.

185. He, K, Liu, K, Daviglus, ML, Morris, SJ, Loria, CM, Van Horn, L, Jacobs, DR, Savage, PJ. Magnesium intake and incidence of metabolic syndrome among young adults. Circulation. 2006 Mar 27 (ahead of print).

186. Huerta, MG, Roemmich, JN, Kington, ML, et al. Magnesium deficiency is associated with insulin resistance in obese children. Diabetes Care 2005; 28:1175–81.

187. Song, Y, Manson, JE, Buring, JE, Liu, S. Dietary magnesium intake in relation to plasma insulin levels and risk of type 2 diabetes in women. Diabetes Care 2004;27:59–65.

188. Ma, J, Folsom, AR, Melnick SL, et al. Associations of serum and dietary magnesium with cardiovascular disease, hypertension, diabetes, insulin, and carotid wall thickness: The ARIC study. J Clin Epidemiol 1985;48:927–40.

189. Lopez-Ridaura, R, Willet, WC, Rimm, EB, et al. Magnesium intake and risk of type 2 diabetes in men and women. Diabetes Care 2004;2:134–40.

190. Nijhoff, WA, Grubben, MJAL, Nagengast, FM. Effects of consumption of brussels sprouts on intestinal and lymphocytic glutathione S-transferases in humans. Carcinogenesis 1995;16:2125–8.

191. Murata, Y, Shumamura, T, Hamuro, J. The polarization of Th1 / Th2 balance is dependent on the intracellular thiol redx status of macrophages due to the distinctive cytokine production. Int Immunol 2002;14:201–12.

192. Hennet, T, Peterhans, E, Stocker, R. Alterations in antioxidant defences in lung and liver of mice infected with influenza A virus. J Gen Virol 1992;73:39–46.

193. Luo, JL, Hammarqvist, F, Andersson, K, Wernermn, J. Skeletal muscle glutathione after surgical trauma. Ann Surg 1996;223:420–7.

194. Cowley, HC, Bacon, PJ, Goode, HF, Webster, NR, et al. Plasma antioxidant potential in severe sepsis: A comparison of survivors and non-survivors. Crit Care Med 1996;24:1179–83.

195. Bernard, GR, Wheeler, AP, Arons, MM, et al. A trial of antioxidants N-acetylcysteine and procysteine in ARDS. Chest 1997;112:164–72.

196. Spapen, H, Zhang, H, Demanet, C, et al. Does N-acetylcysteine influence the cytokine response during early human septic shock? 1998;113:1616–24.

197. Kinscherf, R, Fischbach, T, Mihm, S, et al. Effect of glutathione depletion and oral N-acetylcysteine treatment on CD4+ and CD8+ cells. FASEB J 1994;8:448–51.

198. Newsholme, P. Why is L-glutamine metabolism important to cells of the immune system in health, post-injury, surgery, or infection? J Nutr 2001;131: 2515S–2522S.

199. Vesali, RF, Klaude, M, Rooyackers, O, Wernerman, J. Amino acid metabolism in leg muscle after an endotoxin injection in healthy volunteers. Am J Physiol Endocrinol Metab 2005;288:E360–E364.
200. Costa Rosa, LFBP, Curi, R, Murphy, C, Newsholme, P. The effect of adrenaline and phorbol myristate or bacterial lipopolysaccharie on stimulation of pathways of macrophage glucose, glutamine, and 2 metabolism: Evidence for cyclic AMP-dependent protein kinase-mediated inhibition of glucose-6-phosphate dehydrogenase and activation of NADP+-dependent 'malic' enzyme. Biochem J 1995;310:709–714.
201. Malaguarnera, M, Cammalleri, L, Gargante, MP, et al. L-Carnitine treatment reduces severity of physical and mental fatigue and increases cognitive functions in centenarians: A randomized and controlled clinical trial. Am J Clin Nutr. 2007;86(6):1738–44.
202. Pistone, G, et al. Levocarnitine administration in elderly subjects with rapid muscle fatigue: Effect on body composition, lipid profile and fatigue. Drugs Aging 2003;20(10):761–7.
203. Bellmann-Weiler, R, Schroecksnadel, K, Holzer, C, Larcher, C, Fuchs, D, Weiss, G. IFN-gamma mediated pathways in patients with fatigue and chronic active Epstein Barr virus-infection. J Affect Disord. 2007.
204. Russo, S, Kema, IP, Fokkema, R, et al. Tryptophan as a link between psychopathology and somatic states. Psychosom Med 2003;65:665–71.
205. Serhan, CN. Resolution phase of inflammation: Novel endogenous anti-inflammatory and proresolving lipid mediators and pathways. Annu Rev Immunol 2007;25:101–37.
206. Erride, C, Attina, T, Spickett, CM, Webb, DJ. A high-fat meal induces low-grade endotoxemia: Evidence of a novel mechanism of postprandial inflammation. Am J Clin Nutr 2007;86:1286–92.
207. Lee, JY, Plakidas, A, Lee, WH. Differential modulation of Toll-like receptors by fatty acids: Preferential inhibition by n-3 polyunsaturated fatty acids. J Lipid Res 2003;44:479–486.
208. Rees, D, Miles, EA, Banerjee, T, et al. Dose-related effects of eicosapentaenoic acid on innate immune function in healthy humans: A comparison of young and older men. Am J Clin Nutr 2006;83:331–42.
209. Paddon-Jones, D, Sheffield-Moore, M, Urban, RJ, et al. Essential amino acid and carbohydrate supplementation ameliorates muscle protein loss during 28 days bedrest. J Clin Endocrinol Metab 2004;89:4351–8.

210. Wolfe, RR. The underappreciated role of muscle in health and disease. Am J Clin Nutr 2006;84:475–82.
211. Duncan, SH, Belenguer, A, Holtrop, G, et al. Reduced dietary intake of carbohydrates by obese subjects results in decreased concentrations of butyrate and butyrate-producing bacteria in feces. App Environm Microbiol 2007;73(4):1073–78.
212. Holt, SHA, Brand-Miller, JC. International tables of glycemic index and glycemic load values. Am J Clin Nutr 2002;62: 5–56.
213. Strothers, L. A randomized trial to evaluate effectiveness and cost-effectiveness of naturopathic cranberry products against urinary tract infections in women. Can J Urol 2002;9:1558–62.
214. Avorn, J, Monane, M, Gurwitz, JH, et al. Reduction of bacteriuriua and pyuria after ingestion of cranberry juice. JAMA 1994;271:751–54.
215. McMurdo, ME, Bissett, LY, Price, RJG, Phillips, G. Does ingestion of cranberry juice reduce symptoms of urinary tract infections in older people in hospital? A double-blind, placebo-controlled trial. Age Ageing 2005;34:256–61.
216. Youn, HS, Lee, JY, Saitoh, SI, et al. Suppression of MyD88- and TRIF-dependent signaling pathways of toll-like receptor by epigallocatechin-3-gallate, a polyphenol component of green tea. Biochem Pharmacol 2006;72(7): 850–59.
217. Youn, HS, Saitoh, SI, Miyake, K, Hwang, DH. Inhibition of homodimerization of Toll-like receptor 4 by curcumin. Biochem Pharmacol 2006;72(1): 62–9.
218. Youn, HS, Lim, HJ, Lee, HJ, et al. Garlic (Allium sativum) extract inhibits lipopolysaccharide-induced toll-like receptor 4 dimerization. Biosci Biotechnol Biochem 2008;72(2):368–75.
219. Campos, FA, Flores, H, Underwood, BA. Effect of an infection on vitamin A status of children as measured by the relative dose response (RDR). Am J Clin Nutr 1987;46:91–4.
220. Frieden, TR, Sowell, AL, Henning, KJ, Huff, DL, Gunn, RA. Vitamin A levels and severity of measles. Am J Dis Child 1992;146:182–86.
221. Horrobin, DF. Essential fatty acids and the post-viral fatigue syndrome. In Jenkins, R, Mowbray, J. (eds), Post-viral fatigue syndrome. New York: John Wiley & Sons, 1991;393–404.
222. Anonymous. Says food allergy seems important cause of otitis. Family Pract News 1991;21(5):14.

223. Juntti, H, Tikkanen, S, Kokkonen, J, Alho, OP, Niinimaki, A. Cow's milk allergy is associated with recurrent otitis media during childhood. Acta Otolaryngol 1999;119(8):867–73.
224. Naunton, E. Miami Herald, 1988, Nov. 12.
225. Hijazi, Z, Molla, AM, Al-Habashi, H, Muawad, WM, Molla, AM, Sharma, PN. Intestinal permeability is increased in bronchial asthma. Arch Dis Child 2004;89(3):227–9.
226. Chandra, RK. Prospective studies of the effect of breastfeeding on incidence of infection and allergy. Acta. Pediatr. Scand. 1979;68(5):691–4.
227. Chandra, RK, 691–4.
228. Chandra, RK, 691–4.
229. Saarinen, U.; Breastfeeding Prevents Otitis Media, Nutrition Reviews 41(8): 241, 1983.
230. Sassen, ML, Brand, R., Grote, JJ. Breast-feeding and acute otitis media. Am. J. Otolaryngol. 1994;15(5):351–357.
231. Paradise, JL, Elster, BA, Tan, L. Evidence in Infants with Cleft Palate that Breast Milk Protects Against Otitis Media. Pediatrics 1994;(6 Pt 1):853–860.
232. Hanson, LA, et al: Breast Feeding: Overview and Breast Milk Immunology. Acta. Paediatr. Jpn. 1994;36(5):557–561.
233. Hanson, Breast Feeding, 557–561.
234. Mead, PS, Slutsker, L, Dietz, V, et al. Food-related illness and death in the United States. Emerg Infect Dis 1999;5(5):607–25.
235. Shecter, J, Love, D. Consumer reports finds nearly half of chickens tested contaminated: Analysis of bacteria shows significant resistance to important human antibiotics. Consumer Reports, December 10, 2002.
236. http://www.cdc.gov/ncidod/dbmd/diseaseinfo/foodborneinfections_g.htm#mostcommon.
237. FAO/WHO. Guidelines for the evaluation of probiotics in food. 2002. Internet: http://www.who.int/foodsafety/fs_management/en/probiotic_guidelines.pdf.
238. Kluytmans, JA. Reduction of surgical site infections in major surgery by elimination of nasal carriage of *Staphylococcus aureus*. J Hosp Infect 1998;40 (Supple):25–9.
239. Chang, FY, Singh, N, Gakowski, T, et al. *Staphylococcus aureus* nasal colonization in patients with cirrhosis: Prospective assessment of association with infection. Nephrol Dial Transplant 1998;13:1256–8.
240. Gluck, U, Gebbers, JO. Ingested probiotics redue nasal colonization with

pathogenic bacteria (*Staphylococcus aureus, Streptococcus pneumoniae,* and ,-hemolytic streptococci). Am J Clin Nutr 2003;77:517–20.

241. Alberda, C, Gramlich, L, Meddings, J, et al. Effects of probiotic therapy in critically ill patients: A randomized double-blind, placebo-controlled trial. Am J Clin Nutr 2007;85:816–23.
242. Gill, HS, Rutherfurd, KJ, Cross, JL, Gopal, PK. Enhancement of immunity in the elderly by dietary supplementation with the probiotic *Bifidobacterium lactis* HN019. Am J Clin Nutr 2001;74:833–9.
243. Saavedra, JM, Abi-Hanna, A, Moore, N, Yolken, H. Long-term consumption of infant formulas containing live probiotic bacteria: Tolerance and safety. Am J Clin Nutr 2004;79:261–7.
244. Tano, K, Grahn-Hakansson, E, Holm, SE, Hellstrom, S. Inhibition of OM pathogens by alpha-hemolytic streptococcu from healthy children, children with SOM, and children with rAOM. Intl J Pediatr Otorhinolaryngol 2000;56:185–90.
245. Tano, K, Grahn-Hakansson, E, Holm, SE, Hellstrom, S. A nasal spray with alpha-haemolytic streptococci as long-term prophylaxis against recurrent otitis media. Intl J Pediatri Otorhinolaryngol 2002;122:78–85.
246. Hatakka, K, Blomgren, K, Pohajavuori, S, et al. Treatement of acute otitis media with probiotics in otitis-prone children: A double-blind, placebo-controlled randomized study. Clin Nutr 2007;26(3):314–21.
247. Wilson, M. Microbial Inhabitants of Humans. Their Ecology and Role in Health and Disease. Cambridge, UK: Cambridge University Press, 2005. 410.
248. Kalliomäki, M, Salminen, S, Arvilommi, H, Kero, P, Koskinen, P, Isolauri, E. Probiotics in primary prevention of atopic disease: A randomised placebo-controlled trial. Lancet 2001;7;357(9262):1076–9.
249. Larsson, PG, Stray-Pedersen, B, Ryttig, KR, Larsen, S. Human lactobacilli as supplementation of clindamycin to patients with bacterial vaginosis reduce the recurrence rate; A 6-month, double-blind, randomized, placebo-controlled study. BMC Wom Hlth 2008;8:3.
250. Gershwin, ME, Nestel, P, Keen, CL. Handbook of Nutrition and Immunity. New Jersey: Humana Press, 2004. 220.
251. Boyle, RJ, Robins-Browne, RM, Tang, MLK. Probiotic use in clinical practice: What are the risks? Am J Clin Nutr 2006;83:1256–64.
252. Reid, G. Probiotics to prevent the need for, and augment the use of, antibiotics. Can J Infect Dis Med Microbiol 2006;17(5):291–5.
253. Cani, PD, Neyrinck, AM, Fava, F, et al. Selective increases of bifidobacte-

ria in gut microflora improve high-fat-diet-induced diabetes in mice through a mechanism associated with endotoxaemia. Diabetologia 2007;50(11): 2374–83.
254. Bouhnik, Y, Achour, L, Paineau, D, Riottot, M, Attar, A, Bornet, F. Four-week short chain fructo-oligosaccharides ingestion leads to increasing fecal bifidobacteria and cholesterol excretion in healthy elderly volunteers. Nutr J 2007;5;6:42.
255. Lindsay, JO, Whelan, K, Stagg, AJ. Clinical, microbiological, and immunological effects of fructo-oligosaccharide in patients with Crohn's disease. Gut 2006;55(3):348–55.
256. Schiffrin, EJ, Thomas, DR, Kumar, VB, et al. Systemic inflammatory markers in older persons: The effect of oral nutritional supplementation with prebiotics. J Nutr Health Aging 2007;11(6):475–9.
257. Olakanmi, O, Schlesinger, LS, Britigan, BE. Hereditary hemochromatosis results in decreased iron acquisition and growth by *Mycobacterium tuberculosis* within human macrophages. J Leuk Biol 2007; 81: 195–204.
258. Khan, FA, Fisher, MA, Khakoo, RA. Association of hemochromatosis with infectious diseases: expanding spectrum. Int J Infect Dis 2007;11:482–7.
259. Naik, S. The human HLA system. J Indian Rheumatol Assoc 2003;11:79–83.
260. Baudouin, SV et al. Mitochondrial DNA and survival after sepsis: A prospective study. Lancet 2005;366(9503):2118–21.
261. Hall, MA, Ahmadi, KR, Norman, P, et al. Genetic influence on peripheral blood T lymphocyte levels. Genes Immun 2000;1:423–7.
262. Casselbrant, ML, Mandel, EM, Fall, PA, et al. The heritability of otitis media: A twin and triplet study. JAMA 1999;282(22):2125–30.
263. Rovers, M, Haggard, M, Gannon, M, et al. Heritability of symptom domains in otitis media: A longitudinal study of 1,373 twin pairs. Am J Epidemiol 2002;155(10):958–64.
264. Kvestad, E, Kvaerner, KJ, Toysamb, E, et al. Heritability of recurrent tonsillitis. Arch Otolaryngol Head Neck Surg 2005;131:383–7.
265. Lykken, D, Tellegen, A. Happiness is a stochastic phenomenon. Psychol Sci 1996;7:186–9.
266. Kendler, KS, Neale, MC, Kessler, RC, et al. The lifetime history of major depression in women. Arch Gen Psych 1993;50:863–70.
267. Kendler, KS, Neale, M, Kessler, R, et al. Stressful life events, genetic liability, and onset of an episode of major depression in women. Am J Psych 1995;152:833–42.

268. Plomin, R, Lichtenstein, P, Pderesen, NL, et al. Genetic influence on life events dring the last half of the life span. Psychol Aging 1990;5:25–30.
269. Brown, SM et al. A regulatory variant of the human tryptophan hydroxylase-3 gene biases amygdala reactivity. Mol Psychiatr 2005;10(9):884–88.
270. Ni, X, et al. Association between serotonin transporter gene and borderline personality disorder. J Psych Tres 2006;40(5):448–53.
271. Meyer-Lindenberg, A, et al. Neural mechanisms of genetic risk for impulsivity and violence in humans. Proc Nat Acad Sci 2006;103(16):6269–74.
272. Xu, K, Ernst, M,Goldman, D. Imaging genomics applied to anxiety, stress response, and resiliency. Neuroinformatics 2006;4(1):51–64.
273. Xu, Ernst, and Goldman, Imaging genomics, 51–64.
274. Sen, S, et al. A BDNF coding variant is associated with the NEO personality inventory domain neuroticism: a risk factor for depression. Neropsychopathopharmacoloy 2003;28(2):397–401.
275. Watters, E. DNA is not destiny: The new science of epigenetics rewrites the rules of disease, heredity, and identity. 2006.
276. Fraga, MF, Ballestar, E, Paz, MF, et al. Epigenetic differences arise during the lifetime of monozygotic twins. PNAS 2005;102:10604–9.
277. Liu, D, Diorio, J, Tannenbaum, B, et al. Maternal care, hippocampal glucocorticoid receptors, and hypothalamic-pituitary-adrenal responses to stress. Science 1997;277(5332):1659–62.
278. Buss, C, Wadiwalla, M, Hellhammer, DH, et al. Maternal care modulates the relationship between prenatal risk and hippocampal volume in women but not in men. J Neurosci 2007;7;27(10):2592–5.
279. Weaver, ICG, Meaney, M, Szyf, M. Maternal care effects on the hippocampal transcriptome and anxiety-mediated behaviors in the offspring that are reversible in adulthood. PNAS 2006;103:3480–3485.
280. Pilegaard, H, Ordway, GA, Saltin, B, Neufer, PD. Transcriptional regulation of gene expression in human skeletal muscle during recovery from exercise. Am J Physiol Endocrinol Metab 2000;279(4):E806–14.
281. Büttner, P, Mosig, S, Lechtermann, A, Funke, H, Mooren, FC. Exercise affects the gene expression profiles of human white blood cells. J Appl Physiol 2007;102(1):26–36.
282. Nieman, DC, Henson, DA, Davis, JM, Dumke, CL, Utter, AC, Murphy, EA, Pearce, S, Gojanovich, G, McAnulty, SR, McAnulty, LS. Blood leukocyte mRNA expression for IL-10, IL-1Ra, and IL-8, but not IL-6, increases after exercise. J Interferon Cytokine Res 2006;26(9):668–74.

283. Sureda, A, Ferrer, MD, Tauler, P, Maestre, I, Aguiló, A, Córdova, A, Tur, JA, Roche, E, Pons, A. Intense physical activity enhances neutrophil antioxidant enzyme gene expression: Immunocytochemistry evidence for catalase secretion. Free Radic Res 2007;41(8):874–83.
284. Simon, P, Fehrenbach, E, Niess, AM. Regulation of immediate early gene expression by exercise: Short cuts for the adaptation of immune function. Exerc Immunol Rev 2006;12:112–31.
285. Schauber, J, Dorschner, RA, Yamasaki, K, Brouha, B, Gallo, RL. Control of the innate epithelial antimicrobial response is cell-type specific and dependent on relevant microenvironmental stimuli. Immunology 2006;118(4):509–19.
286. Schauber, J et al, 509–19.
287. Han, SN, Adolfsson, O, Lee, CK, Prolla, TA, Ordovas, J, Meydani, SN. Age and vitamin E-induced changes in gene expression profiles of T cells. J Immunol. 2006;177(9):6052–61.
288. Gorjao, R, Verlengia, R, Lima, TM, et al. Effect of docosahexaenoic acid-rich fish oil supplementation on human leukocyte function. Clin Nutr 2006;(6):923–38.
289. Nair, MP, Mahajan, S, Reynolds, JL, Aalinkee, R, Nair, H, Schwartz, SA, Kandaswami, C. The flavonoid quercetin inhibits proinflammatory cytokine (tumor necrosis factor alpha) gene expression in normal peripheral blood mononuclear cells via modulation of the NF-kappa beta system. Clin Vaccine Immunol 2006;13(3):319–28.
290. Nair, MP, Kandaswami, C, Mahajan, S, Chadha, KC, Chawda, R, Nair, H, Kumar, N, Nair, RE, Schwartz, SA. The flavonoid, quercetin, differentially regulates Th-1 (IFNgamma) and Th-2 (IL4) cytokine gene expression by normal peripheral blood mononuclear cells. Biochim Biophys Acta 2002;1593(1):29–36.
291. Prasad, AS. Zinc: Mechanisms of host defense. J Nutr 2007;137(5):1345–9.
292. Bierhaus, A, Wolf, J, Andrassy, M, et al. A mechanism converting psychosocial stress into mononuclear cell activation. Proc Natl Acad Sci 2003;100(4):1920–5.
293. Cole, S, Hawkley, LC, Arevalo, JM, et al. Social regulation of gene expression in human leukocytes. Genome Biol 2007;138(9):R189.
294. Clarke, SD. Polyunsaturated fatty acid regulation of gene transcription: A mechanism to improve energy balance and insulin resistance. Br J Nutr 2000;83(Suppl 1):S59–66.
295. Clarke, S. Polyunsaturated fatty acid regulation of gene transcription: A

molecular mechanism to improve the metabolic syndrome. J Nutr 2001;131: 1129–32.

296. Ames, BN, Elson-Schwab, I, Silver, EA. High-dose vitamin therapy stimulates variant enzymes with decreased coenzyme binding affinity (increased Km): Relevance to genetic disease and polymorphisms. Am J Clin Nutr 2002; 75:616–58.

297. Lange, T, Dimitrov, S, Fehm, HL, et al. Shift of monocyte function toward cellular immunity during sleep. Arch Inter Med 2006;166:1695–1700.

298. Lange, T, et al, 1695–1700.

299. Irwin, MR, Wang, M, Campomayor, CO, et al. Sleep deprivation and activation of morning levels of cellular and genomic markers of inflammation. Arch Intern Med 166;1756–1762.

300. Everson, CA, Toth, LA. Systemic bacterial invasion induced by sleep deprivation. Am J Physiol Integrative Comp Physiol 2000;278:R905–R916.

301. Everson, CE. Clinical assessment of blood leukocytes, serum cytokines, and serum immunoglobulins as responses to sleep deprivation in laboratory rats. Am J Physiol Rgul Integr Comp Physiol 2005;289:R1054–63.

302. Nieman, DC, Nehlsen-Cannarella, SL, Markoff, PA, et al. The effects of moderate exercise training on natural killer-cells and acute upper respiratory tract infections. Int J Sports Med 1990;11(6):467–73.

303. Chubak, A, McTiernan, B, Sorensen, M. Moderate-intensity exercise reduces the incidence of colds among postmenopausal women. Am J Med 2006; 119(11):937–942.

304. Hippocrates News 1991;10(2).

305. Peters, EM, Bateman, ED. Ultramarathon running and upper respiratory tract infections: an epidemiology survey. SA Med J 1983;64:582–584.

306. Surridge, C. Science tracks down training dangers. Nature 1996;382:14–15.

307. Krack, A, Sharma, R, Figulla, HR, Anker, SD. The importance of the gastrointestinal system in the pathogenesis of heart failure. Europ Heart J 2005; 26:2368–2374.

308. Brock-Utne, JG, Gaffin, SL, Wells, MT, Gathiram, P, Sohar, E, James, MF, Morrell, DF, Norman, RJ. Endotoxemia in exhausted runners after a long-distance race. S Afr Med J 1988;73:533–536.

309. Jeukendrup, AE, Vet-Joop, K, Sturk, A, Stegen, JH, Senden, J, Saris, WH, Wagenmakers, AJ. Relationship between gastro-intestinal complaints and endotoxaemia, cytokine release and the acute-phase reaction during and after a long-distance triathlon in highly trained men. Clin Sci (Lond) 2000;98:47–55.

310. Stewart, LK, Flynn, MG, Campbell, WW. Influence of exercise training and age on CD14+ cell-surface expression of toll-like receptor 2 and 4. Brain Behav Immun. 2005;19(5):389–97.

311. Amar, S, Zhou, Q, Shaik-Dasthagirisaheb, Y, Leeman, S. Diet-induced obesity in mice causes changes in immune responses and bone loss manifested by bacterial challenge. PNAS 2007;104(51):20466–20471.

312. Zaldivar, F, McMurray, RG, Nemet, D, Galassetti, P, Mills, PJ, Cooper, DM. Body fat and circulating leukocytes in children. Int J Obes 2006;30(6):906–11.

313. McMurray, RG, Zaldivar, F, Galassetti, P, Larson, J, Eliakim, A, Nemet, D, Cooper, DM. Cellular immunity and inflammatory mediator responses to intense exercise in overweight children and adolescents. J Investig Med 2007;55(3):120–9

314. Curat, CA, Miranville, A, Sengenes, C, et al. From blood monocytes to adipose tissue-resident macrophages: Induction of diapedesis by human mature adipocytes. Diabetes 2004;53:1285–92.

315. Cinti, S, Mitchell, G, Barbatelli, G, et al. Adipocyte death defines macrophage localization and function in adipose tissue of obese mice and humans. J Lipid Res 2005;46:2347–2355.

316. Clement, K, Vigueries, N, Poitou, C, et al. Weight loss regulates inflammation-related genes in white adipose tissue of obese subjects. FASEB J 2004; 18:1657–69.

317. Fontana, L, Eagon, JC, Colonna, M, Klein, S. Impaired mononuclear cell immune function in extreme obesity is corrected by weight loss. Rejuvenation Res 2007;10(1):41–6.

318. Shi, H, Kokoeva, MV, Inouye, K, Tzameli, I, Yin, H, Flier, JS: TLR4 links innate immunity and fatty acid-induced insulin resistance. J Clin Invest 2006;116:3015–3025.

319. Creely, SJ, McTernan, PG, Kusminski, CM, et al. Lipopolysaccharide activates an innate immune system response in human adipose tissue in obesity and type 2 diabetes. Am J Physiol Endocrinol Metab 2007;292: E740–E747.

320. Hollwich, F, Dieckhues, B. The effect of natural and artificial light via the eye on the hormonal and metabolic balance of animal and man. Opthalmologica 1980;180(4):188–197.

321. Belyayev, II, et al. Combined use of ultraviolet radiation to control acute respiratory disease. Vestn Akad Med Nauk 1975;SSSR3:37.

322. Dantsig, NM. Ultraviolet radiation. In Russian Language Book. Moscow: 1966.

323. Zabaluyeva, AP. General immunological reactivity of the organism in prophylactic ultraviolet irradiation of children in northern regions. Vestn Akad Med Nauk 1975;3:23.
324. Harmon, DB. The Coordinated Classroom. Grand Rapids, Michigan: American Seating Company, 1951.
325. White, CG, Shinder, FS, Shinder, AL, Dyer, DL. Reduction of illness absenteeism in elementary schools using an alcohol-free instant hand sanitizer. J Sch Nurs 2001;17(5):258–65.
326. White, C, Kolble, R, Carlson, R, Lipson, N, Dolan, M, Ali, Y, Cline, M. The effect of hand hygiene on illness rate among students in university residence halls. Am J Infect Control 2003;31(6):364–70.
327. Ryan, MA, Christian, RS, Wohlrabe, J. Handwashing and respiratory illness among young adults in military training. Am J Prev Med 2001;21(2): 79–83.
328. Roberts, L, Jorm, L, Patel, M, Smith, W, Douglas, RM, McGilchrist, C. Effect of infection control measures on the frequency of diarrheal episodes in child care: A randomized, controlled trial. Pediatrics 2000;105(4 Pt 1):743–6.
329. Always wash your hands. Mayo Clinic Health Letter (online). http://www.mayoclinic.com/health/hand-washing/HQ00407.
330. Schectman, G, Byrd, J, Hoffmann, R. Ascorbic acid requirements for smokers: analysis of a population survey. Am J Clin Nutr 1991;53:1466–70.
331. New Age Journal 1990;Nov/Dec:9–10.
332. Montague, A. Touching: The Human Significance of the Skin. New York: Harper & Row, 1978. 188.
333. Montague, A, Touching. 188.
334. Tisserand, R. Aromatherapy: To Heal and Tend the Body. Santa Fe, New Mexico: Lotus Press, 1988. 56–57.
335. Cohen, S. Sound effects on behavior. Psychology Today 1981;10:38–49.
336. Weatherford, J. Indian Givers: How the Indians of the Americas Transformed the World. New York: Fawcett Columbine, 1988. 189–90.
337. Kauppinen, K, Vuori, I. Man in the sauna. Ann Clin Res 1986;18:173–85.
338. Koplin, DW, Furlong, ET, Meyer, MT, et al. Pharmaceuticals, hormones, and other organic wastewater contaminants in U.S. streams, 1999–2000: A national reconnaissance Environ. Sci. Technol. 2002;36:1202–1211.
339. Hughes, S, Denver, J, North, KD. Environmental Emergence of Triclosan. White Paper prepared by the Emerging Contaminants Workgroup of the Santa Clara Basin Watershed Management Initiative. 2006.

340. Allmyr, M, Adolfsson-Erici, McLachlan, MS, et al. Triclosan in plasma and milk from Swedish nursing mothers and their exposure via personal care products. Sci Tot Env 2006;372(1):87–93.
341. Dantas, G, Sommer, MOA, Oluwasegun, RD, Church, GM. Bacteria Subsisting on Antibiotics. Science 2008:320(5872):100–3.
342. Leslie, M. Germs take a bite out of antibiotics. Science 2008:320(5872):33.
343. Alonso, A, Sanchez, P, Martinez, JL. Environmental selection of antibiotic resistance genes. Env Microbiol 2001;3(1):1–9.
344. Lewis, M., et al. Prenatal exposure to heavy metals. Pediatrics 1992; 89 (6): 1011–15.
345. Lutz, PM, Bauer, S, Gale, N, et al. Immunity in children with exposure to environmental lead: II. Effects on humoral immunity. Environmental Geochemistry and Health 1994;16(3–4):179–89.
346. Ahmed, SB, Ibrahim, KS. Effect of lead on immune status of occupationally exposed workers. CEJOEM 2004;10(4):295–303.
347. Ayatollahi, M. Study of the impact of blood lead level on humoral immunity in humans. Toxicol Industr Health 2002;18(1):39–44.
348. Soleo, L, Colosio, C, Alinovi, R, et al. Immunologic effects of exposure to low levels of inorganic mercury. Med Lav 2002;93(3):225–32.
349. Summers, AO, Wireman, J, Totis, PA, Blankenship, J, Vimy, MF, Lorscheider, FL. Mercury released from dental "silver" fillings increases the incidence of multiply resistant bacteria in the oral and intestinal normal flora. American Society for Microbiology Annual Meeting, Dallas, TX 1991;A–137.
350. Ready, D, Pratten, J, Mordan, N, Watts, E, Wilson, M. The effect of amalgam exposure on mercury- and antibiotic-resistant bacteria. Int J Antimicrob Agents 2007;30(1):34–9.
351. Pike, R, Lucas, V, Petrie, A, Roberts, G, Stapleton, P, Rowbury, R, Richards, H, Mullany, P, Wilson, M. Effect of restoration of children's teeth with mercury amalgam on the prevalence of mercury- and antibiotic-resistant oral bacteria. Microb Drug Resist 2003;9(1):93–7.
352. Pike, R, Lucas, V, Stapleton, P, Gilthorpe, MS, Roberts, G, Rowbury, R, Richards, H, Mullany, P, Wilson, M. Prevalence and antibiotic resistance profile of mercury-resistant oral bacteria from children with and without mercury amalgam fillings. J Antimicrob Chemother 2002;49(5):777–83.
353. Mendell, MJ, Smith, AH. Consistent pattern of elevated symptoms in air-conditioned office buildings: A reanalysis of epidemiologic studies. Am J Pub Hlth, 1990;80:1193–1199.

354. Dales, RE, et al. Respiratory health effects of home dampness and molds among Canadian children. Am J Pub Hlth 1991;134(2):196–203.
355. Groth, Benbrook, Lutz. Do you know what you're eating: An analysis of U.S. government data on pesticide residues in foods. Consumer's Union of the United States, February, 1999. 14–15.
356. Baker, BP, Benbrook, CM, Groth, E. Benbrook, KL. Pesticide residues in conventional, IPM-grown and organic foods: Insights from three U.S. data sets. Food Add Contam 2002;19(5):427–446.
357. Kutz, FW, Cook, BT, Carter-Pokras, OD, Brody, D, Murphy, RS. Selected pesticide residues and metabolites in urine from a survey of the U.S. general population. J Toxicol Environ Health 1992;37(2):277–91.
358. Rea, W. Chemical Sensitivity. Boca Raton, FL: CRC Press, 1992.
359. Gerhard, I, Derner, M, Runnebaum, B. Prolonged exposure to wood preservatives induces endocrine and immunologic disorders in women. Am J Obstet Gynecol 1991;165(2):487–8.
360. Tretjak, Z, Shields, M, Beckman, S. PCB reduction and clinical improvement by detoxification: An unexploited approach. Human Experim Toxicol 1990;9:235–44.
361. Aggozzoti, G. Plasma chloroform concentrations in swimmers using indoor swimming pools. Arch Env Hlth 1990;45(3):175–179.
362. Hertz-Picciotto, I, Croen, LA, Hansens, R, et al. The CHARGE study: An epidemiologic investigation of genetic and environmental factors contributing to autism. Environ Hlth Persp 2006;114:1119–25.
363. Duramad, P, Harley, K, Lipsett, M, et al. Early environmental exposures and intracellular Th1 / Th2 cytokine profiles in 24-month-old children living in an agricultural area. Environ Hlth Perspect 2006;114:1916–22.
364. Duramad, P, Tager, IB, Holland, NT. Cytokines and other immunological biomarkers in children's environmental health studies. Toxicol Let 2007;172: 48–59.
365. Chilmonczyk, B. Environmental tobacco smoke exposure during infancy. Am J Pub Hlth 1990;80(10):1205–08.
366. Laseter, JL, DeLeon, IR, Rea, WJ, Butler, JR. Chlorinated hydrocarbon pesticides in environmentally sensitive patients. Clinical Ecology 1983;2(1):10.
367. Lowen, AC, Mubareka, S, Steel, J, Palese, P. Influenza virus transmission is dependent on relative humidity and temperature. PLoS Pathogens 2007; 3(10):1470–76.

368. Becker, RO, Selden, G. The Body Electric: Electromagnetism and the Foundation of Life. New York: William Morrow Company, 1985. 293.
369. Becker, The Body Electric, 293.
370. Beasley, J, Swift, J. The Kellogg report: The impact of environment & lifestyle on the health of Americans. Annandale-on-Hudson, NY: The Bard College Center, 1989;243.
371. Locke, S, Colligan, D. The Healer Within. New York: New American Library, 1986. 71.
372. Ferguson, M, Coleman, W, Perrin, P. PragMagic. New York: Pocket Books, 1990. 151.
373. Sehnert, KW. Stress/Unstress. Minneapolis: Augsburg Publishing House, 1981. 19.
374. Locke and Colligan, The Healer Within, 68.
375. Boyce, TW, et al. Influence of life events and family routines on childhood respiratory tract illness. Pediatrics 1977;60(4):609–615.
376. Meyer, RJ, Haggerty, RJ. Streptococcal infections in families. Pediatrics 1962;4:539–49.
377. Caserta, MT, O'Connor, TG, Wyman, PA, et al. The associations between psychosocial stress and the frequency of illness, and innate and adaptive immune function in children. Brain Behav Immun 2008 Feb 26 [Epub ahead of print].
378. Boyce, WT, Chesney, M, Ailon, A, et al. Psychophysiologic reactivity to stress and childhood respiratory illness: Results of two prospective studies. Psychosomatic Medicine 1993;57:411–22.
379. Phillips, AC, Carroll, D, Evans, P, et al. Stressful life events are associated with low secretion rates of immunoglobulin A in saliva in the middle aged and elderly. Brain, Behavior, Immunity 20006;20:191–197.
380. Selye, H. The Stress of Life. New York: McGraw Hill, 1978. 299.
381. Cohen, S, Tyrrell, D, Smith, A. Psychological stress and susceptibility to the common cold. New Engl J Med 1991;325:606–12.
382. Cohen, S, et al., 606.
383. Women abused as kids found in poorer health. The New York Times, August 1990.
384. Epel, ES, Blackburn, EH, Lin, J, Dhabhar, FS, et al. Accelerated telomere shortening in response to life stress. Proc Natl Acad Sci 2004;101(49):17312–5.
385. Vulliamy, T, Marrone, A, Goldman, F, et al. The RNA component of telom-

erase is mutated in autosomal dominant dyskeratosis congenital. Nature 2001;413:432–35.

386. Brouilette, S, Singh, RK, Thompson, JR, et al. White cell telomere length and risk of myocardial infarction. Arteroscler Thromb Vasc Biol 2003; 23:842–46.

387. Miller, GE, Cohen, S, Pressman, S, et al. Psychological stress and antibody response to influenza vaccination: When is the critical period for stress, and how does it get inside the body? Psychosom Med 2004;66:215–23.

388. Kasl, SV, Evans, AS, Neiderman, JC. Psychosocial risk factors in the development of infectious mononucleosis. Psychosomatic Medicine 1979;41:445–66.

389. Velin, AK, Ericson, A-C, Braaf, Y, et al. Increased antigen and bacterial uptake in rats. Gut 2004;53:494–500.

390. Solderholm, JD, Yates, DA, Gareau, MG, et al. Neonatal maternal separation predisposes adult rats to colonic barrier dysfunction in response to mild stress. Am J Physiol Gastrointest Liv Physiol 2002;283(6):G1257–63.

391. Zareie, M, Johnson-Henry, K, Jury, J, et al. Probiotics prevent bacterial translocation and improved intestinal barrier function in rats following chronic psychological stress. Gut 2006;55(11):1553–60.

392. Holdeman, LV, Good, IJ, Moore, WE. Human fecal flora: Variation in bacterial composition within individuals and a possible effect of emotional stress. Appl Environ Microbiol 1976;31:359–375.

393. Jemmott, JB 3rd, McClelland, DC. Secretory IgA as a measure of resistance to infectious disease: Comments on Stone, Cox, Vladimarsdottir, and Neale. Behav Med 1989;15:63–71.

394. Eisenhofer, G, Aneman, A, Hooper, D, et al. Mesenteric organ production, hepatic metabolism, and renal elimination of norepinephrine and its metabolites in humans. J Neurochem 1996;66:1565–1573.

395. Cogan, TA, Thomas, AO, Rees, LE. Norepinephrine increases the pathogenic potential of *Campylobacter jejuni*. Gut 2007;56(8):1060–5.

396. Walters, M, Sperandio, V. Quorum sensing in *Escherichia coli* and Salmonella. Int J Med Microbiol 2006;296(2–3):125–31.

397. Alverdy, J, Zaborina, O, Wu, L. The impact of stress and nutrition on bacterial–host interactions at the intestinal epithelial surface. Curr Opin in Clin Nutr Metab Care 2005;8:205–209.

398. Elenkov, IJ. Glucocorticoids and the Th1/Th2 balance. Ann NY Acad Sci 2004;1024:138–46.

399. Segal, BM, Dwyer, BK, Shevach, EM. An interleukin (IL)-10/IL-12 immunoregulatory circuit controls susceptibility to autoimmune disease. J Exp Med 1998;187:537–46.
400. Maes, M, Kubera, M, Leunis, JC. The gut-brain barrier in major depression: intestinal mucosal dysfunction with an increased translocation of LPS from gram negative enterobacteria (leaky gut) plays a role in the inflammatory pathophysiology of depression. Neuro Endocrinol Lett 2008;29(1):117–24.
401. Maes, M, Mihaylova, I, Leunis, JC. Increased serum IgA and IgM against LPS of enterobacteria in chronic fatigue syndrome (CFS): Indication for the involvement of gram-negative enterobacteria in the etiology of CFS and for the presence of an increased gut–intestinal permeability. J Affect Dis 2007;99(1–3):237–40.
402. Maes, M, Coucke, F, Leunis, J. Normalization of the increased translocation of endotoxin from gram negative enterobacteria (leaky gut) is accompanied by a remission of chronic fatigue syndrome Neuroendocrinol Lett 2007;28(6):739–744.
403. Davis, MM. Panning for T-cell gold. The Scientist 2004;18:28–29.
404. Pennebaker, JW, Burnam, MA, Schaeffer, MA, Harper, DC. Lack of control as a determinant of perceived physical symptoms. J Personal Soc Psych 1977;35(3):167–74.
405. Bandura, A. Self-efficacy mechanism in human agency. American Psychologist 1982;37:122–47.
406. Slovut, G. Great expectations: Elderly who call selves healthy may live longer. Star Tribune 1991;April 16.
407. Idler, E, Kasl, S. Journal of Gerontology: Social Sciences, March 1991.
408. Campbell, RS, Pennebaker, JW. The secret life of pronouns: flexibility in writing style and physical health. Psychol Sci 2003;14(1):60–5.
409. Temoshok, L. Biopsychosocial studies on cutaneous malignant melanoma: Psychosocial factors associated with prognostic indicators, progression, psychophysiology, and tumor-host response. Soc Sci Med 1985;20:833–40.
410. Temoshok, L, Heller, B, Sagebiel, R, Blois, M, Sweet, D, DiClemente, R, Gold, M. The relationship of psychosocial factors to prognostic indicators in cutaneous malignant melanoma. J Psychosom Res 1985;2:139–53.
411. Petri, KJ, Booth, RJ, Pennebaker, JW. The immunological effects of thought suppression. J Pers Soc Psychol 1998;75(5):1264–72.
412. Justice, B. Who Gets Sick: How Thoughts, Moods, and Beliefs Can Affect Your Health. Los Angeles: J.P. Tarcher, 1988.

413. Sobel, D, Ornstein, R. Healthy Pleasures. Massachusetts: Addison Wesley, 1989. 168.

414. Seligman, MEP. Learned Optimism. New York: Alfred A. Knopf, 1991. 167–184.

415. Segerstrom, SC. Optimism and immunity: Do positive thoughts always lead to positive effects? Brain Behav Immun. 2005;19(3):195–200.

416. Cohen, S, Doyle, WJ, Turner, RB, Alper, CM, Skoner, DP. Emotional style and susceptibility to the common cold. Psychosom Med 2003;65:652–657.

417. Cohen, S, Alper, CM, Doyle, WJ, Treanor, JJ, Turner, RB. Positive emotional style predicts resistance to illness after experimental exposure to rhinovirus or influenza virus. Psychosom Med 2006;68(6):809–15.

418. McKay, JR. Assessing aspects of object relations associated with immune function: Development of the Affiliative Trust-Mistrust Coding system. Psychological Assessment 1991;3(4):1991.

419. McClelland, D. Motivational factors in health and disease. American Psychologist 1989;44(4):675–683.

420. Moskowitz, H. Hiding in the Hammond Report. Hospital Practice 1975; 8:35–39.

421. Marmot, M, Syme, SL. Acculturation and coronary heart disease in Japanese-Americans. American Journal of Epidemiology 1976;104:107–23.

422. Cohen, S, Doyle, WJ, Sliner, EP, et al. Social ties and susceptibility to the common cold. JAMA 1997;277:1940–44.

423. Russek, LG, Schwartz, GE. Narrative descriptions of parental love and caring predict health status in mid-life: A 35-year follow-up of the Harvard Mastery of Stress study. Alternative Therapies in Health and Medicine 1996; 2:55–62.

424. Wolf, S. Predictors of myocardial infarction over a span of 30 years in Roseto, Pennsylvania. Integrative Phys and Behav Sci 1992;27(3):246–57.

425. O'Donnell, K, Badrick, E, Kumari, M, Steptoe, A. Psychological coping styles and cortisol over the day in healthy older adults. Psychoneuroendocrinol 2008 (in press).

426. Cole, S, Hawkley, LC, Arevalo, JM, et al. Social regulation of gene expression in human leukocytes. Genome Biol 2007;138(9):R189.

427. Sobel, D, Ornstein, R. Healthy Pleasures. Massachusetts: Addison Wesley, 1989.

428. Thomsen, J, Bretlau, P, et al. Placebo effect for surgery for Meniere's disease. Arch Otolaryngol 1981;107;271–77.

429. Thomsen, Bretlau, et al. Placebo effect in surgery for Meniere's disease: Three-year follow-up. Otolaryngology Head Neck Surgery 1983;91:183.
430. Wolf, S. The pharmacology of placebos. Pharmacological Reviews 1959; 11:689–704.
431. Adler, G. The physician and the hypochondrial patient. New Engl J Med 1981;June 4:1394–96.
432. Giving Mirth. Mothering 1990;Winter.
433. The American Heritage Dictionary of the English Language. Boston: Houghton Mifflin Company, 1976.
434. Cousins, N. Anatomy of an Illness. New York: WW Norton, 1979.
435. Mind-Body-Health Digest 1990;2:5.
436. Dillon, KM, Minchoff, B, Baker, KH. Positive emotional states and enhancement of the immune system. International Journal of Psychiatry in Medicine 1985–86;15:13–17.
437. Kimata H. Increase in dermcidin-derived peptides in sweat of patients with atopic eczema caused by a humorous video. J Psychosom Res. 2007; 62(1):57–9.
438. Chopra, D. Quantum Healing. New York: Bantam Books, 1989. 67.
439. McCullough, ME. Beyond Revenge: The Evolution of the Forgiveness Instinct. San Francisco, CA: Jossey-Bass, 2008. 27.
440. Rosenberg, M. Personal communication, 2006.
441. Trainer, M. Forgiveness: Intrinsic, role-expected, expedient, in the context of divorce. PhD dissertation, Boston University, 1981.
442. Worthington, EL, Witvliet, CV, Pietrini, P, Miller, AJ. Forgiveness, health, and well-being: A review of evidence for emotional versus decisional forgiveness, dispositional forgiveness, and reduced unforgiveness. J Behav Med 2007;30(4):291–302.
443. Strasser, JA. The relation of general forgiveness and forgiveness type to reported health in the elderly. PhD dissertation, Catholic University of America, 1984.
444. Ciras, HJ. First give thanks, then do no harm. Science Theology News 2005;1.
445. Frederickson, BL, Tugade, MM, Waugh, CE, Larkin, GR. What good are positive emotions in crisis: A prospective study of resilience and emotions following the terrorist attacks on the Unid States on September 11th, 2001. J Personal Soc Psych 2003;84:365–76.
446. Kendler, KS, Liu, XQ, Garnder, CO, et al. Dimensions of religiousity and

their relationship to lifetime psychiatric and substance use disorders. Am J Psychiatry 2003;160:496–503.

447. Segerstrom, SC, Miller, GE. Psychological stress and the human immune system: A meta-analytic study of 30 years of inquiry. Psychological Bulletin 2004:130(4):601–30.
448. Berg, RD, Wommack, E, Deitch, EA. Immunosuppression and intestinal bacterial overgrowth synergistically promote bacterial translocation. Arch Surg 1988;123:1359–1364.
449. Nucera, C, Lupascu, AM, Gabrielli, M, et al. Sugar intolerance in irritable bowel syndrome: The role of small bowel bacterial overgrowth. Gastroenterology 2004; 126(4, suppl 2):A511.
450. Monteleone, P, Carratù, R, Cartenì, M, et al. Intestinal permeability is decreased in anorexia nervosa. Mol Psychiatry 2004;9(1):76–80.
451. Linder, JA, Bates, DW, Lee, GM, Finkelstein, JA. Antibiotic treatment of children with sore throat JAMA 2005 ;294(18):2315–2322.
452. Putto A. Febrile exudative tonsillitis: Viral or streptococcal? Pediatrics 1987; 80: 6–12.
453. Poses, RM, Cebul, RD, Collins, M, et al. The accuracy of experienced physicians' probability estimates for patients with sore throat: Implications for decision making. JAMA 1985;254:925–29.
454. Denson MR. Viral pharyngitis. Semin Pediatr Infect Dis 1995;6:62–68.
455. American Academy of Pediatrics. Group A streptococcal infections. In: Pickering LK, ed. 2000 Red Book: Report of the Committee on Infectious Diseases, 25th ed. Elk Grove, IL: American Academy of Pediatrics 2000:528.
456. Cooper, RJ, et al. Principles of appropriate antibiotic use for acute pharyngitis in adults: Background. Annals of Internal Medicine 2001;134(6):509–17.
457. McCaig, LF, Besser, RE, Hughes, JM. Trends in antimicrobial prescribing rates for children and adolescents. JAMA. 2002;287:3096–3102.
458. Mah, TF, O'Toole, GA. Mechanisms of biofilm resistance to antimicrobial agents. Trends Microbiol 2001;9:34–39.
459. Hall-Stoodley, H, Hu, FZ, Gieseke, A, et al. Direct detection of bacterial biofilms on the middle-ear mucosa of children with chronic otitis media. JAMA 2006;296:202–211.
460. Dohar, JE. Evidence that otitis media is not a biofilm disease. Ear Nose Throat J 2007.
461. Dowell, SF, Editor. Principals of judicious use of antimicrobial agents for children's upper respiratory infections. Pediatrics 1998;1. Supplement.

462. American Academy of Pediatrics and American Academy of Family Physicians, Subcommittee on Management of Acute Otitis Media. Diagnosis and management of acute otitis media. Pediatrics 2004;113:1451–1.
463. McConaghy, JR, Smith, SR. Controversy in otitis media management: Should we follow the CDC recommendations? 2000;61(2).
464. Cantekin, EI; McGuire, TW; Griffith, TL: Antimicrobial therapy for otitis media with effusion (secretory otitis media). JAMA 1991;266(23):3309–3317.
465. Bailar, J. The practice of meta-analysis. J Clin Epidemiol 1995;48:149–157.
466. Prellner, K. Personal communication with Professor E. Cantekin, 1995.
467. Ruben, RJ. Sequelae of surgical and medical interventions for otitis media with effusion. Presented at: Second Extraordinary International Symposium on Recent Advances in Otitis Media. Oita, Japan, March 31–April 3, 1993.
468. Stool SE, Berg AO, Berman S, et al. Otitis media with effusion in young children. Clinical practice guideline. AHCPR Publication 94–0622 1994.
469. Pshetizky, Y, Naimer, S, Shvartzman, P. Acute otitis media: A brief explanation to parents and antibiotic use. Fam Pract 2003;20:417–19.
470. Bucher, HC, Tshudi, P, Young, J, et al. Effect of amoxicillin-clavulanate in clinically diagnosed acute rhinosinusitis. A placebo-controlled, double-blind, randomized trial in general practice. Arch Intern Med 2003;163:1793–8.
471. Chapman, RS, Henderson, FW, Clyde, WA, Collier, AM, Denny, FW. The epidemiology of tracheobronchitis in pediatric practice. Am J Epidemiol 1981;114:789–797.
472. Orr, PH, Scherer, K, Macdonald, A, Moffatt, MEK. Randomized placebo-controlled trials of antibiotics for acute bronchitis: A critical review of the literature. J Fam Pract 1993;36:507–512.
473. Gadomski, AM. Potential interventions for preventing pneumonia among young children: Lack of effect of antibiotic treatment for upper respiratory infections. Pediatr Infect Dis J 1993;12:115–120.
474. Wald, E. Management of sinusitis in infants and children. Pediatr Infect Dis J 1988;7:449–452.
475. Denny, FW, Clyde, WA, Glezen, WP. Mycoplasma pneumoniae disease clinical spectrum, pathophysiology, epidemiology and control. J Infect Dis 1971;123:74–92.
476. Metlay, JP, Kapoor, WN, Fine, MJ. Does this patient have community-acquired pneumonia? JAMA 1997;278:1440–5
477. Wenzel, RP, Fowler, AA. Acute bronchitis. N Engl J Med 2006;355(20): 2125–2130.

478. Bent, S, Saint, S, Vittinghoff, E, Grady, D. Antibiotics in acute bronchitis: A meta-analysis. Am J Med 1999;107:62–67.
479. Monto, AS, Ullman, BM. Acute respiratory illness in an American community. JAMA 1974;227:164–169.
480. Bagshaw, SM, Kellner, JD. Beliefs and behaviours of parents regarding antibiotic use by children. Can J Infect Dis 2001;12(2):93–97.
481. Steinman, MA, Landefeld, CS, Gonzales, R. Predictors of broad-spectrum antibiotic prescribing for acute respiratory tract infections in adult primary care. JAMA. 2003;289:719–725.
482. Gonzales, R, Malone, DC, Maselli, JH, Sande, MA. Excessive antibiotic use for acute respiratory infections in the United States. Clin Infect Dis. 2001; 33:757–762.
483. Pichichero, ME. Understanding antibiotic overuse for respiratory tract infections in children. Pediatrics 1999;104(6):1384–88.
484. Lexomboon, U, Duangmani, C, Kusalasai, V, Sunakorn, P, Olson, LC, Noyes, HE. Evaluation of orally administered antibiotics for treatment of upper respiratory infections in Thai children. J Pediatr. 1971;78:772–778.
485. Ambulatory Care Visits to Physician Offices, Hospital Outpatient Departments, and Emergency Departments: United States, 1999–2000. Vital and Health Statistics. Series 13, No. 157. Hyattsville, MD: National Center for Health Statistics, Centers for Disease Control and Prevention, U.S. Dept. of Health and Human Services; September 2004.
486. Avorn, J. The effect of cranberry juice on the presence of bacteria and white blood cells in the urine of elderly women: What is the role of bacterial adhesion. Adv Exp Med Biol 1996;408:185–6.
487. Crook, WG. The Yeast Connection. New York: Vintage Books, 1986. 214.
488. Geddes, R. Minocycline-induced lupus in adolescents: Clinical implications for physical therapists. J Orthop Sports Phys Ther 2007;37(2):65–71.
489. Lawrenson, RA, Seaman, HE, Sundström, A, Williams, TJ, Farmer, RD. Liver damage associated with minocycline use in acne: A systematic review of the published literature and pharmacovigilance data. Drug Saf 2000; 23(4):333–49.
490. Wilson, W, Taubert, KA, Gewitz, M. Prevention of infective endocarditis: Guidelines from the American Heart Association. JADA 2008;139(1):3S–24S.
491. http://www.ada.org/prof/resources/topics/infective_endocarditis.asp
492. Ibid.
493. Bartzokis, G, Tishler, TA, Shin, IS, et al. Brain ferritin iron as a risk factor

for age at onset in neurodegenerative diseases. Ann NY Acad Sci 2004; 224–236.

494. Bralley, JA, Lord, RS. Laboratory Evaluations in Molecular Medicine. Georgia: Institute for Advances in Molecular Medicine. 2001. 222.

495. Lin, HC. Small intestinal bacterial overgrowth: A framework for understanding irritable bowel syndrome. JAMA 2004;292(7):852–58.

496. Perron, G, Zasloff, M, Bell, G. Experimental evolution of resistance to an antimicrobial peptide. Proc Royal Soc: B (biology) 2006;273:251–56.

497. Blackhed, F, et al. Proc Natl Acad Sci USA 2004;101:15718–23.

498. Ley, RE, et al. Proc Natl Acad Sci USA 2005;102:11070–75.

499. Marchesi, J, Shanahan, F. The normal intestinal microbiota. Cur Opin Infect Dis 2007;20:508–13.

500. Backhed, F, Ding, H, Wang, T, et al. The gut microbiota as an environmental factor that regulates fat storage. Proc Natl Acad Sci USA 2004;101: 15718–23.

501. Turnbaugh, PJ, Ley, RE, Mahowald, MA, et al. An obesity-associated gut microbiome with increased capacity for energy harvest. Nature 2006; 444:1027–31.

502. Newburg, D. Innate immunity and human milk. J Nutr 2005;135:1308–1312.

503. Phadke, SM, Deslouches, B, Hileman, et al. Antimicrobial peptides in mucosal secretions: The importance of local secretions in mitigating infection. J Nutr 2005;135:1289–1293.

504. Weinberg, ED. Iron loading and disease surveillance. Emerg Infect Dis 1999;5:346–352.

505. Ashrafian, H. Hepcidin: The missing link between hemochromatosis and infections. Infect Immun 2003;71(12):6693–6700.

Index

D

M

N

Q

R

S

About the Author

MICHAEL A. SCHMIDT, PhD, did his doctoral research in molecular medicine and biochemistry within the Life Sciences Division at NASA Ames Research Center in Moffett Field, California.

His work is focused on a systems biology approach to complex problems of enhancing human performance. He applies these same complexity models to disease biomarker discovery, development of personalized medicine systems, and development of health recovery systems.

His current research includes collaborations in metabolomics and functional genomics at the University of Cambridge (UK) and the University of Manchester (UK). He also teaches postgraduate medicine through a fellowship in regenerative medicine sponsored by the University of South Florida.

Dr. Schmidt is a professional member of the Society for Neuroscience, the Epigenetics Society, and the Metabolomics Society.

He resides in Boulder, Colorado.